2018

PHYSICIAN CODING EXAM REVIEW

The Certification Step

D1541162

Carol J. Buck
MS, CPC, CCS-P

Jackie Grass Koesterman
CPC

2018

PHYSICIAN CODING
EXAM REVIEW
The Certification Step

Carol J. Buck
MS, CPC, CCS-P

Jackie Grass Koesterman
CPC

Former Program Director
Medical Secretary Programs
Northwest Technical College
East Grand Forks, Minnesota

Lead Technical Collaborator
Coder III/Reimbursement Specialist
Grand Forks, North Dakota

ELSEVIER

ELSEVIER

3251 Riverport Lane
St. Louis, Missouri 63043

PHYSICIAN CODING EXAM REVIEW 2018:
THE CERTIFICATION STEP

ISBN: 978-0-323-43078-4

Notice

Knowledge and best practice in this field are constantly changing. As new research and experience broaden our understanding, changes in research methods, professional practices, or medical treatment may become necessary.

Practitioners and researchers must always rely on their own experience and knowledge in evaluating and using any information, methods, compounds, or experiments described herein. In using such information or methods they should be mindful of their own safety and the safety of others, including parties for whom they have a professional responsibility.

With respect to any drug or pharmaceutical products identified, readers are advised to check the most current information provided (i) on procedures featured or (ii) by the manufacturer of each product to be administered, to verify the recommended dose or formula, the method and duration of administration, and contraindications. It is the responsibility of practitioners, relying on their own experience and knowledge of their patients, to make diagnoses, to determine dosages and the best treatment for each individual patient, and to take all appropriate safety precautions.

To the fullest extent of the law, neither the Publisher nor the authors, contributors, or editors, assume any liability for any injury and/or damage to persons or property as a matter of products liability, negligence or otherwise, or from any use or operation of any methods, products, instructions, or ideas contained in the material herein.

International Standard Book Number: 978-0-323-43078-4

Director, Private Sector Education: Jennifer Janson
Content Strategist: Brandi Graham
Content Development Manager: Luke Held
Senior Content Development Specialist: Joshua S. Rapplean
Publishing Services Manager: Julie Eddy
Project Manager: Abigail Bradberry
Senior Book Designer: Maggie Reid

Printed in Canada

Last digit is the print number: 9 8 7 6 5 4 3 2 1

Working together
to grow libraries in
developing countries

www.elsevier.com • www.bookaid.org

To coding instructors,
who each day strive to enhance the lives
of their students and provide the next generation
of knowledgeable medical coders.

Carol J. Buck
Jackie Grass Koesterman

About the Author

Carol J. Buck, MS, CPC, CCS-P, is a leading coding author and educator. Her *Step* series of textbooks were the first in the market to help coders and coding students develop their skills to advanced and specialized levels. Carol has dedicated herself to the growth and advancement of the coding profession.

Carol has a Master's degree in Education, as well as CPC and CCS-P national coding certifications. She began authoring textbooks when she was Program Director of the Medical Secretarial programs at Northwest Technical College in Minnesota, recognizing the need for classroom texts that could be used to teach medical coding. It was then that she began developing classroom lectures, abstracting medical reports, and compiling materials to prepare her students for careers as medical coders. These materials later became *Step-by-Step Medical Coding*.

Carol has expanded on the original text with a line of annual products for advanced coding, certification, specialization, and reference manuals, providing quality educational materials from the first day of a coding program to preparation for national certification.

To meet the needs of practicing coders, Carol and Elsevier produce professional editions of ICD-10-CM, ICD-10-PCS, and HCPCS references, designed by coders for coders, with unique features such as color tables and the *Official Guidelines for Coding and Reporting*.

From the classroom to the workplace, from application to certification, Carol J. Buck and Elsevier are the trusted names for coding education, practice, and professionalism.

Jackie Grass Koesterman, CPC, has been a Certified Professional Coder and Medical Assistant for over 20 years. Jackie has also served as an instructor at the Minnesota Northland Technical College in the medical clerical and medical assistant programs. Jackie is employed by a large medical health system as a Senior Coder III and Reimbursement Specialist, specializing in multi-specialty coding and multi-payer denial review in both the inpatient and outpatient settings. She also serves as a trainer and mentor to the coders.

Since the inception of *Step-by-Step Medical Coding*, Jackie has been involved in the development and review of the texts, serving as both a developer and reviewer. Jackie is now the Senior Lead Technical Collaborator for the entire line of Buck books.

Acknowledgments

There are so many, many people who participated in the development of this text, and only through the effort of all of the team members has it been possible to publish this text.

Brandi Graham, Content Strategist, who maintains an excellent sense of humor and is a valued member of the team who can always be depended upon for reasoned judgment. **Josh Rapplean,** Senior Content Development Specialist, who assumed the responsibility of shepherding this project with steady fortitude. **Megan Chandler,** Project Manager at Graphic World, who assumed responsibility for many projects while maintaining a high degree of professionalism. The employees of Elsevier have participated in the publication of this text and demonstrated exceptional professionalism and competence.

Preface

Thank you for purchasing *Physician Coding Exam Review 2018: The Certification Step*, the latest guide to the outpatient physician coding certification exam. This 2018 edition has been carefully reviewed and updated with the latest content, making it the most current guide for your review. The author and publisher have made every effort to equip you with skills and tools you will need to succeed on the exam. To this end, this review guide presents essential information about all health care coding systems, anatomy, terminology, and pathophysiology, as well as sample examinations for practice. No other review guide on the market brings together such thorough coverage of all necessary examination material in one source.

Organization of This Textbook

Following a basic outline approach, this text takes a practical approach to assisting you with your examination preparations. The text is divided into five parts—Anatomy, Terminology, and Pathophysiology; Reimbursement Issues; CPT and HCPCS Coding; ICD-10-CM Coding; and Coding Challenge—and there are several appendices for your reference. Additionally, Part 3 includes Practice Exercises, while examinations are provided on the companion Evolve website to help assist you in your preparation.

> **NOTE**
>
> Some of the CPT code descriptions for physician services include physician extender services. Physician extenders, such as nurse practitioners, physician assistants, and nurse anesthetists, etc., provide medical services typically performed by a physician. Within this educational material the term "physician" may include "and other qualified health care professionals" depending on the code. Refer to the official CPT® code descriptions and guidelines to determine codes that are appropriate to report services provided by non-physician practitioners.

Part 1, Anatomy, Terminology, and Pathophysiology, covers all the essential body systems and terms you'll need to get certified. Organized by body systems to follow the CPT codes, the sections also include illustrations to review each major anatomical area and quizzes to check your understanding and recall. (Answers are located in Appendix B.)

Part 2, Reimbursement Issues, provides a review of important insurance and billing information to help you review the connections between medical coding, insurance, billing, and reimbursement.

Part 3, CPT and HCPCS Coding and Part 4, ICD-10-CM Coding, contain comprehensive coverage of the different coding systems and their applications, making other references unnecessary! Simplified text and clear examples are the highlights of these parts, and illustrations are included to clarify difficult concepts.

Part 5, Coding Challenge, contains the Exam Format A—Final Examination to be taken at the end of your complete program of study. To help you quantify the examination, this is meant to be taken using paper and pencil.

About the Outpatient Certification Examinations

The AAPC (www.aapc.com) and the American Health Information Management Association (AHIMA, www.ahima.org) offer outpatient, physician-based coding certifications:

AAPC CPC® (Certified Professional Coder)
AHIMA CCS-P® (Certified Coding Specialist-Physician)
AAPC: The choice of date and location to take the examination is to be made from the AAPC website at www.aapc.com/certification/cpc. Click the orange button in the middle of the page labeled "Locate/Schedule an Exam."

AHIMA: The choice of date and location to take the examination is to be made from the AHIMA website at www.ahima.org/certification/ccsp. Click the "Applying" tab, then the "Register Online" link.

About the Practice Examinations

The companion Evolve website contains valuable resources to assist you with your preparation for the **Physician** coding certification examination. (To access the Exams along with your free Evolve resources, follow the instructions located on the inside front cover of this book.) For the purposes of this text, two practice exam formats have been developed. It's recommended that the learner focus on the exam format that most closely resembles the certification exam chosen:

Exam Format A
Pre-/Post-Examination (150 multiple-choice questions)
Final Examination (150 multiple-choice questions)
Exam Format B
Pre-/Post-Examination (97 multiple-choice and 8 cases)
Final Examination (97 multiple-choice and 8 cases)

The Pre-Examination on the Evolve website should be completed at the start of your study, and the Post-Examination, also on the Evolve website, should be taken after your study is complete. By comparing the results of these examinations, you can see your improvement after using the review guide! Once you check your scores, you are ready to take the Final Examination.

Exam Sessions Screen

After choosing your exam format, the Exam Sessions screen serves as home base. Here you can find information relating to your progress and performance in different subject areas. From this screen, you can choose an examination mode, submit an examination, check your progress, and review your results.

In addition to displaying your scores for completed sections and tracking the total elapsed time, this screen also shows the total, attempted, and correct questions in each subsection. You can return to the Exam Sessions screen at any point while taking or reviewing an examination, and all information related to your answers and position is saved.

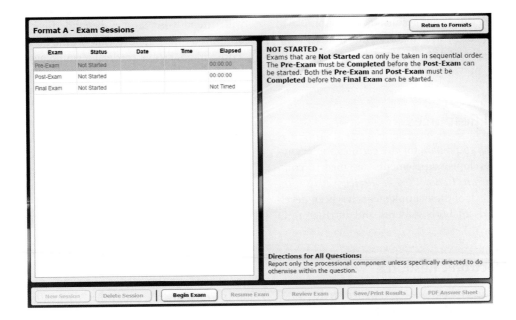

Taking the Examination

While taking the examination, click on the letter of your answer choice, and the circle will appear in red to the left. Click on the "Next" button at the bottom of the screen to proceed to the next question. At the top of the screen, the Quick Jump feature is a pull-down menu that allows you to jump to any question in the current section. Additionally, the Bookmark button at the bottom of the screen allows you to mark questions for later reference.

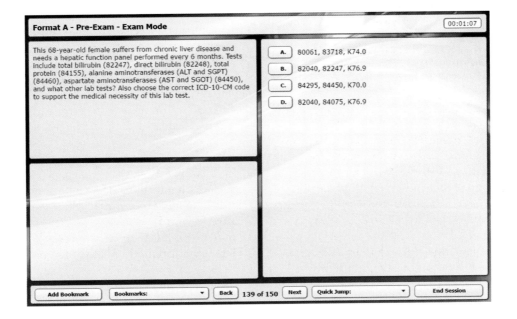

Reviewing Your Results

Once you have taken the Post-Examination on the companion Evolve website, you have the option to review all the Pre- and Post-Examination questions with rationales, even the ones you answered correctly, by clicking the "Review Exam" button at the bottom of the summary screen. The correct answer is shown for each question, and a rationale is given for each answer option. Or, if you prefer, you can review the answers and rationales using a PDF answer sheet. You can also compare your results on the Pre- and Post-Examinations by clicking on each exam on the Exam Sessions screen and viewing your results in the "Completed Exams" on the right or by printing out your results.

Once you have completed the Final Examination, the software will then provide you with all the answers and rationales.

Supplemental Resources

However you decide to prepare for the certification examination, we have developed supplements designed to complement the *Physician Coding Exam Review 2018: The Certification Step.* Each of these supplements has been developed with the needs of both students and instructors in mind.

Instructor's Electronic Resource

No matter what your level of teaching experience, this total-teaching solution, located on the companion Evolve website, will help you plan your lessons with ease, and the author has developed all the curriculum materials necessary to use the textbook in the classroom. This includes extra quizzes, a course calendar and syllabus, lesson plans, ready-made tests for easy assessment, and PDF files with the questions and answers for the Pre-/Post- and Final Examinations. Also included is a comprehensive PowerPoint collection for the entire text, and ExamView test banks. The PowerPoint slides can be easily customized to support your lectures or formatted as overhead transparencies or handouts for student note-taking. The ExamView test generator will help you quickly and easily prepare quizzes and exams from the ready-made test questions, and the test banks can be customized to your specific teaching methods.

Additional Evolve Resources

The Evolve companion website offers many resources that will extend your studies beyond the classroom. Mobile-optimized quick quizzes offer on-the-go practice and review with 380 additional medical terminology, pathophysiology, CPT, ICD-10-CM, and HCPCS questions. Related Web-Links offer you the opportunity to expand your knowledge base and stay current with this ever-changing field, and additional material is available for help and practice.

A Course Management System (CMS) is also available free to instructors who adopt this textbook. This web-based platform gives instructors yet another resource to facilitate learning and to make medical coding content accessible to students. In addition to the Evolve Resources available to both faculty and students, there is an entire suite of tools available that allows for communication between instructors and students. Students can log on through the Evolve portal to take online quizzes and practice examinations, participate in threaded discussions, post assignments to instructors, or chat with other classmates, while instructors can use the online grade book to follow class progress.

To access this comprehensive online resource, follow the instructions located on the inside front cover of this book. You will need the course ID number provided by your instructor. If your instructor has not set up a Course Management System, you can still access the free Evolve resources at http://evolve.elsevier.com/Buck/physicianexam/.

Reviewers

Contents

Success Strategies

This review was developed to help you as you prepare for your certification examination. First, congratulations on your initiative. Preparing for a certification examination can seem like a daunting and formidable task. You have already taken the first and hardest step: you have made a commitment. Your steely determination and organizational skills are your best tools as you prepare to complete this exciting journey successfully.

How do you prepare for a certification examination? The answers to that question are as varied as the persons preparing for it. Each person comes to the preparation with different educational, coding, and personal experiences. Therefore, each must develop a plan that meets his or her individual needs and preferences. Success Strategies will help you to develop your individual plan.

The Certification Examination

This text has been developed to serve as a tool in your preparation for the outpatient (physician-based) certification examination.

AAPC: For AAPC, the CPC® (Certified Professional Coder) certification examination consists of a total of 150 multiple-choice questions covering medical terminology, anatomy, pathophysiology, CPT, ICD-10-CM, HCPCS, coding guidelines, and compliance and regulatory. You have 5 hours and 40 minutes to complete the examination. Exam results are reported with scores and your top three areas of weakness. Visit the AAPC website (www.aapc.com/certification/cpc) for the latest information on the CPC® examination.

AHIMA: For AHIMA, the CCS-P® (Certified Coding Specialist-Physician) certification examination consists of a total of 105 questions: 97 multiple-choice and 8 coding scenarios. Questions cover medical terminology, anatomy, pathophysiology, coding for CPT, ICD-10-CM, and HCPCS, and reimbursement and health information management concepts. You will have 4 hours to complete the examination. Exam results are reported with score percentages for each "domain" tested, as well as the total possible score and the individual's score. Visit the AHIMA website (www.ahima.org/certification/ccsp) for the latest information on the CCS-P® exam.

To be successful on either certification examination, you will have to know how to assign medical codes to patient services and diagnoses. This textbook focuses on providing you with that coding practice as well as anatomy, terminology, pathophysiology, reimbursement, and health information management concepts in preparation for the examination.

Date and Location

Although every journey begins with the first step, you have to know where you are going to make a plan to get there.

- Choose the **date and location** for taking the certification examination.

  AAPC: The website www.aapc.com/certification/cpc contains detailed information about examination sites and dates. The exams are sponsored by local chapters or instructors licensed through AAPC. You may choose from those listed. The test is administered on paper.

  AHIMA: The website www.ahima.org/certification/ccsp contains detailed information about registering for the examination.

- **AAPC:** The AAPC has information that can be downloaded from their website at www.aapc.com/certification/cpc or sent for by contacting:
  AAPC
  2233 S. Presidents Dr., Suite F
  Salt Lake City, UT 84120
  Telephone: 800-626-2633

- **AHIMA:** The American Health Information Management Association has a Candidate Guide that includes eligibility requirements, information on applying for the examination, test center restrictions, and sample examination screens. The Candidate Guide can be downloaded from their website at www.ahima.org/certification/ccsp, or sent for by contacting:
  American Health Information Management Association (AHIMA)
  233 N. Michigan Avenue, 21st Floor
  Chicago, IL 60601-5809
  Telephone: (312) 233-1100

- After you have obtained the candidate information and examination materials, read all the information carefully. Review all competencies outlined in the material to ensure that your study plan contains strategies to address each of these competencies. Check for the latest information on acceptable forms of identification, coding rules to follow, and passing scores.

- The questions within this textbook are not the same questions that are in the certification examination, but the skill and knowledge that you gain through analysis, coding, and recall will increase your ability to be successful on examination day.

Managing Your Time

Role strain! That is what you get when you have so many different roles in your life and you cannot find time for all of them! Know that feeling? Are you a daughter/son, mother/father, wife/husband, student, friend, worker, volunteer, hobbyist—the list is endless. Each takes time from your schedule, and somehow you now need to fit into the role of successful learner. Because you have only 24 hours in your day, being a successful learner requires a time-balancing act. Maybe you will have to be satisfied with dust bunnies under your bed, dishes in your kitchen sink, or fewer visits with your friends. Whatever you have to do to juggle the time around to give yourself ample time to devote to this important task of examination preparation, you must do and make a plan for in advance; otherwise, life just takes over and you find you do not have adequate study time.

If you are planning a big event in your life—moving, a trip, and so on—think about postponing it until after the examination. Your focus right now has to be on yourself. Make your motto **"It's All About Me!"** Sounds self-centered, I know, and most likely very different from who you are, but just this once, you need to carve out the time you need to accomplish this important goal. This time is for yourself. Make it happen for yourself. Move everything you can out of the way, focus on this preparation, and give this preparation your best effort.

Schedule

Each person has an individual learning style. The coding profession seems to attract those most influenced by logic and facts. The best way for a logical and factual person to learn is to problem-solve and apply the information. Hands-on practice is how you will build your skill and confidence for the examination.

- Choose a location to be your Study Central.
- Gather into Study Central the following study resources:
  - Certification packet or handbook from the certifying organization
  - CPT, designated edition
  - ICD-10-CM, designated edition
  - HCPCS, designated edition
  - ICD-10-CM *Official Guidelines for Coding and Reporting* (Can be accessed by following the Evolve Resources link provided in Appendix A of this text)
  - Medical dictionary
  - Coding textbooks, professional journals, and magazines
  - Terminology, anatomy, or pathology text, as needed
  - See Appendix H for Further Text Resources

Make Study Central your special place where you can get away from all other responsibilities. Make it a quiet, calm getaway, even if it is a corner of your bedroom. In this quiet place have a comfortable chair, adequate lighting, supplies, and sufficient desktop surface to use all your coding books. This is your place to focus all your attention on preparation for the examination, without distractions.

- Plan your **schedule** from now until the certification examination using a calendar. Make weekly goals so that you have definite tasks to accomplish each week and you can check the tasks off—a great feeling of accomplishment comes from being able to check off a task. In this way, you can see your progress on your countdown to success.
- Choose a specific **time** each day or several times a week when you are going to study and mark them on your calendar. Make this commitment in writing. After each study session, you should check off that date on the calendar as a visual reminder that you are sticking to your plan and are one step closer to your goal.
- You should plan your study time in advance, know what you are going to be studying the next session, and **be prepared** for that upcoming study session. This will greatly increase the amount of material you are able to cover during the session. At the end of each session, decide what you are going to study next session and ensure that you have all the material and references you will need readily available. At the end of each session, you should be ready for the next study session.
- Your plan should include those areas where you know you will need improvement. For example, when is the last time you read, not referenced or reviewed, but really read, the CPT Anesthesia Guidelines? You probably do not code anesthesia services often, if ever, and as such are not familiar with the information in these guidelines. That is an area of improvement, and your plan should include a thorough reading of all the CPT section guidelines.
- **DO THIS BEFORE YOU BEGIN YOUR STUDY: Assess** your strengths and weaknesses. By making this assessment, you will know where to concentrate your efforts and where to focus your study schedule. You know those areas where you already have strong skills and knowledge and will not need to spend as much time preparing in these areas. The **Pre-Examination,** found on the Evolve website, is an examination that you can use as a tool to assess your current skill level. This examination should be taken before you begin your study and then again (as the Post-Examination) immediately after you have completed your entire study schedule. Do not analyze the questions by reviewing the Pre-Examination rationales (located on the Evolve website); rather, wait until after you have completed your studies and have taken this same examination a second time as the Post-Examination. If you review the rationales after the first time you take the examination, you will know the answers too well to provide a valid comparison between examinations. See Part 5 of this textbook for further information.
- After you have completed your course of study, take the **Post-Examination** on the companion Evolve website. You should plan to cover the examination in the same

amount of time as will be given for the certification examination you are going to take. Compare your scores to those from the first time you took this examination. Note the areas where you did not demonstrate sufficient skills and knowledge.

- Develop a **second plan** to improve the specific areas where you believe you need further study.
- You are now ready to take the **Final Examination**. Take the examination in the same amount of time that will be allocated for the certification examination. It is best if you do this final in one sitting, thereby mimicking the actual examination. If your schedule does not allow for taking the examination in one sitting, plan to take it in several sessions, but always keep track of the time used to ensure that you take the examination in the same amount of time allowed for the official examination. Learning to work within the time allocated is part of the skill you are developing. Remember the certification examinations assess not only your coding knowledge but also your efficiency in completing the examination within the allocated time.

Using This Text

This text is divided into:
- Success Strategies
- Part 1, Anatomy, Terminology, and Pathophysiology
- Part 2, Reimbursement Issues
- Part 3, CPT and HCPCS Coding
- Part 4, ICD-10-CM Coding
- Part 5, Coding Challenge
- Appendix A, Resources (Web-Based)
- Appendix B, Answers
- Appendix C, Medical Terminology
- Appendix D, Combining Forms
- Appendix E, Prefixes
- Appendix F, Suffixes
- Appendix G, Abbreviations
- Appendix H, Further Text Resources

Appendices C–G are combined lists of Medical Terminology, Combining Forms, Prefixes, Suffixes, and Abbreviations used within Part 1, Anatomy, Terminology, and Pathophysiology.

The material in this review features the following:
- Comprehensive guide in outline format
- Photos and drawings to illustrate key points
- Practice examinations

For the purposes of this text, two practice exam formats have been developed so you can focus on the exam format that most closely resembles the certification exam you've chosen to take:

Exam Format A
Pre-/Post-Examination (150 multiple-choice questions)
Final Examination (150 multiple-choice questions)

Exam Format B
Pre-/Post-Examination (97 multiple-choice and 8 case scenarios)

Final Examination (97 multiple-choice and 8 case scenarios)

- **Part 1** is a review of the anatomy, terminology, and pathophysiology by organ systems designed to provide you with a quick review of that organ system. In addition, there is a list of combining forms, prefixes, suffixes, and abbreviations that are often used in that organ system. At the end of each organ system, there is a quiz that will give you an opportunity to assess your knowledge. (Answers are located in Appendix B.)
- **Part 2** is a review of reimbursement issues and terminology. A quiz is located at the end of the part to assess your knowledge. (Answers are located in Appendix B.)
- **Part 3 and Part 4** review CPT, HCPCS, and ICD-10-CM. The CPT and ICD-10-CM material follows the order of the manuals. Practice exercises are located throughout this part. (Answers are located in Appendix B.)
- **Part 5** contains instructions regarding the practice examinations, including the Final Examination for Exam Format A.

> **NOTE**
>
> To enable the learner to calculate an examination score, the minimum of 70% has been identified as "passing" within this text; however, this may not be the percentage identified by the certifying organization as a "passing" grade. It is your responsibility to review all certification information published by the certifying organization.

There are many ways you could use this text. However you decide to prepare, you should take the Pre-Examination before you begin your study to ensure that you develop a study plan that includes time and activities that will increase your knowledge in those areas where your test scores indicate areas of weakness. You could then take the parts in the order they are presented, or you may want to review the anatomy, terminology, and pathophysiology for a body system and then review the CPT material for that body system. There is no one best way to approach the use of this text because each individual will have a personal learning style and preferences that will direct how the material is used. Your skills may be very strong in one or more coding or knowledge areas, and you will want to delete those areas from your individual study plan.

This text is not meant to be the only study source but only one tool of many that you will use. For example, if your terminology skills need a complete overhaul, the brief overview in this text may not meet your needs. You may want to supplement this text with a terminology text and an in-depth study of terminology.

- **Appendices** are a resource for you as you prepare your study plan.
  - **Appendix A,** Resources, is an Evolve Resources link (web-based) to the *ICD-10-CM Official Guidelines for Coding and Reporting*. This link provides the rules for use of ICD-10-CM codes and will be referenced in Part 4 when reviewing the use of ICD-10-CM codes.

- **Appendix B,** Answers, Part 1 and Part 2 Quiz Answers, and Part 3 Practice Exercises Answers and Rationales.
- **Appendix C,** Medical Terminology, is a complete alphabetic list of all the medical terms listed in the Medical Terminology portion of the organ system reviews used in Part 1.
- **Appendix D,** Combining Forms, is a complete alphabetic list of the combining forms used in Part 1.
- **Appendix E,** Prefixes, is a complete alphabetic list of the prefixes used in Part 1.
- **Appendix F,** Suffixes, is a complete alphabetic list of the suffixes used in Part 1.
- **Appendix G,** Abbreviations, is a complete list of the abbreviations referenced in Part 1.
- **Appendix H,** Further Text Resources, is a list of texts that you may want to obtain to supplement your study plan.

Day Before the Examination

- No cramming! Your study time is now over, and cramming the day before the test is not a good idea because it just increases your anxiety level. This day is your day to prepare yourself. Do some things you enjoy this day. Take your mind off the examination. Pamper yourself: you deserve it.
- Review the certification packet information one last time to ensure that you have all the required material.
- Listen to the weather and traffic reports. Plan your route to the examination site. If it is in a new location, drive to the location before the big day.
- Eat a light supper and get to bed early. Set the alarm in plenty of time to arrive at the site early. It is a good idea to have a friend or family member give you an early wake-up call to ensure that you do not oversleep.
- Bring a copy of any official errata associated with your CPT, HCPCS or ICD-10-CM manual.
- **AAPC:** Prepare pencils (no. 2), erasers, picture identification, CPT (AMA standard or professional version only), ICD-10-CM, HCPCS code manuals, and examination admission card. For a paper/pencil examination, take a ruler so that if you skip a question and want to mark that question to return to later, you can use the ruler to make certain you return to the correct question.
- **AAPC:** Although writing, sticky notes, labels, etc., are allowed in your code books, make sure to check the AAPC examination information to ensure that your books meet the specifications identified by the testing organization.
- **AAPC:** Pack quiet snacks and bottled water sufficient for 5 hours and 40 minutes.
- **AHIMA:** Bring two forms of ID. One must be a government-issued picture ID. The other may be a credit card. Your identification will be checked multiple times during your exam experience.

- **AHIMA:** Your test will be administered at a computer terminal. If you wear special glasses when working on a computer, plan to bring them.
- **AHIMA:** No food or snacks will be permitted at the exam. Everything except your code books and identification will be stowed in a locker.
- **AHIMA:** Plan to bring your examination confirmation form with you to the exam.
- **AHIMA:** AHIMA designates the year of CPT, HCPCS, and ICD-10-CM code books used for the exam. Be sure you possess the right year. You are also allowed to bring a medical dictionary into the exam, and you should plan to do so. You will still be admitted to the exam if you do not have a medical dictionary, but you must have all three designated-year code books. The code books must be free of excessive writing, additional papers, or sticky notes.

Day of the Examination

- Wear comfortable clothes and be prepared for any room temperature. A short-sleeved shirt with a sweater is a good plan. Dress in layers so you can ensure that you will be comfortable in any environment.
- Eat a good breakfast. Avoid caffeine because it initially stimulates you, but in the long run will decrease your concentration.
- Arrive early. The doors are locked to those who arrive late. This is a day to be early.
- Ensure that you have the correct room for your examination. Often there are several examinations being administered at one time, so be certain you are in the correct room for your examination.
- **AAPC:** Bring a watch with you so that you can pace yourself during the exam.
- **AHIMA:** No phones or watches are allowed into the exam room but should be left at home or placed in the locker provided to you. The computer will have a clock embedded in it so you can manage your time during the test.

The Certification Examination

You are ready for this! You have planned your work and have worked your plan. Now it is time to reap the rewards for all that hard work.

- **AAPC:** Choose a good location in which to sit. Choose a location that will not get a lot of traffic from those leaving the room. Place all your supplies on the table.
- **AHIMA:** You will be taken to an assigned seat to begin your exam. Have all your books available to you. The exam table is small, so plan how best to access your books quickly in this space.
- Have faith in yourself, and visualize yourself being successful. Say to yourself "I can do this," and then take several deep breaths before you begin to help relax you.
- **AAPC:** Some prefer to take the parts of the examination out of order, taking those questions they are most

confident of first. Others prefer to start at the beginning and work through all questions in order. The approach that you use will depend on your individual test-taking style.

- **AAPC:** When you come to a question for which you are unsure of the answer, you may wish to skip over and come back to all those ones you were unsure of at the end of the examination, depending on the time available. Or you may want to attempt each question and note those you are unsure of to return to when you have finished the exam section. Again, the approach you will use depends on your individual style.

- **AHIMA:** One question will be displayed at a time. You must answer a question before moving to the next. If the answer is not immediately apparent to you, select your "best guess" and flag this question for review once you have completed the entire exam. In this way, you will be able to manage your time more effectively.

- Read the directions. This may sound too simple, but many persons do not completely read the directions, only to find that the directions gave specific directions about what or what not to code on a certain case (for example, "code only this certain portion of the proce-dure"). Yet the choices for answers included the full coding of the case as a selection; if you did not read all the directions, you would choose the response with codes for all the items listed in the report. For example, the question may have directed you to code the service only, not the diagnosis, and yet one of the choices would be the correct service and diagnosis codes, which of course would be an incorrect answer based on the directions. So read all of the directions.

- Your speed and accuracy are being tested. You do not have time to labor over each question for a long time if you intend to complete all the questions. Read the directions, read the question, put down your best assessment of the answer, and then move on to the next question.

- Words such as *always, every, never,* and *all* generally indicate broad terms that, with true/false questions, usually indicate a false question.

- If you do not know the answer to the question, try eliminating those that you know are incorrect first and then select that answer that seems more likely to be correct.

- Judge the time as you are moving through the examina-tion. Keep assessing whether you are making sufficient progress or whether you can slow down or need to speed up.

- **AAPC:** Answer all questions. Even if you have to guess quickly, at least fill in an answer. The best situation is that you answer all questions and have time left to go back over the questions about which you are in doubt.

- **AAPC:** Be certain to carefully complete the information sheet that accompanies the examination. This sheet will include your name, address, and other information that ensures that your test results are accurately recorded.

- Use every minute of the test time, but it is not a good idea to begin second-guessing yourself. Do not return to those questions for which you did not have serious doubts about the correct answer. Usually, your first answer is the best.

- **AAPC:** When the time is finished, hand in your exami-nation, and pat yourself on the back! You have done an excellent job.

- **AHIMA:** When your time is up, the computer will gen-erate a score that will be printed out and given to you before you leave. You will know that day whether you passed the exam.

- Now it is time to go get a good supper and a good night's sleep.

Days After the Examination

- You will miss the preparation! Okay, maybe not miss it exactly, but your life will be different now without that constant preparation.

- **AAPC:** Relax and await the results in confidence. You have done your best. That is always good enough!

- **Be proud of yourself;** this was no small undertaking, and you did it.

  My personal best wishes to you as you prepare for your certification. You can do this!

  Best regards,

  Carol J. Buck, MS, CPC, CCS-P

  Our goals can only be reached through a vehicle of a plan, in which we must fervently believe, and upon which we must vigorously act. There is no other route to success.
  Stephen A. Brennen

PART 1

Anatomy, Terminology, and Pathophysiology

1

Integumentary System

The skin and accessory organs (nails, hair, and glands)

Layers

(Fig. 1.1)

Two Layers Make Up Skin: Epidermis and Dermis

Epidermis. Outermost layer; containing keratin
Stratum corneum, most superficial layer of four layers called stratum
Basal layer, deepest region of epidermis (stratum germinativum or stratum basale), is growth layer
Dermis. The second layer of skin

Two layers are papillary and reticular and contain:

Fibrous connective tissue or skin appendages
Blood vessels
Nerves
Hair
Nails
Glands
Subcutaneous Tissue or Hypodermis. Not considered a layer of skin
Contains fat tissue and fibrous connective tissue
AKA: superficial fascia
Connects skin to underlying muscle

Nails

Keratin plates covering dorsal surface of each finger and toe
Lunula—semilunar or half-moon

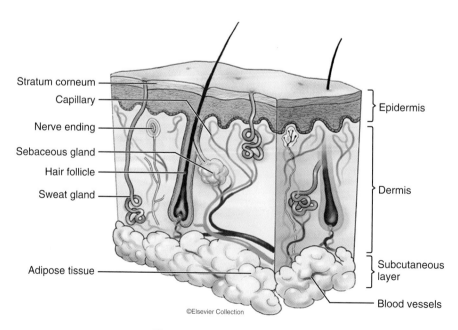

Stratum corneum
Capillary
Nerve ending
Sebaceous gland
Hair follicle
Sweat gland

Adipose tissue

Epidermis

Dermis

Subcutaneous layer

Blood vessels

©Elsevier Collection

• **Figure 1.1** Integumentary system.

White area at base of nail plate is growth area
Thickens and lengthens nail
Eponychium or cuticle: narrow band of epidermis at base
and sides of nail
Paronychium: soft tissue around nail border

TABLE 1-1
Combining Forms

Combining Form	Meaning
1. aden/o	in relationship to a gland
2. adip/o	fat
3. albin/o	white
4. aut/o	self
5. bi/o	life
6. caus/o	burning sensation
7. cauter/o	burn
8. crypt/o	hidden
9. cutane/o	skin
10. cyan/o	blue
11. derm/o, dermat/o	skin
12. diaphor/o	profuse sweating
13. eosin/o	rosy
14. erythem/o	red
15. erythr/o	red
16. heter/o	different
17. hidr/o	sweat
18. ichthy/o	dry/scaly
19. jaund/o	yellow
20. kerat/o	hard
21. leuk/o	white
22. lip/o	fat
23. lute/o	yellow
24. melan/o	black
25. myc/o	fungus
26. necr/o	death
27. onych/o	nail
28. pachy/o	thick
29. phyt/o	plant
30. pil/o	hair
31. poli/o	gray matter
32. py/o	pus
33. rhytid/o	wrinkle
34. rube/o	red
35. seb/o	sebum/oil
36. staphyl/o	clusters
37. steat/o	fat
38. strept/o	twisted chain
39. steat/o	fat
40. squam/o	flat/scalelike
41. trich/o	hair
42. ungu/o	nail
43. xanth/o	yellow
44. xer/o	dry

Glands

Sebaceous glands located in dermal layer
Secrete sebum that lubricates skin/hair
Influenced by sex hormones so they hypertrophy in adolescence and atrophy in old age
Sudoriferous glands originate in dermis. See Fig. 1.1.
AKA: sweat glands
Extend up through epidermis opening as pores
Secrete mostly water and salts to cool body

TABLE 1-2
Prefixes

Prefix	Meaning
1. epi-	on/upon
2. hyper-	over
3. hypo-	under
4. intra-	within
5. para-	beside
6. per-	through
7. peri-	surrounding
8. sub-	under

TABLE 1-3
Suffixes

Suffix	Meaning
1. -coccus	spherical bacterium
2. -ectomy	removal
3. -ia	condition
4. -malacia	softening
5. -opsy	view of
6. -plasty	surgical repair
7. -rrhea	discharge
8. -tome	an instrument to cut
9. -tomy	to cut

TABLE 1-4
Medical Abbreviations

Abbreviation	Meaning
1. bx	biopsy
2. ca	cancer
3. derm	dermatology
4. I&D	incision and drainage
5. subcu, subq, SC, SQ	subcutaneous
6. PPD	tuberculin skin test

TABLE 1-5

Medical Terms

Term	Meaning	Term	Meaning
Absence	Without	Hematoma	A localized collection of blood, usually result of a break in a blood vessel
Adipose	Fatty		
Albinism	Lack of color pigment		
Allograft	Homograft, same species graft	Homograft	Allograft, same species graft
Alopecia	Condition in which hair falls out	Ichthyosis	Skin disorder characterized by scaling
Anhidrosis	Deficiency of sweat		
Autograft	From patient's own body	Incise	To cut into
Avulsion	Ripping or tearing away of part either surgically or accidentally	Island pedicle flap	Contains a single artery and vein that remains attached to origin temporarily or permanently
Biopsy	Removal of a small piece of living tissue for diagnostic purposes		
		Leukoderma	Depigmentation of skin
Causalgia	Burning pain	Leukoplakia	White patch on mucous membrane
Collagen	Protein substance of skin	Lipocyte	Fat cell
Debridement	Cleansing of or removal of dead tissue from a wound	Lipoma	Fatty tumor
		Melanin	Dark pigment of skin
Delayed flap	Pedicle of skin with blood supply that is separated from origin over time	Melanoma	Tumor of epidermis, malignant and black in color
Dermabrasion	Planing of skin by means of sander, brush, or sandpaper	Mohs surgery or Mohs micrographic surgery	Removal of skin cancer in layers by a surgeon who also acts as a pathologist during surgery
Dermatologist	Physician who treats conditions of skin	Muscle flap	Transfer of muscle from origin to recipient site
Dermatoplasty	Surgical repair of skin	Neurovascular flap	Contains artery, vein, and nerve
Electrocautery	Cauterization by means of heated instrument	Pedicle	Growth attached with a stem
		Pilosebaceous	Pertains to hair follicles and sebaceous glands
Epidermolysis	Loosening of epidermis		
Epidermomycosis	Superficial fungal infection	Sebaceous gland	Secretes sebum
Epithelium	Surface covering of internal and external organs of body	Seborrhea	Excess sebum secretion
		Sebum	Oily substance
Erythema	Redness of skin	Split-thickness graft	All epidermis and some of dermis
Escharotomy	Surgical incision into necrotic (dead) tissue	Steatoma	Fat mass in sebaceous gland
		Stratified	Layered
Fissure	Cleft or groove	Stratum (strata)	Layer
Free full-thickness graft	Graft of epidermis and dermis that is completely removed from donor area	Subungual	Beneath nail
		Xanthoma	Tumor composed of cells containing lipid material, yellow in color
Furuncle	Nodule in skin caused by *Staphylococcus* entering through hair follicle	Xenograft	Different species graft
		Xeroderma	Dry, discolored, scaly skin

Chapter 1: Anatomy and Terminology Quiz

(Quiz Answers Are Located in Appendix B)

1. This is the outermost layer of skin:
   a. basal
   b. dermis
   c. epidermis
   d. subcutaneous

2. Which of the following is/are NOT a part of skin or accessory organs?
   a. sudoriferous glands
   b. sebaceous gland
   c. nail
   d. arterioles

3. This prefix means beside:
   a. para-
   b. intra-
   c. per-
   d. epi-
4. This combining form means hair:
   a. xanth/o
   b. trich/o
   c. ichthy/o
   d. kerat/o
5. Lunula is the:
   a. narrow band of epidermis at base of nail
   b. opening of pores
   c. outermost layer of epidermis
   d. white area at base of nail plate
6. Subcutaneous tissue is also known as:
   a. dermal
   b. adipose
   c. hypodermis
   d. stratum corneum
7. Which of the following combining forms does NOT refer to a color?
   a. cyan/o
   b. jaund/o
   c. eosin/o
   d. pachy/o
8. This medical term means surgical incision into dead tissue:
   a. onychomycosis
   b. escharotomy
   c. keratotomy
   d. curettage
9. This suffix means surgical repair:
   a. -opsy
   b. -rrhea
   c. -plasty
   d. -tome
10. Soft tissue around nail border is the:
    a. cuticle
    b. lunula
    c. paronychium
    d. corium

PATHOPHYSIOLOGY

Lesions and Other Abnormalities (Fig. 1.2)

Macule

Flat area of color change (mostly reddened)

No elevation or depression
Example: flat moles, freckles

Papule

Solid elevation
  Less than 1.0 cm in diameter
  May run together and form plaques
  Example: warts, lichen planus, elevated mole

Nodule

Solid elevation 1-2 cm in diameter

Extends deeper into dermis than papule
Example: lipoma, erythema nodosum, enlarged lymph nodes

Pustule

Elevated area

Filled with purulent fluid
Example: pimple, impetigo, abscess

Tumor

Solid mass

Uncontrolled, progressive growth of cells
Example: hemangioma, neoplasm, lipoma

Plaque

Flat, elevated surface

Equal or greater than 1.0 cm
Example: psoriasis, seborrheic keratosis

Wheal

Temporary localized elevation of skin
  Results in transient edema in dermis
  Example: insect bite, allergic reaction

Vesicle

Small blister
  Less than 1 cm in diameter
  Filled with serous fluid in epidermis
  Example: herpes zoster (shingles), varicella (chickenpox)

Bulla

Large blister
  Greater than 1.0 cm in diameter
Example: blister

Scales

Flakes of cornified skin layer
Example: dry skin

Crust

Dried exudate on skin
  Example: scab

MACULE
Flat area of color change; no elevation or depression

©Elsevier Collection

BULLA
Larger blister; greater than 1.0 cm in diameter

©Elsevier Collection

PAPULE
Solid elevation; less than 1.0 cm in diameter

©Elsevier Collection

SCALES
Flakes of cornified skin layer

©Elsevier Collection

NODULE
Solid elevation 1-2 cm in diameter; extends deeper into dermis than papule

©Elsevier Collection

CRUST
Dried exudate on skin

©Elsevier Collection

PUSTULE
Elevated, superficial lesion; similar to a vesicle but filled with purulent fluid

©Elsevier Collection

FISSURE
Cracks in skin

©Elsevier Collection

TUMOR
Solid mass; larger than 2.0 cm

©Elsevier Collection

EROSION
Loss of epidermis that does not extend into dermis

©Elsevier Collection

PLAQUE
Flat elevated surface found where papules, nodules, or tumors cluster

©Elsevier Collection

SCAR
Excess collagen production following injury

©Elsevier Collection

WHEAL
Temporary localized elevation of the skin; result is transient edema in dermis

©Elsevier Collection

ATROPHY
Loss of some portion of the skin

©Elsevier Collection

VESICLE
Small blister; fluid within or under epidermis

©Elsevier Collection

ULCER
Area of destruction of entire epidermis

©Elsevier Collection

• **Figure 1.2** Lesions of skin.

Fissure

Cracks in skin
Example: athlete's foot, openings in corners of mouth

Erosion

Loss of epidermis
Does not extend into dermis
Example: blisters

Scar

Excess collagen production following surgery or trauma
Example: healed surgical wound

Atrophy

Loss of some portion of skin and appears translucent
Example: aged skin
• Not a lesion, but a physiologic response in aging process

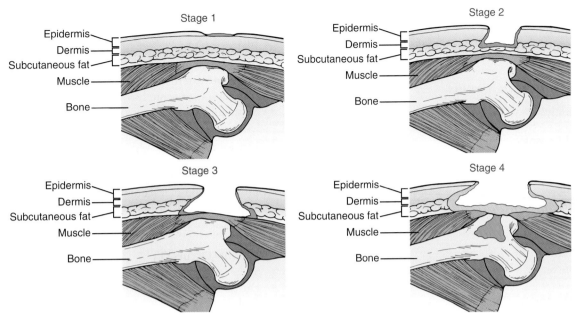

• **Figure 1.3** Stages 1, 2, 3, and 4 of pressure ulcers.

Ulcer

Area of destruction of entire epidermis
Example: missing tissue on heel, decubitus bedsore (pressure sore)

Pressure Ulcer (Decubitus Ulcer) *(Fig. 1.3)*

Result of Pressure or Force
Occludes blood flow, causing ischemia and tissue death
  Develops over bony prominence

Locations
- Coccygeal (end of spine)
- Sacral (between hips)
- Heel
- Elbow
- Ischial (lower hip)
- Trochanteric (outer hip)

Staging or Classification System
- Stage 1: erythema (redness) of skin
- Stage 2: partial loss of skin (epidermis or dermis)
- Stage 3: full-thickness loss of skin (up to but not through fascia)
- Stage 4: full-thickness loss (extensive destruction and necrosis)
  Deep ulcers may require surgical debridement

Keloids

Sharply elevated, irregularly shaped scars that progressively enlarge
  Due to excessive collagen in corneum during connective tissue repair
  Result of tissue repair or trauma
  Familial tendency for formation

Cicatrix

Normal scar left after wound healing

Inflammatory Disorders

Atopic Dermatitis

Unknown etiology
  Exogenous (External) Causes Include
Irritant dermatitis
  Allergic contact dermatitis
  Endogenous (Internal) Cause Includes. Seborrheic dermatitis
  Results in Activation Of
- Mast cells
- Eosinophils
- T lymphocytes
- Monocytes

Greater in Those With Family History Of
- Asthma
- Dry skin
- Eczema
- Allergic rhinitis

Common In
- Children
- Infants

Results In
- Chronic inflammation
- Scratching
- Erythema
- Thickened, leathery skin (lichenification)
- Secondary *Staphylococcus aureus* infection

Treatment
- Topical steroid
- Antibiotic for secondary infection
- Antihistamines

Allergic Contact Dermatitis
Most common in infants and children

Potential Causes
- Hypersensitivity to allergens
  - Microorganisms
  - Drugs
  - Foreign proteins
  - Chemicals
  - Latex
  - Metals
  - Plants

Manifestations
- Scaling
- Lichenification (leathery, thickened skin)
- Erythema
- Itching (pruritus)
- Vesicular lesions
- Edema

Diagnosis and Treatment
- Check medical history
- Patch test
- Avoidance of irritant
- Skin lubrication and hydration
- Steroids
  - Topical
  - Systemic
- Topical tacrolimus (immunosuppressive agent)

Irritant Contact Dermatitis
Response To
- Chemical
- Exposure to irritant

Treatment
- Removal of irritant
- Topical agents

Stasis Dermatitis
Usually on the legs from venous stasis

Associated With
- Phlebitis
- Vascular trauma
- Varicosities

Progress
- Begins with erythema and pruritus
- Progresses to scaling, hyperpigmentation, petechiae (small hemorrhagic areas)
- Lesion becomes ulcerated

Treatment
- Elevate legs
- Reduce standing
- No constricting clothes
- Eliminate external compression
- Antibiotics for acute lesions
- Silver nitrate or Burow's solution dressings for chronic lesions

Seborrheic Dermatitis
Common chronic inflammation of sebaceous glands—cause unknown
Periods of remission and exacerbation

Commonly Occurs On
- Scalp (cradle cap in infants)
- Ear canals
- Eyelids
- Eyebrow
- Nose
- Axillae
- Chest
- Groin

Lesions Are
- Scaly (dry or greasy)
- White or yellowish
- Mildly pruritic

Treatment of Mild Cases
- Soap/shampoo of
  - Coal tar
  - Sulfur
  - Salicylic acid

Treatment of More Severe Cases
- Corticosteroid

Papulosquamous Disorders
Conditions Associated With
- Scales
- Papules
- Plaque
- Erythema

Three Types
- Psoriasis
- Pityriasis
- Lichen planus

Psoriasis
Chronic, relapsing, proliferating skin disorder
Usually begins by age 20

Cause Unknown, Suggested to Be
- Exacerbated by anxiety; appears to run in families
- Immunologic

- Biochemical alterations
- Triggering agent

Commonly Occurs On
- Face
- Scalp
- Forearms and elbows
- Knees and legs

Results In
- Thickened dermis and epidermis
- Well-demarcated plaque
- Cell hyperproliferation/scaly
- Inflammation (pruritus)
- Deep red lesions

Treatment
- Only palliative (treatment of symptoms)
  Mild cases
- Keratolytic agents
- Corticosteroids
- Emollients
  Moderate cases
- Interleukin-2 inhibitors
- Psoralens and ultraviolet A (PUVA) light therapy
- Coal tar
- Cyclosporin
- Vitamin D analogs
  Severe cases
- Topical agents
- Systemic corticosteroids
- Antimetabolic
- Hospitalization

Pityriasis Rosea

Unknown cause
  Self-limiting inflammatory disorder
  Occurs most often in young adults

Primary Lesion
- Begins with herald patch 3 to 4 cm
- Salmon-pink colored
- Circular and well-defined lesions

Secondary Lesions
- 14 to 21 days
  Trunk and upper extremities
- Oval lesions
- Severe pruritus

Diagnosis
May be confused with
- Secondary syphilis
- Seborrheic dermatitis
- Psoriasis

Treatment
- Antipruritics

- Antihistamines
- Corticosteroids
- Ultraviolet light
- Sunlight

Lichen Planus

Occurs on skin and mucous membranes
  Unknown cause (idiopathic)
  Autoimmune inflammatory disorder
  Onset ages 30 to 70

Lesions
- Begin as pink lesions that turn into violet-colored pruritic papules
- Result in hyperpigmentation
- 2- to 10-mm flat lesions with central depression
- Last 12 to 18 months
- Tend to reoccur

Treatment
- Antihistamines
- Corticosteroids
  Topical
  Systemic

Acne Vulgaris

Site of lesion is sebaceous (pilosebaceous) follicles

Primarily on face and upper trunk
Occurs in 85% of the population between the ages of 12 and 25
Exact cause: unknown
Causative factor: sebum accumulation/inflammation in pores of skin

Types
Noninflammatory acne
- Whiteheads
- Blackheads
Inflammatory acne
- Follicle walls rupture
- Sebum expels into dermis
- Inflammation begins
- Pustules, cysts, and papules result

Cause
Unknown

Treatment
Topical
- Antibiotics
- Salicylic acid
- Benzoyl peroxide
- Tretinoin
Systemic
- Antibiotic
- Hormones
- Corticosteroids
- Isotretinoin

Diaper Dermatitis

Variety of disorders

Causes

Urine
Feces
Plastic diaper cover
Allergic reaction
Secondary *Candida albicans* infection

Treatment

Clean, dry area
Expose to air
Topical antifungal medications
Topical steroids

Pruritus (Itching)

Symptom of skin disorder/dermatitis

Can be localized or generalized and is a condition, not an inflammation
Results from stimulation of nerves of skin reacting to an allergen or irritation from substances in blood or foreign bodies

Causes

Primary skin disorder
    Example: eczema or lice
    Systemic disease
    Example: chronic renal failure
    Opiates
    Allergic reaction

Treatment Is for Underlying Condition

Antihistamines
Minor tranquilizers
Application of emollients (lotions)
Topical steroids

Skin Infections

Bacterial

Impetigo

Most common in infants and children

Usually on face and begins as small vesicles
Caused primarily by *Staphylococcus*
   • Sometimes by group A beta-hemolytic *Streptococcus*
It is a highly contagious pyoderma

Treatment in Mild Cases

Topical antibiotics
Topical antiseptics

Treatment in Moderate Cases

Systemic antibiotics

Local compresses
Analgesics

Cellulitis

Caused primarily by *Staphylococcus*
Often secondary to an injury

Results In

Erythema, usually of lower trunk and legs
Fever
Localized pain
Lymphangitis

Treatment

Systemic antibiotics
Burow's soaks for pain relief

Furuncles (Boils)

Infected hair follicle

Usually caused by *Staphylococcus*
Developed boil drains pus and necrotic tissue
Squeezing spreads infection
Collection of furuncles that have merged is a carbuncle

Folliculitis

Infection of hair follicles

Results In

Erythema
Pustules

Causes

Skin trauma, such as irritation or friction
Poor hygiene
Excessive skin moisture

Treatment

Cleansing of area
Topical antibiotics

Erysipelas

Infection of skin

Cause

Group A beta-hemolytic *Streptococcus*
Common occurrence: face, ears, lower legs
    Prior to outbreak, presents with
   • Fever
   • Malaise
   • Chills

Lesions Appear As

Bright red and hot
   • Develop raised borders
   • Itching

- Burning
- Tenderness

Acute Necrotizing Fasciitis

Flesh-Eating Disease

Virulent strain of gram-positive, group A beta-hemolytic *Streptococcus*
  Mortality rate of over 40%

Causes

Skin trauma
Skin infection

Areas Secrete Tissue-Destroying Enzyme, Proteases

Extreme inflammation and pain

Rapidly increasing
Dermal gangrene develops

Systemic Toxicity May Develop With

Fever
Disorientation
Hypotension
Tachycardia (fast heart rate)
  May lead to organ failure

Treatment

Antimicrobial therapy
Fluid replacement
Removal of areas of infection

Viral

Herpes Simplex (Cold Sores)

Causes

Herpes simplex virus type 1 (HSV-1)
- Most common type
- Results in fever blisters or cold sores on or near lips or canker sores of the mouth
Herpes simplex virus type 2 (HSV-2)
- Genital and oral type
- Prominent sexually transmitted disease
Primary infections may show no symptoms (asymptomatic)
Virus remains in nerve tissue to later reactivate

Reactivation May Be Triggered By

Stress
Common cold
Exposure to sun

Presents With

Burning or tingling

Develops Painful Vesicles That Rupture

Causes spreading
  May cause secondary infection of eye

- Episode lasts several weeks
- Treatment may include antiviral medication
  - No permanent cure exists

Herpes Zoster (Shingles)

Usually older adult

Caused by Varicella-Zoster Virus (VZV)

Virus was dormant and then reactivates
Result of varicella or chickenpox, usually in childhood

Affects

One cranial nerve or one dermatome (an area of skin supplied with afferent nerve fibers by a posterior spinal root)

Results In

Pain
Rash (unilateral)
Paresthesia (abnormal touch sensation, such as burning)

Course

Several weeks
Pain may continue even after lesion disappears

Treatment

Clears spontaneously
Antiviral medications provide symptomatic relief
Sedatives
Analgesic
Antipruritics

Warts (Verrucae)

Verruca vulgaris (common wart)

Caused by human papillomavirus (HPV)
  - Numerous types of HPV
Spread by contact
Appear anywhere on body
Present with a grayish appearance
Variety of shapes and sizes
Transmitted by touch
Plantar warts (verrucae) are located on pressure points of body (such as feet; *plantar* means the bottom surface of foot)
Painful when pressure is applied
Juvenile warts occur on feet and hands of children
Venereal warts occur on genitals/anus

Treatment

Liquid nitrogen
Topical keratolytics
Laser
Electrocautery
Often persist even with treatment

Fungal (Mycoses)

Usually superficial dermatophytes (fungus)
  Fungus lives off dead cells

Tinea
Superficial skin infections

Tinea capitis
- Infection of scalp
- Common in children
- Treatment with oral antifungal medication

Tinea corporis (ringworm)
- Infection of body
- Presents as a red ring
- Produces burning sensation and pruritus
- Treatment with topical antifungal medication

Tinea pedis (athlete's foot)
- Involves feet and toes
- Produces pain, inflammation, fissures, and foul odor
- Treatment with topical antifungal medication

Tinea unguium (onychomycosis)
- Nail infection
- Usually toenails
- Nail turns white then brown, thickens and cracks
- Spreads to other nails

Candidiasis
Caused by *Candida albicans*

Normally on mucous membranes of gastrointestinal tract and vagina

Poor health and certain conditions predispose individuals to overarching infection by *Candida*
- Antibiotic therapy, which changes the balance of the normal flora in the body

Treatment is topical or oral antifungal medications

Tumors of Skin

Benign Tumors
Keratosis(es)
Seborrheic Keratosis
Proliferation of basal cells
Dark-colored lesion
Found on trunk and face

Actinic Keratosis
Pigmented, scaly patch
Often caused by exposure to sun
Often in fair-skinned individuals
Premalignant lesion
May develop into squamous cell carcinoma
    Treatment with cryosurgery (freezing area) or excision

Keratoacanthoma
Occurs in hair follicles
Usually in those over 60

Often on face, neck, back of hands, and other locations exposed to the sun

Resolve spontaneously or are excised

Moles (Nevi)
Located on any body part
Various shapes and sizes
May become malignant
- Especially if located in area of continual irritation

Malignant Tumors
Squamous Cell Carcinoma
Similar to basal cell carcinoma
    Grows wherever squamous epithelium is located (skin, mouth, pharynx, esophagus, lungs, bladder)

Most often appears in areas exposed to sun (actinic keratosis—precancerous)
Scaly appearance
Rarely metastatic (spreading)
Easily treated with good prognosis
Surgical excision
    Cryotherapy
    Curettage
    Electrodesiccation
    Radiotherapy

Basal Cell Carcinoma
Common type of skin cancer
    Developed in deeper skin layers (basal cells) than squamous cell carcinoma
    Often occurs with sun exposure in fair-skinned individuals
    Shiny appearance and slow growing
    Easily treated with good prognosis

Malignant Melanoma
Originates in cells that produce pigment (melanocytes) or nevi

Increased Incidence With
Sun exposure
Fair hair and skin, freckles
Genetic predisposition
Skin nevus (mole) often brown and evenly colored with irregular borders
Grow downward into tissues
- Metastasize quickly

Treatment is removal with extensive border excision
- Depending on extent, chemotherapy or radiation therapy may be used

Kaposi's Sarcoma
Rare form of vascular skin cancer

Associated With

Human immunodeficiency virus (HIV)

Acquired immunodeficiency syndrome (AIDS)

Herpes virus may be found in lesions

    Cells originate from endothelium in small blood vessels

    Painful lesions develop rapidly, appearing as purple papules;
        spread quickly to lymph nodes and internal organs

    Treatment

Radiation

Chemotherapy

Merkel Cell Carcinoma

Neuroendocrine carcinoma of skin

    Rare and very aggressive

Associated With

Sun-exposed skin in elderly patients

    Treatment with excision, radiation, and chemotherapy

Chapter 1: Pathophysiology Quiz

(Quiz Answers Are Located in Appendix B)

1. A pimple is an example of a:
   a. papule
   b. vesicle
   c. pustule
   d. nodule

2. A Stage III pressure ulcer involves:
   a. erythema of skin
   b. partial loss of epidermis and dermis
   c. full thickness loss of skin up to but not through fascia
   d. full thickness loss of skin with extensive destruction and necrosis

3. This type of dermatitis may be exogenous or endogenous and is common in children and infants:
   a. atopic
   b. irritant contact
   c. stasis
   d. seborrheic

4. Psoriasis, pityriasis, and lichen planus are three types of this disorder:
   a. dermatitis
   b. inflammatory
   c. acne
   d. papulosquamous

5. This condition begins with a herald spot:
   a. psoriasis
   b. pityriasis
   c. lichen planus
   d. dermatitis

6. This skin infection is caused by group A beta-hemolytic *Streptococcus*, and the lesions appear as firm red spots with itching, burning, and tenderness:
   a. furuncles
   b. folliculitis
   c. erysipelas
   d. fasciitis

7. This type of herpes produces cold sores:
   a. herpes zoster
   b. shingles
   c. VZV
   d. herpes simplex

8. This condition is caused by human papillomavirus:
   a. mycoses
   b. verrucae
   c. shingles
   d. folliculitis

9. This type of tumor occurs in hair follicles:
   a. keratoses
   b. nevi
   c. Kaposi's sarcoma
   d. keratoacanthoma

10. This type of superficial carcinoma is rarely metastatic:
    a. squamous cell
    b. basal cell
    c. melanoma
    d. Kaposi's sarcoma

2
Musculoskeletal System

Skeletal System

Comprises 206 bones, cartilage, and ligaments
  Provides organ protection, movement, framework, stores calcium, hematopoiesis (formation of blood cells)

Classification of Bones

Long Bones (Tubular)
Length exceeds width of bone
  Broad at ends, such as thigh, lower leg, upper arm, and lower arm

Short Bones (Cuboidal)
Cubelike bones, such as carpals (wrist) and tarsals (ankle)

Flat
Thin—flattened with curved surfaces
  Cover body parts, such as skull, scapula, sternum, ribs

Irregular
Varied shapes, such as zygoma of face or vertebrae

Sesamoid
Rounded
  Found near joint, such as patella (kneecap)
  Patella is largest sesamoid bone in body

Structure

Long Bones (Fig. 2.1)
Diaphysis: shaft

Epiphysis: both ends of long bones—bulbular shape with muscle attachments
  • Articular cartilage covers epiphyses and serves as a cushion
Epiphyseal line or plate: growth plate that disappears when fully grown
Metaphysis: flared portion of bone near epiphyseal plate
Periosteum: dense, white outer covering (fibrous)
Cortical or compact bone: hard bone beneath periosteum mainly found in shaft

  • Medullary cavity contains yellow marrow (fatty bone marrow)
Cancellous bones: spongy or trabecular
  • Contains red bone marrow (blood cell development)
Endosteum is thin epithelial membrane lining medullary cavity of long bone

Two Skeletal Divisions

Axial (trunk)
  Appendicular (appendages)

Axial Skeleton, Comprised of 80 Bones

Skull, hyoid bone, vertebral column, sacrum, ribs, and sternum

Skull
(Fig. 2.2)

Cranial
Frontal (forehead)
  Parietal (sides and top)
  Temporal (lower sides)
  Occipital (posterior of cranium)

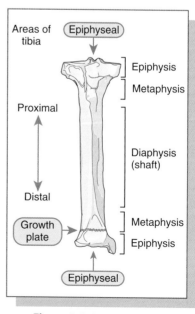

• **Figure 2.1** Structure of bones.

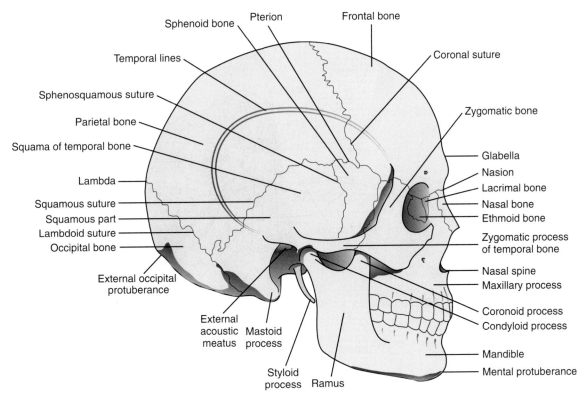

• **Figure 2.2** Lateral view of skull.

Sphenoid (floor of cranium)
Ethmoid (area between orbits and nasal cavity)
Styloid process (below ear)
Zygomatic process (cheek)

Middle Ear Bones (Fig. 2.3)
Malleus (hammer)
  Incus (anvil)
  Stapes (stirrup)

Face (Fig. 2.4)
Nasal (bridge of nose)
Maxilla (upper jaw)
Zygomatic (arch of cheekbone)
Mandible (lower jawbone)
Lacrimal (near orbits)
Palate (separates oral and nasal cavities)
Vomer (base, nasal septum)
Nasal conchae (turbinates)
  Interior
  Middle
  Superior

Hyoid
Supports tongue
  U-shaped
  Attached by ligaments and muscles to larynx and skull

Spine (33 Vertebrae) (Fig. 2.5)
Cervical vertebrae (7)
  • C1-7

• (C1)-atlas
• (C2)-axis
Thoracic vertebrae (12) (T1-12)
Lumbar vertebrae (5) (L1-5)
Sacrum (5)—fused in adults
Coccyx (4)—fused in adults

Thorax (Fig. 2.6)
Ribs, 12 pairs
  • True ribs, 1-7
  • False ribs, 8-10
  • Floating ribs, 11 and 12
Sternum

Appendicular Skeleton, Comprised of 126 Bones (Fig. 2.7)

Shoulder, Girdle, Pelvic Girdle, and Extremities, Pelvis
Ilium (uppermost part), wing shaped
• Acetabulum, depression on lateral hip surface into which head of femur fits
  Ischium (posterior part)
  Pubis (anterior part)
  Pubis symphysis (cartilage between pubic bones)

Lower Extremities, Femur (Thighbone)
Trochanter (processes at neck of femur)
  Head fits into acetabulum
  Patella (kneecap)
  Tibia (shinbone)
  Fibula (smaller lateral bone in lower leg)

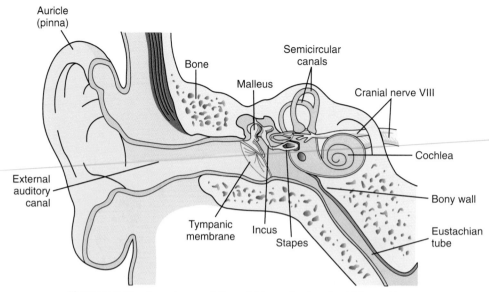

• **Figure 2.3** Structure of ear and three divisions of external, middle, and inner ear.

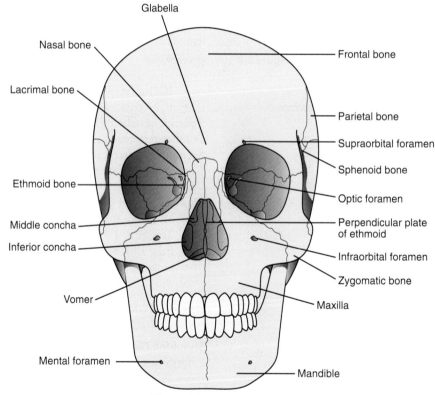

• **Figure 2.4** Frontal view of skull.

Talus (ankle bone)
Calcaneus (heel bone)
Metatarsals (foot instep)
Phalanges (toes)
Lateral malleolus (lower part of fibula)
Medial malleolus (lower part of tibia)

Upper Extremities
Clavicle (collarbone)
  Scapula (shoulder blade)

Humerus (upper arm)
Radius (forearm, thumb side)
Ulna (forearm, little finger side)
Olecranon (projection of ulna at elbow)
Carpals (wrist)—eight bones bound by ligaments in two
  rows with four bones in each
Metacarpals (hand)—framework or palm of hand (five
  bones)
Phalanges (finger)
Olecranon (tip of elbow)

Joints (Articulations)

Condyle, rounded end of bone
  Classified by degree of movement
- Synarthrosis (immovable and fibrous)
  Example: joint between cranial bones
- Amphiarthrosis (slightly movable and cartilaginous)

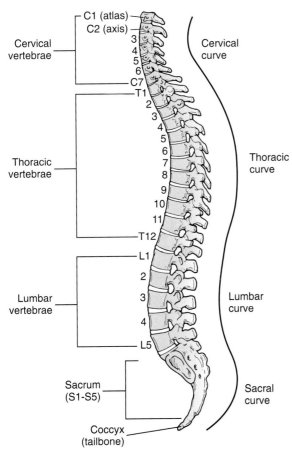

- **Figure 2.5** Anterior view of vertebral column.

Example: intervertebral (joint between bodies of vertebra)
- Diarthrosis (considerably movable and synovial)
  Types
- Uniaxial—hinge and pivot joints
  Example—elbow (hinge and pivot) and cervical 2 (axis) (pivot)
- Biaxial—saddle and condyloid joints
  Example—thumb and joints between radius and carpal bones
- Multiaxial—ball and socket, gliding
  Example—shoulder and hip joints between articular surfaces of vertebrae
  Example: elbow, hip
- Bursa, sac of synovial fluid located in the tissues to prevent friction

Muscular System

Functions

Heat production
  Movement
  Posture
  Protection
  Shape

Muscle Tissue Types

Skeletal—600 Muscles Constituting 40% to 50% of Body Weight

Striated (cross-striped) (Figs. 2.8 and 2.9)
Move body
Voluntary
Attaches to bones
- Most attach to two bones with a joint in between
- Origin, point where muscle attaches to stationary bone
- Insertion, where muscle attaches to movable bone
- Body of muscle, main part of muscle

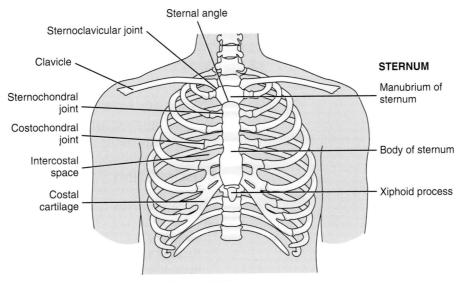

- **Figure 2.6** The thoracic cage.

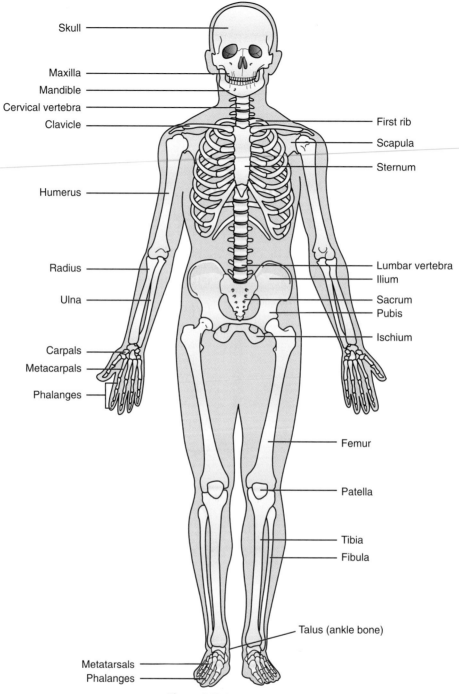

Skull

Maxilla

Mandible

Cervical vertebra

Clavicle

First rib

Scapula

Sternum

Humerus

Radius

Ulna

Lumbar vertebra

Ilium

Sacrum

Pubis

Ischium

Carpals

Metacarpals

Phalanges

Femur

Patella

Tibia

Fibula

Talus (ankle bone)

Metatarsals

Phalanges

• **Figure 2.7** Skeletal system.

Cardiac/Heart Muscle

Striated and smooth muscle
  Specialized cells that interlock so that muscle cells contract together
  Involuntary
  Moves blood by means of contractions

Smooth/Visceral

Linings such as bowel, urethra, blood vessels
Nonstriated
Involuntary

Tendons and Ligaments

Tendons Anchor Muscle to Bone
Ligaments Anchor Bones to Bones

Muscle Action

Muscle Capabilities
Stretches
  Contracts
  Receives and responds to stimulus
  Returns to original shape and length

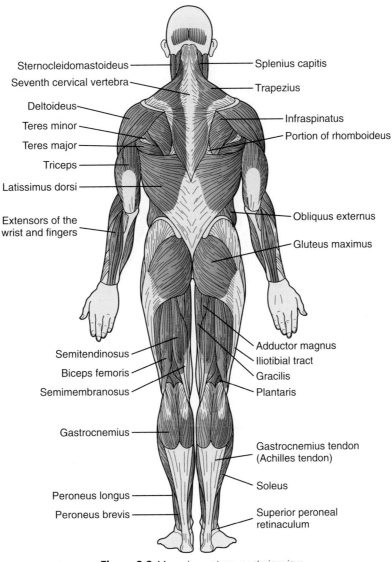

Sternocleidomastoideus
Seventh cervical vertebra
Deltoideus
Teres minor
Teres major
Triceps
Latissimus dorsi
Extensors of the wrist and fingers
Semitendinosus
Biceps femoris
Semimembranosus
Gastrocnemius
Peroneus longus
Peroneus brevis

Splenius capitis
Trapezius
Infraspinatus
Portion of rhomboideus
Obliquus externus
Gluteus maximus
Adductor magnus
Iliotibial tract
Gracilis
Plantaris
Gastrocnemius tendon (Achilles tendon)
Soleus
Superior peroneal retinaculum

• **Figure 2.8** Muscular system, posterior view.

Muscle Movement

Prime mover, responsible for movement (agonist)
   Synergist, assists prime mover
   Antagonist, relaxes as prime mover and synergists con-
      tract, resulting in movement
   Fixator, acts as joint stabilizer

Terms of Movement—From Midline of Body

Flexion (bend)
   Extension (straighten)
   Abduction (away)
   Adduction (toward)
   Rotation (turn on axis)
   Circumduction (circular)
   Supination (turning palm upward or forward [anteri-
      orly] or lying down with face upward)

Pronation (turning palm downward or backward or act
   of lying face down)
Hyperextension (overextension)
Inversion (inward)
Eversion (outward)

Names of Muscles

Head and Neck

Facial expression
• Occipitofrontalis (raises eyebrows and wrinkles forehead
   horizontally)
• Corrugator supercilii (wrinkles forehead vertically)
• Orbicularis oris (opens mouth)
• Zygomaticus (elevates corners of mouth)
• Orbicularis oculi (opens and closes eyelid)
• Buccinator (smiling and blowing)
   Mastication (chewing)

Cranial muscles

Facial muscles

Sternocleidomastoideus

Trapezius

Deltoideus

Pectoralis major

Biceps brachii

Linea alba

Serratus anterior

Rectus abdominis

Aponeurosis of the biceps

Obliquus externus

Extensors of the wrist and fingers

Adductors of thigh

Flexors of the wrist and fingers

Flexor retinaculum

Tensor fasciae latae

Sartorius

Rectus femoris

Vastus medialis

Vastus lateralis

Patellar tendon

Patella

Gastrocnemius

Tibialis anterior

Extensor digitorum longus

Soleus

Peroneus longus

Peroneus brevis

Extensor hallucis longus tendon

Superior extensor retinaculum

• **Figure 2.9** Muscular system, anterior view.

- Masseter (used to chew closing jaw)
- Temporalis (closes jaw)
- Pterygoids (grates teeth)
  Muscles moving head
- Sternocleidomastoid (flexes head)
- Semispinalis capitis (complexus) (extends head)
- Splenius capitis (extends head, bends and rotates head to side where muscle is contracting)
- Longissimus capitis (trachelomastoid muscle) (extends head, bends and rotates to contracting side)
- Trapezius (extends head)

Upper Extremities
Biceps brachii (flexes elbow)
   Triceps brachii and anconeus (extends elbow)
   Brachialis (flexes prone forearm)
   Brachioradialis (flexes semi-prone/supinated forearm)
   Deltoid (abducts upper arm)
   Latissimus dorsi (extends upper arm)

Pectoralis major (flexes upper arm)
Trapezius (raises/lowers shoulder)

Trunk
External oblique (compresses abdomen)
   Internal oblique (compresses abdomen)
   Transversus abdominis (compresses abdomen)
   Rectus abdominis (flexes trunk)
   Quadratus lumborum (flexes vertebral column laterally)

Respiratory
Diaphragm (enlarges thorax/inspiration)
   External intercostals (raise ribs)
   Internal intercostal (depress ribs)

Lower Extremities
Thigh
- Gluteus group, maximus, medius, minimus (abducts thigh)

TABLE 2-1

Combining Forms

Combining Form	Meaning	Combining Form	Meaning
1. acetabul/o	hip socket	32. myel/o	bone marrow
2. ankyl/o	bent, fused	33. my/o, muscul/o	muscle
3. aponeur/o	tendon type	34. olecran/o	olecranon (elbow)
4. arthr/o	joint	35. orth/o	straight
5. articul/o	joint	36. oste/o	bone
6. burs/o	fluid-filled sac in a joint	37. patell/o	patella (kneecap)
7. calc/o, calci/o	calcium	38. pelv/i	pelvis (hip)
8. calcane/o	calcaneus (heel)	39. perone/o	fibula
9. carp/o	carpals (wrist bones)	40. petr/o	stone
10. chondr/o	cartilage	41. phalang/o	phalanges (finger or toe)
11. clavic/o, clavicul/o	clavicle (collar bone)	42. plant/o	sole of foot
12. cost/o	rib	43. pub/o	pubis
13. crani/o	cranium (skull)	44. rachi/o	spine
14. disc/o	intervertebral disc	45. radi/o	radius (lower arm)
15. femor/o	thighbone	46. rhabdomy/o	skeletal (striated muscle)
16. fibul/o	fibula	47. rheumat/o	watery flow (collection of fluids in joints)
17. humer/o	humerus (upper arm bone)		
18. ili/o	ilium (upper pelvic bone)	48. sacr/o	sacrum
19. ischi/o	ischium (posterior pelvic bone)	49. scapul/o	scapula (shoulder)
20. kinesi/o	movement	50. scoli/o	bent
21. kyph/o	hump	51. spondyl/o	vertebra
22. lamin/o	lamina	52. stern/o	sternum (breast bone)
23. lord/o	curve	53. synovi/o	synovial joint membrane
24. lumb/o	lower back	54. tars/o	tarsal (ankle/foot)
25. malleol/o	malleolus (process on lateral ankle)	55. ten/o	tendon
26. mandibul/o	mandible (lower jawbone)	56. tend/o	tendon (connective tissue)
27. maxill/o	maxilla (upper jawbone)	57. tendin/o	tendon (connective tissue)
28. menisc/o	meniscus	58. tibi/o	shin bone
29. menisci/o	meniscus	59. uln/o	ulna (lower arm bone)
30. metacarp/o	metacarpals (hand)	60. vertebr/o	vertebra
31. metatars/o	metatarsals (foot)		

- Tensor fasciae latae (abducts thigh)
- Abductor group, brevis, longus, magnus (adducts thigh)
- Gracilis (adducts thigh)
- Iliopsoas (flexes thigh)
- Rectus femoris (flexes thigh)
  Hamstring group, biceps femoris, semitendinosus, semi-
    membranosus (extends thigh)
  Quadriceps group, rectus femoris, vastus lateralis, vastus
    medialis, vastus intermedius (extends lower leg)
  Sartorius (flexes, abducts, and rotates leg)
  Lower leg
  Tibialis anterior (dorsiflexes foot)
  Peroneus group, longus, brevis, tertius (everts foot)
  Gastrocnemius (calf, with soleus extends foot, also flexes
    knee)

TABLE 2-2

Prefixes

Prefix	Meaning
1. inter-	between
2. supra-	above
3. sym-	together
4. syn-	together

Soleus (calf, extends foot)
Extensor digitorum longus (extends toes, flexes foot)
Achilles tendon (largest tendon, extending from gastroc-
  nemius to calcaneus)

TABLE 2-3
Suffixes

Suffix	Meaning
1. -asthenia	weakness
2. -blast	embryonic
3. -clast, -clasia, -clasis	break
4. -desis	bind together
5. -listhesia	slipping
6. -malacia	softening
7. -physis	to grow
8. -porosis	passage, cavity formation
9. -schisis	split
10. -stenosis	narrowing
11. -tome	instrument that cuts
12. -tomy	incision

TABLE 2-4
Medical Abbreviations

Abbreviation	Meaning
1. ACL	anterior cruciate ligament
2. AKA	above-knee amputation
3. BKA	below-knee amputation
4. C1-C7	cervical vertebrae
5. CTS	carpal tunnel syndrome
6. fx	fracture
7. L1-L5	lumbar vertebrae
8. OA	osteoarthritis
9. RA	rheumatoid arthritis
10. T1-T12	thoracic vertebrae
11. TMJ	temporomandibular joint

TABLE 2-5
Medical Terms

Term	Meaning
Arthrocentesis	Injection and/or aspiration of joint
Arthrodesis	Surgical immobilization of a joint
Arthrography	Radiography of joint
Arthroplasty	Reshaping or reconstruction of a joint
Arthroscopy	Use of scope to view inside joint
Arthrotomy	Incision into a joint
Articular	Pertains to a joint
Aspiration	Use of a needle and a syringe to withdraw fluid
Atrophy	Wasting away
Bunion	Hallux valgus, abnormal increase in size of metatarsal head that results in displacement of great toe
Bursitis	Inflammation of bursa (joint sac)
Carpal tunnel syndrome	Compression of medial nerve
Chondral	Referring to the cartilage
Closed fracture repair	Not surgically opened with/without manipulation and with/without traction
Closed treatment	Fracture site that is not surgically opened and visualized
Colles' fracture	Fracture at lower end of radius that displaces bone posteriorly
Dislocation	Placement in a location other than original location
Endoscopy	Inspection of body organs or cavities using a lighted scope that may be inserted through an existing opening or through a small incision
Fasciectomy	Removal of band of fibrous tissue
Fissure	Groove
Fracture	Break in a bone
Ganglion	Knot or knotlike mass
Internal/External fixation	Application of pins, wires, screws, placed externally or internally to immobilize a body part
Kyphosis	Humpback
Lamina	Flat plate
Ligament	Fibrous band of tissue that connects cartilage or bone
Lordosis	Anterior curvature of the spine
Lumbodynia	Pain in lumbar area
Lysis	Releasing
Manipulation or reduction	Alignment of a fracture or joint dislocation to normal position
Open fracture repair	Surgical opening (incision) over or remote opening as access to a fracture site
Osteoarthritis	Degenerative condition of articular cartilage
Osteoclast	Absorbs or removes bone
Osteotomy	Cutting into bone
Percutaneous	Through skin
Percutaneous fracture repair	Repair of a fracture by means of pins and wires inserted through the fracture site
Percutaneous skeletal fixation	Considered neither open nor closed; fracture is not visualized, but fixation is placed across fracture site under x-ray imaging

TABLE 2-5

Medical Terms—cont'd

Term	Meaning	Term	Meaning
Reduction	Replacement to normal position	Synchondrosis	Union between two bones (connected by cartilage)
Scoliosis	Lateral curvature of the spine		
Skeletal traction	Application of pressure to bone by means of pins and/or wires inserted into bone	Tendon	Attaches a muscle to a bone
		Tenodesis	Suturing of a tendon to a bone
		Tenorrhaphy	Suture repair of tendon
Skin traction	Application of pressure to bone by means of tape applied to the skin	Traction	Application of pressure to maintain normal alignment
Spondylitis	Inflammation of vertebrae	Trocar needle	Needle with a cannula that can be removed; used to puncture and withdraw fluid from a cavity
Subluxation	Partial dislocation		
Supination	Supine position—lying on back, face upward		

Chapter 2: Anatomy and Terminology Quiz

(Quiz Answers Are Located in Appendix B)

1. Tubular is another name for these bones:
   a. short
   b. long
   c. flat
   d. irregular
2. These bones are found near joints:
   a. irregular
   b. flat
   c. sesamoid
   d. broad
3. Zygoma is an example of this type of bone:
   a. irregular
   b. flat
   c. sesamoid
   d. broad
4. Diaphysis is this part of bone:
   a. end
   b. surface
   c. shaft
   d. marrow
5. Which is NOT a part of cranium?
   a. condyle
   b. sphenoid
   c. ethmoid
   d. parietal

6. This is NOT an ear bone:
   a. malleus
   b. stapes
   c. incus
   d. styloid
7. This term describes growth plate:
   a. endosteum
   b. epiphyseal
   c. metaphysis
   d. periosteum
8. This is a depression on lateral hip surface into which head of femur fits:
   a. ilium
   b. ischium
   c. patella
   d. acetabulum
9. Tip of elbow is the:
   a. olecranon
   b. trapezium
   c. humerus
   d. tarsal
10. This term describes an immovable joint:
    a. amphiarthrosis
    b. diarthrosis
    c. synarthrosis
    d. ischium

PATHOPHYSIOLOGY

Injuries

Fractures

Classification of Fractures

Open/Closed

Open (compound): broken bone penetrates skin
   Closed (simple): broken bone does not penetrate skin

Complete/Incomplete

Complete: bone is broken all way through
   Example: oblique, linear, spiral, and transverse
   Incomplete: bone is not broken all way through
   Example: greenstick, bowing, torus, stress, and transchondral

Treatment

Closed reduction (realignment of bone fragments by manipulation)

• **Figure 2.10** Skeletal traction uses patient's bones to secure internal devices to which traction is attached.

• **Figure 2.11** Skin traction utilizes strapping, wraps, or tape to which traction is attached.

Reduction (the returning of the bone to normal alignment)

Immobilization (returns to normal alignment and holds in place)

Traction (application of pulling force to hold bone in alignment)

- Skeletal traction uses internal devices (pins, screws, wires, etc.) inserted into bone with ends sticking out through skin for attachment of traction device (Fig. 2.10)
- Skin traction is use of strapping, elastic wrap, or tape attached to skin to which weights are attached (Fig. 2.11)

Improper Union

Nonunion: failure of bone ends to grow together

Malunion: incorrect alignment of bone ends

Delayed union: delay of bone union 8 or 9 months

Dislocations

Bone and soft tissue damage usually caused by trauma

Any part of bone is displaced

Can result in nerve and tissue damage

Treatment

Reduction

Immobilization

Sprains and Strains

Soft tissue damage usually caused by trauma to tendons and ligaments

Strain: partial tear of a tendon

Sprain results from overuse or overextension/tearing or rupture of some part of musculature

Bone Disorders

Osteomyelitis

Bone infection

Usually caused by bacteria

- Exogenous osteomyelitis is caused by bacteria that enter from outside body
- Hematogenous osteomyelitis (endogenous) is caused by a bacterial infection within body

Osteoporosis

Common disorder in postmenopausal women and elderly and most common metabolic disease

- Malabsorption of calcium and magnesium; certain trace elements and vitamins C and D contribute to bone loss

Decreased bone mass and density

- Fractures more common due to decrease in strength of bone

Treatment

Increased intake of calcium, magnesium, and vitamin D

Increased weight-bearing activity

Osteomalacia and Rickets

Osteomalacia is softened adult bones, whereas rickets is softened growing bones in children

Caused by vitamin D and phosphate deficiency

Osteitis Deformans (Paget's Disease)

Abnormal bone remodeling and resorption resulting in enlarged, soft bones

Unknown cause but strong genetic considerations

Treatment

Calcitonin and biophosphates

Spinal Curvatures

Lordosis: swayback

- Inward curvature of spine

Kyphosis: humpback

- Outward curvature of spine

Scoliosis

- Lateral curvature of spine

Spina Bifida

Congenital abnormality in which vertebrae do not close correctly around the spinal cord

Joint Disorders

Bursitis: inflammation of bursa (joint sac)
  Arthritis: inflammation of joints

Osteoarthritis (OA)

This is degenerative or wear/tear arthritis
- DJD, degenerative joint disease
  Chronic inflammation of joint
  Increased pain on weightbearing or movement
  Affects weight-bearing joints
- Loss of articular cartilage
- Sclerosis of bone—eburnation
  Turning bone into ivorylike mass—polished
- Osteophytes (bone spurs)

Symptoms

Pain and stiffness
Crepitation (bone on bone creates characteristic grinding sound)

Classifications

Primary (idiopathic)
- No known cause
  Secondary
- Associated with joint instability, joint stress, or congenital abnormalities

Treatment

Symptomatic
  Arthroplasty

Rheumatoid Arthritis (RA)

Progressive inflammatory connective tissue disease of the joints

Systemic autoimmune disease
- Can invade arteries, lungs, skin, and other organs with inflammation or nodules
Affects small joints
- Destroys synovial membrane, articular cartilage, and surrounding tissues
Leads to loss of function due to fixation and deformity

Treatment

Pharmaceuticals to modify autoimmune and inflammatory processes
Gene therapy and stem cell transplantation are being researched
Symptomatic
Arthroplasty

Infectious and Septic Arthritis

Infectious process

Usually affects single joint
Without antimicrobial intervention, permanent joint damage results
Example: Lyme disease

Treatment

Antibiotics—early intervention

Gout (Gouty Arthritis)

Inflammatory arthritis
  Often affects the joint of the great toe
  Caused by excessive amounts of uric acid that crystallizes in connective tissue of joints
  Leads to inflammation and destruction of joint

Treatment

Pharmaceuticals—nonsteroidal anti-inflammatory drugs

Ankylosing Spondylitis (AS)

Inflammatory disease that is progressive
Affects vertebral joints and insertion points of ligaments, tendons, and joint capsules
Leads to rigid spinal column and sacroiliac joints

Treatment

Nonsteroidal anti-inflammatory drugs relieve symptoms
Analgesics for pain

Tendon, Muscle, and Ligament Disorders

Muscular Dystrophy—Familial Disorder

Progressive degenerative muscle disorder
Multiple types of muscular dystrophy
Most often affects boys
- Genetic predisposition—Duchenne muscular dystrophy

Primary Fibromyalgia Syndrome

Symptoms

Generalized aching and pain
Tender points
Fatigue
Depression

Usually Appears in

Middle-aged women

Polymyositis

General muscle inflammation causing weakness
- With skin rash = dermatomyositis

Tumors

Bone Tumors

Origin of Bone Tumors

Osteogenic (bone cells)

Chondrogenic (cartilage cell)
Collagenic (fibrous tissue cell)
Myelogenic (marrow cell)

Osteoma
Benign
Abnormal outgrowth of bone

Chondroblastoma
Rare
Usually benign

Osteosarcoma
Malignant tumor of long bones
Usually in young adults
Typically causes bone pain

Multiple Myeloma
Malignant plasma cells in skeletal system and soft tissue
Progressive and generally fatal
Usually in those over 40

Chondrosarcoma
Malignant cartilage tumor
Usually in middle-aged and older individuals
In late stages, symptoms include local swelling and pain
  • Worsens with time
Surgical excision is usually treatment of choice
If diagnosed in early stages, it is treatable with long-term
    survival possible

Muscle Tumors

Rare
  Rhabdomyosarcoma
  Aggressive, invasive carcinoma with widespread
    metastasis

Chapter 2: Pathophysiology Quiz

(Quiz Answers Are Located in Appendix B)

1. A compound fracture is also known as:
  a. complete
  b. incomplete
  c. closed
  d. open
2. This is a common bone disorder in postmenopausal women resulting from lower levels of calcium and potassium:
  a. Paget's disease
  b. lordosis
  c. osteoporosis
  d. rheumatoid arthritis
3. This inflammatory disease is progressive and leads to a rigid spinal column:
  a. polymyositis
  b. ankylosing spondylitis
  c. primary fibromyalgia syndrome
  d. septic arthritis of spine
4. This type of tumor arises from bone cells:
  a. osteogenic
  b. chondrogenic
  c. collagenic
  d. myelogenic
5. This type of tumor is the most common type of malignant bone tumor that occurs in those over 40 and is progressive and generally fatal:
  a. rhabdomyosarcoma
  b. chondrosarcoma
  c. osteosarcoma
  d. multiple myeloma

6. A general muscle inflammation with an accompanying skin rash is:
  a. muscular dystrophy
  b. dermatologic arthritis
  c. ankylosing spondylitis
  d. dermatomyositis
7. A cartilage tumor that usually occurs in middle-aged and older individuals:
  a. chondrosarcoma
  b. osteosarcoma
  c. chondroblastoma
  d. rhabdomyosarcoma
8. Returning of bone to normal alignment is:
  a. immobilization
  b. traction
  c. reduction
  d. manipulation
9. Result of overuse or overextension of a ligament is:
  a. strain
  b. sprain
  c. fracture
  d. displacement
10. Primary osteoarthritis is also known as:
  a. secondary
  b. functional
  c. congenital
  d. idiopathic

3

Respiratory System

ANATOMY AND TERMINOLOGY

Supplies oxygen to body and helps clean body of waste (carbon dioxide)

Two tracts (Fig. 3.1A)
- Upper respiratory tract (nose, pharynx, and larynx)
- Lower respiratory tract (trachea, bronchial tree, and lungs)

Lined with ciliated mucosa
- Purifies air by trapping irritants

Warms and humidifies air

Upper Respiratory Tract (URT)

Nose

Sense of smell (olfactory)

Moistens and warms air

Nasal septum divides interior

Sinuses (Paranasal or Accessory Sinuses) (4 Pair)

Frontal

Ethmoid

Maxillary

Sphenoid

Turbinates (Conchae)

Bones on inside of nose

Divided into inferior, middle, and superior (Fig. 3.1B)

Warms and humidifies air

Pharynx (Throat)

Passageway for both food and air

Nasopharynx contains adenoids

Oropharynx contains tonsils

Laryngopharynx leads to larynx

Larynx (Voice Box) (Opening to Trachea)

Contains vocal cords
- Cartilages of larynx, thyroid, epiglottis, and arytenoid

Lower Respiratory Tract (LRT)

Trachea (Windpipe)—Air-Conducting Structure

Mucus-lined tube with C-shaped cartilage rings to hold windpipe open

Segmental Bronchi

Trachea divides into right and left main bronchus, which further divide into lobar bronchii—3 on right, 2 on left

Bronchioles

Branches divide into secondary bronchi, then smaller bronchioles

Alveolar Ducts (Minute Branches of Bronchial Tree)

End in alveoli (sacs) of simple squamous cells
- Primary gas-exchange units

Surrounded by capillaries and where exchange of oxygen and carbon dioxide takes place

Lungs

Covered by pleura

Cone-shaped organs filling thoracic cavity

Base rests on diaphragm and apex (top of lungs) extends to above clavicles

Hilum is medial surface of lung where pulmonary artery, pulmonary veins, nerves, lymphatics, and bronchial tubes enter and exit

Left lung contains two lobes divided by fissures

Right lung contains three lobes

Respiration

Inspiration—oxygen moves in, downward movement of lungs enlarging thoracic cavity

Expiration—carbon dioxide moves out, upward movement of diaphragm decreasing lung space

Upper Respiratory Tract

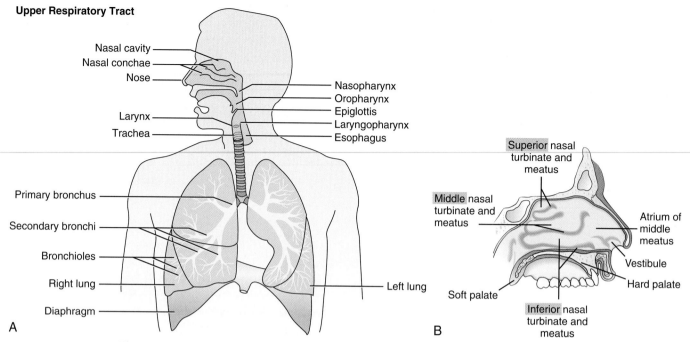

• **Figure 3.1 A.** Upper and lower respiratory system. **B.** Superior, inferior, and middle nasal turbinates.

TABLE 3-1			
Combining Forms			
Combining Form	**Meaning**	**Combining Form**	**Meaning**
1. adenoid/o	adenoid	20. pector/o	chest
2. alveol/o	alveolus	21. pharyng/o	pharynx
3. atel/o	incomplete	22. phon/o	voice
4. bronch/o	bronchus	23. phren/o	diaphragm
5. bronchi/o	bronchus	24. pleur/o	pleura
6. bronchiol/o	bronchiole	25. pneum/o	lung/air
7. capn/o	carbon dioxide	26. pneumat/o	air
8. coni/o	dust	27. pneumon/o	lung/air
9. cyan/o	blue	28. pulmon/o	lung
10. diaphragmat/o	diaphragm	29. py/o	pus
11. epiglott/o	epiglottis	30. rhin/o	nose
12. laryng/o	larynx	31. sept/o	septum
13. lob/o	lobe	32. sinus/o	sinus
14. mediastin/o	mediastinum	33. spir/o	breath
15. muc/o	mucus	34. tel/o	complete
16. nas/o	nose	35. thorac/o	thorax
17. orth/o	straight	36. tonsill/o	tonsil
18. ox/o	oxygen	37. trache/o	trachea
19. oxy/o	oxygen		

TABLE 3-2
Prefixes

Prefix	Meaning
1. a-	not
2. an-	not
3. endo-	within
4. eu-	good
5. dys-	difficult
6. pan-	all
7. poly-	many

TABLE 3-3
Suffixes

Suffix	Meaning
1. -algia	pain
2. -ar	pertaining to
3. -ary	pertaining to
4. -capnia	carbon dioxide
5. -centesis	puncture to remove (drain)
6. -dynia	pain
7. -eal	pertaining to
8. -ectasis	stretching
9. -emia	blood
10. -gram	record
11. -graph	recording instrument
12. -graphy	recording process
13. -itis	inflammation
14. -meter	measurement or instrument that measures
15. -metry	measurement of
16. -osmia	smell
17. -oxia	oxygen
18. -pexy	fixation
19. -phonia	sound
20. -pnea	breathing
21. -ptysis	spitting
22. -rrhage, -rrhagia	abnormal, excessive flow
23. -scopy	to examine
24. -spasm	contraction of muscle
25. -sphyxia	pulse
26. -stenosis	blockage, narrowing
27. -stomy	opening
28. -thorax	chest
29. -tomy	cutting, incision

TABLE 3-4
Medical Abbreviations

Abbreviation	Meaning
1. ABG	arterial blood gas
2. AFB	acid-fast bacillus
3. ARDS	adult respiratory distress syndrome
4. BiPAP	bi-level positive airway pressure
5. COPD	chronic obstructive pulmonary disease
6. CPAP	continuous positive airway pressure
7. DLCO	diffuse capacity of lungs for carbon monoxide
8. FEF	forced expiratory flow
9. FEV_1	forced expiratory volume in 1 second
10. FEV_1: FVC	maximum amount of forced expiratory volume in 1 second
11. FRC	functional residual capacity
12. FVC	forced vital capacity
13. HHN	handheld nebulizer
14. IPAP	inspiratory positive airway pressure
15. IRDS	infant respiratory distress syndrome
16. MDI	metered-dose inhaler
17. MVV	maximum voluntary ventilation
18. PAWP	pulmonary artery wedge pressure
19. PCWP	pulmonary capillary wedge pressure
20. PEAP	positive end-airway pressure
21. PEEP	positive end-expiratory pressure
22. PFT	pulmonary function test
23. PND	paroxysmal nocturnal dyspnea
24. RDS	respiratory distress syndrome
25. RSV	respiratory syncytial virus
26. RV	respiratory volume
27. RV: TLC	ratio of respiratory volume to total lung capacity
28. TLC	total lung capacity
29. TLV	total lung volume
30. URI	upper respiratory infection
31. V/Q	ventilation/perfusion scan

TABLE 3-5

Medical Terms

Term	Meaning	Term	Meaning
Ablation	Removal or destruction by cutting, chemicals, or electrocautery	Laryngoscopy	Direct visualization and examination of interior of larynx with a laryngoscope
Adenoidectomy	Removal of adenoids	Laryngotomy	Incision into larynx
Apnea	Cessation of breathing	Lavage	Washing out
Asphyxia	Lack of oxygen	Lobectomy	Surgical excision of a lobe of lung
Asthma	Shortage of breath caused by contraction of bronchi	Nasal button	Synthetic circular disc used to cover a hole in the nasal septum
Atelectasis	Incomplete expansion of lung, collapse	Orthopnea	Difficulty in breathing, relieved by assuming upright position
Auscultation	Listening to sounds, such as to lung sounds	Percussion	Tapping with sharp blows as a diagnostic technique
Bacilli	Plural of bacillus, a rod-shaped bacteria	Pertussis	Whooping cough—highly contagious bacterial infection of pharynx, larynx, and trachea
Bilobectomy	Surgical removal of two lobes of a lung	Pharyngolaryngectomy	Surgical removal of pharynx and larynx
Bronchiole	Smaller division of bronchial tree	Pleura	Covers lungs and lines thoracic cavity
Bronchoplasty	Surgical repair of bronchi		
Bronchoscopy	Inspection of bronchial tree using a bronchoscope	Pleurectomy	Surgical excision of pleura
		Pleuritis	Inflammation of pleura
Catheter	Tube placed into body to put fluid in or take fluid out	Pneumocentesis/ pneumonocentesis	Surgical puncturing of a lung to withdraw fluid
Cauterization	Destruction of tissue by use of cautery	Pneumonia	Inflammation of lungs with consolidation
Cordectomy	Surgical removal of vocal cord(s)	Pneumonolysis/ pneumolysis	Surgical separation of lung from chest wall to allow lung to collapse
Crackle	Abnormal sound when breathing (heard on auscultation)		
Croup	Acute viral infection (obstruction of larynx), stridor	Pneumonotomy/ pneumotomy	Incision of lung
Cyanosis	Bluish discoloration	Pulmonary edema	Accumulation of fluid in pulmonary tissues and air spaces
Drainage	Free flow or withdrawal of fluids from a wound or cavity		
Dysphonia	Speech impairment	Pulmonary embolism	Thrombus or other foreign material lodged in pulmonary artery or one of its branches
Dyspnea	Shortage of breath, difficult breathing		
Emphysema	Air accumulated in organ or tissue	Rales	An abnormal respiratory sound heard in auscultation, indicating some pathologic condition
Epiglottidectomy	Excision of covering of larynx		
Epistaxis	Nose bleed	Rhinoplasty	Surgical repair of nose
Glottis	True vocal cords	Rhinorrhea	Free discharge of a thin nasal mucus
Hemoptysis	Bloody sputum		
Intramural	Within organ wall	Sarcoidosis	Chronic inflammatory disease with nodules developing in lungs, lymph nodes, other organs
Intubation	Insertion of a tube		
Laryngeal web	Congenital abnormality of connective tissue between vocal cords		
Laryngectomy	Surgical removal of larynx	Segmentectomy	Surgical removal of the smaller subdivisions (segment) of lobes of a lung
Laryngoplasty	Surgical repair of larynx		
Laryngoscope	Fiberoptic scope used to view inside of larynx		

TABLE 3-5

Medical Terms—cont'd

Term	Meaning	Term	Meaning
Septoplasty	Surgical repair of nasal septum	Thoracostomy	Surgical incision into chest wall and insertion of a chest tube
Sinusotomy	Surgical incision into a sinus	Thoracotomy	Surgical incision into chest wall
Spirometry	Measuring breathing capacity	Total pneumonectomy	Surgical removal of an entire lung
Tachypnea	Quick, shallow breathing	Tracheostomy	Creation of an opening into trachea
Thoracentesis/ thoracocentesis (pleuracentesis/ pleurocentesis)	Surgical puncture of thoracic cavity, usually using a needle, to remove fluids	Tracheotomy	Incision into trachea
		Transtracheal	Across trachea
Thoracoplasty	Surgical procedure that removes rib(s) and thereby allows collapse of a lung	Tuberculosis	Infection of the lungs caused by bacteria (tubercle bacillus)
Thoracoscopy	Use of a lighted endoscope to view pleural spaces and thoracic cavity or to perform surgical procedures		

Chapter 3: Anatomy and Terminology Quiz

(Quiz Answers Are Located in Appendix B)

1. This is NOT a part of lower respiratory tract:
   a. trachea
   b. larynx
   c. bronchi
   d. lungs
2. Another name for voice box is:
   a. oropharynx
   b. pharynx
   c. laryngopharynx
   d. larynx
3. This is the windpipe:
   a. pharynx
   b. larynx
   c. trachea
   d. sphenoid
4. Interior of nose is divided by the:
   a. septum
   b. sphenoid
   c. oropharynx
   d. apical
5. This combining form means "incomplete":
   a. atel/o
   b. alveol/o
   c. ox/i
   d. pneumat/o
6. This combining form means "breath":
   a. py/o
   b. lob/o
   c. spir/o
   d. pleur/o
7. This prefix means "all":
   a. a-
   b. an-
   c. pan-
   d. poly-
8. This abbreviation refers to a syndrome that involves difficulty in breathing:
   a. ABG
   b. ARDS
   c. BiPAP
   d. FEF
9. This abbreviation refers to amount of air patient can expel from the lungs in 1 second:
   a. PFT
   b. PND
   c. RDS
   d. FEV_1
10. This suffix means "breathing":
   a. -stenosis
   b. -spasm
   c. -pexy
   d. -pnea

PATHOPHYSIOLOGY

Signs and Symptoms of Pulmonary Disorders

Dyspnea

Difficult breathing (sense of air hunger)
Increased respiratory effort

Hypoventilation

Decreased alveolar ventilation

Hyperventilation

Increased alveolar ventilation

Hemoptysis

Bloody sputum

Hypoxia

Reduced oxygenation of tissue cells

Cough

Caused by irritant
Protective reflex
Acute cough is up to 3 weeks
Chronic cough is over 3 weeks

Tachypnea

Rapid breathing

Apnea

Lack of breathing

Orthopnea

Requiring sitting upright to facilitate breathing

Pulmonary Diseases and Disorders

Hypercapnia

Increased carbon dioxide in arterial blood
Caused by inadequate ventilation of alveoli
Can result in respiratory acidosis

Hypoxemia

Reduced oxygenation of arterial blood

Acute Respiratory Failure

Inadequate gas exchange
Hypoxemia
Can result from trauma or disease

Adult Respiratory Distress Syndrome (ARDS)

Acute injury to alveolocapillary membrane
Results in edema and atelectasis
In infants, infant respiratory distress syndrome (IRDS)

Pulmonary Edema

Accumulation of fluid in lung tissue
Most common cause is left ventricular failure

Aspiration

Passage of fluid and solid particles into lung
Can cause severe pneumonitis
- Localized inflammation of lung

Atelectasis

Collapse of lung
Three most common types are:
- Adhesive
- Compression
- Obstruction
May be chronic or acute
- Acute, such as compression as a result of an automobile accident
- Chronic from structural defect

Absorption Atelectasis

Results from absence of air in alveoli

Caused by
Foreign body
Tumor
Abnormal external pressure

Bronchiectasis

Chronic, irreversible dilation of bronchi

Common Types That Describe Severity of Condition
- Cylindrical
- Varicose
- Saccular or cystic

Respiratory Acidosis

Decreased level of pH
Due to excess retention of carbon dioxide

Bronchiolitis

Inflammation and obstruction of bronchioles
Usually in children younger than 2 years old—preceded by URI
Viral infection (respiratory syncytial virus, or RSV)

Common Types
- Constrictive
- Proliferative
- Obliterative

Pneumothorax

Air collected in pleural cavity
Leads to lung collapse
Communicating pneumothorax is barometric air pressure in pleural space

Spontaneous pneumothorax is spontaneous rupture of visceral pleura

Secondary pneumothorax is a result of trauma to chest

Pneumoconiosis

Dust particles or other particulate matter in lung

Common Types

- Coal
- Asbestos
- Fiberglass

Pleural Effusion–Fluid in Pleural Space

Common Types

- Hemothorax—hemorrhage into pleural cavity
- Empyema—Infectious materials in pleural space
- Exudate—Fluid remaining after infection, inflammation, malignancy

Empyema

Infectious Pleural Effusion

Pus in pleural space
- Complication of respiratory infection
- Commonly follows pneumonia and is treated like pneumonia

Pulmonary Embolism

Air, tissue, or clot occlusion
- Lodges in pulmonary artery or branch of artery
- Risk with congestive heart failure
- Most clots originate in leg veins

Cor Pulmonale

Hypertrophy or failure of right ventricle
- Result of lung, pulmonary vessels, or chest wall disorders
- Acute is secondary to pulmonary embolus
- Chronic is secondary to obstructive lung disease

Pleurisy (Pleuritis)

Inflammation of pleura
- Often preceded by an upper respiratory infection

Infectious Disease

Upper Respiratory Infection (URI)

Acute inflammatory process of mucous membranes in trachea and above

Common Types

- Common cold
- Croup
- Sinusitis
- Laryngitis

Lower Respiratory Infection (LRI)

Pneumonia

Inflammation of lungs with consolidation

Categorized according to causative organism
Can be caused by
- Aspiration
- Bacteria
- Protozoa
- Fungi
- Chlamydia
- Virus

Common Types

Aspiration pneumonia
Bacterial
Chlamydial
Drug resistant
Eosinophil
Fungal
Hospital acquired (nosocomial)
Legionnaires' disease
Mycoplasma
Pneumococcal
Viral

Tuberculosis

Communicable lung disease—airborne droplet
- Caused by *Mycobacterium tuberculosis* (bacilli)

Chronic Obstructive Pulmonary Disease (COPD)

Irreversible airway obstruction that decreases expiration

Includes

Chronic bronchitis
- Bronchial spasms
- Dyspnea
- Wheezing
- Productive cough
- Cyanosis
- Chronic hypoventilation
- Polycythemia
- Cor pulmonale
- Prolonged expiration

Emphysema
- Loss of elasticity and enlargement of alveoli
- Mimics symptoms of chronic bronchitis but more exaggerated

Chapter 3: Pathophysiology Quiz

(Quiz Answers Are Located in Appendix B)

1. Acute injury to alveolocapillary membrane that results in edema and atelectasis:
   a. hypoxemia
   b. adult respiratory distress syndrome
   c. bronchiolitis
   d. pneumoconiosis

2. Condition in which pus is in pleural space and is often a complication of pneumonia:
   a. empyema
   b. cor pulmonale
   c. pneumothorax
   d. atelectasis

3. Which of the following is NOT one of the most common types of atelectasis?
   a. adhesive
   b. compression
   c. obstruction
   d. expansion

4. This condition is a result of accumulation of dust particles in lung:
   a. pleurisy
   b. tuberculosis
   c. chronic obstructive pulmonary disease
   d. pneumoconiosis

5. An irreversible airway obstructive disease in which symptoms are bronchial spasm, dyspnea, and wheezing:
   a. pleurisy
   b. empyema
   c. bronchiolitis
   d. COPD

6. Cylindrical, varicose, and secular/cystic are examples of:
   a. bronchiectasis
   b. cor pulmonale
   c. pneumothorax
   d. atelectasis

7. Condition in which there is a loss of elasticity and enlargement of alveoli:
   a. chronic bronchitis
   b. asthma
   c. emphysema
   d. empyema

8. Definition of a chronic cough is one that lasts for more than this number of weeks:
   a. 2
   b. 3
   c. 4
   d. 5

9. A condition marked by an increase in carbon dioxide in arterial blood and decreased ability to breathe that can result in respiratory acidosis:
   a. hypercapnia
   b. hypoxemia
   c. acute respiratory failure
   d. pulmonary edema

10. This condition often follows a viral infection and occurs in children under 2 years of age. Examples of various types of this condition are constrictive, proliferating, and obliterative.
    a. pneumoconiosis
    b. pulmonary edema
    c. bronchiolitis
    d. bronchiectasis

4

Cardiovascular System

ANATOMY AND TERMINOLOGY

Consists of blood, blood vessels, and heart

Blood (Function Is to Maintain a Constant Environment)

Composed of cells suspended in plasma (clear, straw-colored liquid)

Carries

Oxygen and nutrients to cells
   Waste and carbon dioxide to kidneys, liver, and lungs
   Hormones from endocrine system

Regulates

Temperature by circulating blood

Protection

White cells (leukocytes) produce antibodies

Composed of Two Parts

Liquid Part (Extracellular) Is Plasma
Water 91%
Protein 1%, albumin, globulins, fibrinogen, ferritin, transferrin
2% ions, nutrients, waste products, gases, regulating substances

Cellular Structures
Leukocytes (WBCs)—granular and agranular—fight infections
   • Neutrophils
   • Lymphocytes
   • Monocytes
   • Eosinophils
   • Basophils
Erythrocytes (red blood cells)—hemoglobin carries oxygen
Thrombocytes (platelets)—important for hemostasis
Blood types: A, B, AB, and O are genetically endowed
   • Blood type O negative is known as universal donor (no Rh and no red cell antigens present)

Vessels—Circulatory System

Function

To carry blood delivering nutrients and oxygen (arterial system) and carry away cell waste and carbon dioxide (venous system)

Types

Arteries (Fig. 4.1) Carrying Oxygenated Blood
Inner layer, endothelium
   Lead away from heart
   Branches are arterioles

Capillaries
Connection between arterioles and venules
Exchange structure (oxygen and carbon dioxide, nutrients, and waste)

Veins (Fig. 4.2) Carrying Deoxygenated Blood
Carry blood to heart
   Venules are small branches

Heart

Circulates blood

Four Chambers (Fig. 4.3)

Two Upper
Right and left atria (singular: atrium) receive blood

Two Lower
Right and left ventricles discharge blood (pump)

Chamber Walls

Composed of three layers
   • Endocardium: smooth inner layer
   • Myocardium: middle muscular layer
   • Epicardium: outer layer

Septa (Singular: Septum)

Divide chambers
   • Interatrial septum
      Separates two upper chambers

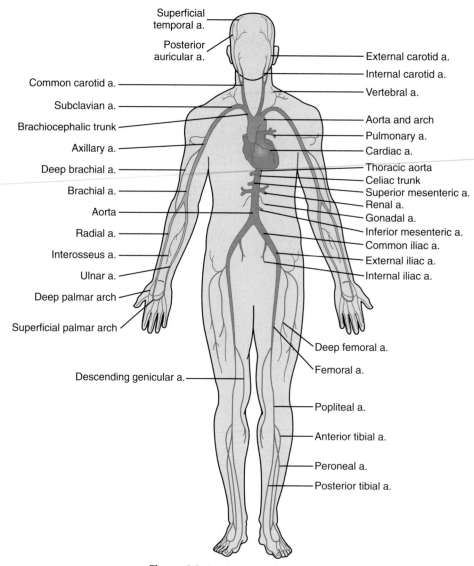

Superficial temporal a.
Posterior auricular a.
Common carotid a.
Subclavian a.
Brachiocephalic trunk
Axillary a.
Deep brachial a.
Brachial a.
Aorta
Radial a.
Interosseus a.
Ulnar a.
Deep palmar arch
Superficial palmar arch
Descending genicular a.

External carotid a.
Internal carotid a.
Vertebral a.
Aorta and arch
Pulmonary a.
Cardiac a.
Thoracic aorta
Celiac trunk
Superior mesenteric a.
Renal a.
Gonadal a.
Inferior mesenteric a.
Common iliac a.
External iliac a.
Internal iliac a.
Deep femoral a.
Femoral a.
Popliteal a.
Anterior tibial a.
Peroneal a.
Posterior tibial a.

• **Figure 4.1** Arteries of circulatory system.

- Interventricular septum
  Separates two lower chambers

Major Blood Vessels

Inferior vena cava—carries deoxygenated blood from lower extremities, pelvic, and abdominal viscera to right atrium

Superior vena cava—drains deoxygenated blood from head, neck, upper extremities, and chest to right atrium

Pulmonary artery bifurcates and becomes right and left pulmonary artery—carries deoxygenated blood from right ventricle to lungs

Right and left pulmonary veins (4)—carry oxygenated blood from lungs to left atrium

Aorta—carries oxygenated blood from left side of heart to body

Pericardium

Sac comprised of two layers that covers heart

- Parietal pericardium: outermost covering

- Visceral pericardium: innermost (epicardium)
- Pericardial cavity: contains about 30 cc of fluid

Valves (4 in Heart)

Tricuspid: between right atrium and right ventricle
  Pulmonary: at entrance of pulmonary artery leading from right ventricle
  Aortic: at entrance of aorta leading from left ventricle
Bicuspid (mitral): between left atrium and left ventricle

Conduction System (Fig. 4.4)

Sinoatrial node: SAN, nature's pacemaker, sends impulses to atrioventricular node

Atrioventricular node (AVN): located on interatrial septum and sends impulses to bundle of His

Bundle of His: divides into right bundle branch (RBB) and left bundle branch (LBB) in septum

Purkinje fibers: merge from bundle branches into specialized cells of myocardium, located in ventricular endocardium

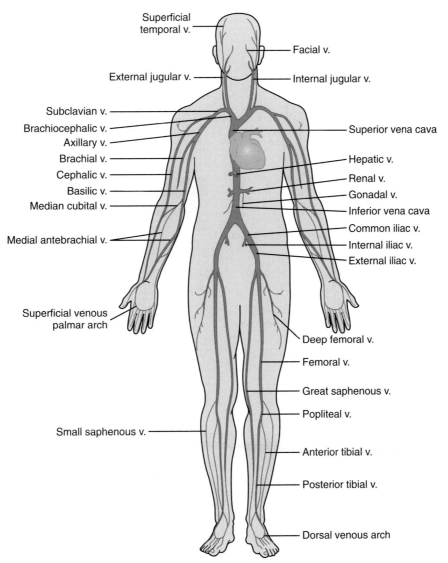

Superficial temporal v.

Facial v.

External jugular v.

Internal jugular v.

Subclavian v.

Brachiocephalic v.

Axillary v.

Brachial v.

Cephalic v.

Basilic v.

Median cubital v.

Superior vena cava

Hepatic v.

Renal v.

Gonadal v.

Inferior vena cava

Common iliac v.

Medial antebrachial v.

Internal iliac v.

External iliac v.

Superficial venous palmar arch

Deep femoral v.

Femoral v.

Great saphenous v.

Popliteal v.

Small saphenous v.

Anterior tibial v.

Posterior tibial v.

Dorsal venous arch

• **Figure 4.2** Veins of circulatory system.

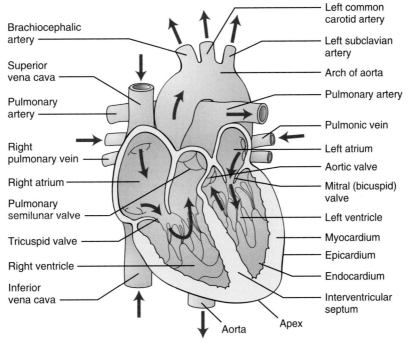

Brachiocephalic artery

Left common carotid artery

Superior vena cava

Left subclavian artery

Pulmonary artery

Arch of aorta

Pulmonary artery

Right pulmonary vein

Pulmonic vein

Left atrium

Right atrium

Aortic valve

Pulmonary semilunar valve

Mitral (bicuspid) valve

Tricuspid valve

Left ventricle

Right ventricle

Myocardium

Epicardium

Inferior vena cava

Endocardium

Interventricular septum

Aorta

Apex

• **Figure 4.3** Internal view of heart.

Heartbeat

Two Phases—Correspond to Blood Pressure Readouts

Systole: contraction—top number reading
   Diastole: relaxation—lower number reading
     Trace a drop of blood from trunk of body (deoxygenated) to trunk of body (oxygenated)

Inferior vena cava to right atrium
Through tricuspid valve to right ventricle
From right ventricle to pulmonary artery to lung capillaries
From lung capillaries to pulmonary veins
To left atrium through mitral (bicuspid) valve to left ventricle
Through aortic valve to aorta

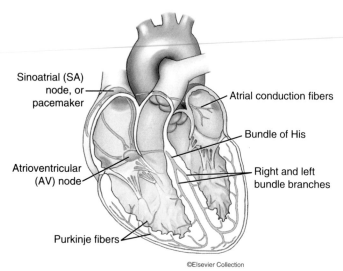

Sinoatrial (SA) node, or pacemaker
Atrial conduction fibers
Bundle of His
Atrioventricular (AV) node
Right and left bundle branches
Purkinje fibers

©Elsevier Collection

• **Figure 4.4** Conduction system of heart.

TABLE 4-1
Combining Forms

Combining Form	Meaning
1. angi/o	vessel
2. aort/o	aorta
3. ather/o	yellow plaque (fat)
4. arter/o	artery
5. arteri/o	artery
6. atri/o	atrium
7. brachi/o	arm
8. cardi/o	heart
9. cholesterol/o	cholesterol
10. coron/o	heart
11. cyan/o	blue
12. my/o, muscul/o	muscle
13. myx/o	mucous
14. ox/o	oxygen
15. pericardi/o	pericardium
16. phleb/o	vein
17. sphygm/o	pulse
18. steth/o	chest
19. thromb/o	clot
20. valv/o	valve
21. valvul/o	valve
22. vascul/o	vessel
23. vas/o	vessel
24. ven/o	vein
25. ventricul/o	ventricle

TABLE 4-2
Prefixes

Prefix	Meaning
1. a-	not
2. an-	not
3. bi-	two
4. brady-	slow
5. de-	lack of
6. dys-	bad, difficult, painful
7. endo-	in
8. hyper-	over
9. hypo-	under
10. inter-	between
11. intra-	within
12. meta-	change, after
13. peri-	surrounding
14. tachy-	fast
15. tetra-	four
16. tri-	three

TABLE 4-3
Suffixes

Suffix	Meaning
1. -dilation	widening, expanding
2. -emia	blood
3. -graphy	recording process
4. -lysis	separation
5. -megaly	enlargement
6. -oma	tumor
7. -osis	condition
8. -plasty	repair
9. -sclerosis	hardening
10. -stenosis	blockage, narrowing
11. -tomy	cutting, incision

TABLE 4-4

Medical Abbreviations

Abbreviation	Meaning
1. ASCVD	arteriosclerotic cardiovascular disease
2. ASD	atrial septal defect
3. ASHD	arteriosclerotic heart disease
4. AV	atrioventricular
5. CABG	coronary artery bypass graft
6. CHF	congestive heart failure
7. CK	creatine kinase
8. CPK	creatine phosphokinase
9. CVI	cerebrovascular insufficiency
10. DSE	dobutamine stress echocardiography
11. HCVD	hypertensive cardiovascular disease
12. LBBB	left bundle branch block
13. LVH	left ventricular hypertrophy
14. MAT	multifocal atrial tachycardia
15. MI	myocardial infarction
16. NSR	normal sinus rhythm
17. PAC	premature atrial contraction
18. PAT	paroxysmal atrial tachycardia
19. PST/PSVT	paroxysmal supraventricular tachycardia
20. PTCA	percutaneous transluminal coronary angioplasty
21. PVC	premature ventricular contraction
22. RBBB	right bundle branch block
23. RSR	regular sinus rhythm
24. RVH	right ventricular hypertrophy
25. SVT	supraventricular tachycardia
26. TEE	transesophageal echocardiography
27. TST	treadmill stress test

TABLE 4-5

Medical Terms

Term	Meaning
Acute coronary syndrome (ACS)	An umbrella term used to cover clinical symptoms compatible with acute myocardial ischemia
Anastomosis	Surgical connection of two tubular structures, such as two pieces of the intestine
Aneurysm	Abnormal dilation of vessels, usually an artery
Angina	Spasmotic, choking, or suffocative pain
Angiography	Radiography of blood vessels
Angioplasty	Procedure in a vessel to dilate vessel opening
Atherectomy	Removal of plaque from an artery (can be done by a percutaneous or open procedure)
Auscultation	Listening for sounds within body
Bundle of His	Muscular cardiac fibers that provide heart rhythm to ventricles
Bypass	To go around
Cardiopulmonary	Refers to heart and lungs
Cardiopulmonary bypass	Blood bypasses heart through a heart-lung machine
Circumflex	A coronary artery that circles heart
Cutdown	Incision into a vessel for placement of a catheter
Edema	Swelling due to abnormal fluid collection in tissue spaces
Electrode	Lead attached to a generator that carries electric current from the generator to atria or ventricles
Electrophysiology	Study of electrical system of heart, including study of arrhythmias
Embolectomy	Removal of blockage (embolism) from vessel
Endarterectomy	Incision into an artery to remove inner lining
Epicardial	Over heart
False aneurysm	Sac of clotted blood that has completely destroyed vessel and is being contained by tissue that surrounds vessel
Fistula	Abnormal opening from one area to another area or to outside of the body
Hematoma	Mass of blood that forms outside vessel
Hemolysis	Breakdown of red blood cells
Hypoxemia	Low level of oxygen in blood
Hypoxia	Low level of oxygen in tissue
Implantable defibrillator	Surgically placed or wearable device that directs an electric shock to the heart to restore rhythm
Intracardiac	Inside heart

Continued

TABLE 4-5

Medical Terms—cont'd

Term	Meaning	Term	Meaning
Invasive	Entering body, breaking skin	Pericardium	Membranous sac enclosing heart and ends of great vessels
Noninvasive	Not entering body, not breaking skin		
Nuclear cardiology	Diagnostic specialty that uses radiologic procedures to aid in diagnosis of cardiologic conditions	Swan-Ganz catheter	A catheter that measures pressure in right side of heart and in pulmonary artery
		Thoracostomy	Incision into chest wall and insertion of a chest tube
Order	Shows subordination of one thing to another; family or class	Thromboendarterectomy	Removal of thrombus and atherosclerotic lining from an artery (percutaneous or open procedure)
Pericardiocentesis	Procedure in which a surgeon withdraws fluid from pericardial space by means of a needle inserted percutaneously	Transvenous	Through a vein

Chapter 4: Anatomy and Terminology Quiz

(Quiz Answers Are Located in Appendix B)

1. These carry blood to the heart:
   a. capillaries
   b. arteries
   c. arterioles
   d. veins
2. Relaxation phase of heartbeat:
   a. diastole
   b. systole
3. Nature's pacemaker is this node:
   a. atrioventricular
   b. Bundle of His
   c. sinoatrial
   d. mitral
4. Node located on interatrial septum:
   a. atrioventricular
   b. Bundle of His
   c. sinoatrial
   d. Purkinje
5. Which of the following is NOT one of the three layers of chamber walls of the heart?
   a. endocardium
   b. myocardium
   c. epicardium
   d. parietal
6. Septum that divides upper two chambers of heart:
   a. intraventricular
   b. interatrial
   c. tricuspid
   d. myocardium
7. Valve between right atrium and right ventricle:
   a. pulmonary
   b. aortic
   c. bicuspid
   d. tricuspid
8. Outer two-layer covering of heart:
   a. pericardium
   b. mitral
   c. myocardium
   d. epicardium
9. These are chambers that receive blood:
   a. right and left ventricle
   b. left ventricle and right atrium
   c. right atrium and right ventricle
   d. right and left atria
10. This combining form means "plaque":
    a. atri/o
    b. brachi/o
    c. cyan/o
    d. ather/o

PATHOPHYSIOLOGY

Vascular Disorders

Coronary Artery Disease (CAD)/Ischemic Heart Disease (IHD)

Thickening and hardening of arterial intima (innermost layer) with lipid and fibrous plaque (atherosclerosis)
- Produces narrowing and stiffening of vessel
  Location of lesions leads to various vascular diseases
- Femoral and popliteal arteries = peripheral vascular disease
- Carotid arteries = stroke
- Aorta = aneurysms (dilation/weakening of vessel walls)
- Coronary arteries = ischemic heart disease or myocardial infarction
  Resulting in decreased oxygen supply
  Risk factors increased by:
- Age
- Family history of CAD
- Hyperlipidemia
- Low HDL-C (good cholesterol)
- Hypertension
- Cigarette smoking
- Diabetes mellitus
- Obesity, particularly abdominal

Ischemia

Deficiency of oxygenated blood
- Often due to constriction or obstruction of blood vessel

Localized Myocardial Ischemia—Most Common Cause: Atherosclerosis of Vessels

Oxygen demand of tissues greater than supply
Presenting symptoms
- Chest pain (angina pectoris)
- Hypotension
- Changes in ECG

Transient Ischemia

Heart muscle begins to perform at a low level due to lack of oxygen (reversible ischemia)

Irreversible Ischemia—Is Cause of an MI (Myocardial Infarction)

Heart muscle dies—necrosis (myocardial infarction)
- Prolonged ischemia of 30 minutes or more
- Reestablishment of blood flow reduces residual necrosis
- Thrombolytic agents to dissolve or split up thrombus
- Primary percutaneous transluminal coronary angioplasty (PTCA)

Cardiac enzymes are released from damaged cells
- Blood test reveals elevation of enzymes, confirming myocardial infarction

Classification of blood pressure for adults aged 18 years or older[1]

Category	Systolic (mm Hg)	Diastolic (mm Hg)
Normal	<120	<80
Prehypertension (stays between)	120–139	80–89
Hypertension[2]		
Stage 1 (mild)	140–159	90–99
Stage 2 (moderate)	160–179	100–109
Stage 3 (severe)	≥180	≥110

[1] Not taking antihypertensive drugs and not acutely ill. When systolic and diastolic pressures fall into different categories, the higher category should be selected.

[2] Based on the average of two or more readings taken at each of two or more visits after an initial screening.

• **Figure 4.5** Classification of blood pressure.

Hypertension (HTN)

Normal is less than 120/80 for adults
- Fig. 4.5 illustrates new hypertension classifications

Leading cause of death in United States due to damage to brain, heart, kidneys, eyes, and arteries of the lower extremities

Cause is unknown in 95% of cases
- Known as
  - Primary hypertension
  - Essential hypertension

5% of cases are secondary to underlying disease
Increased resistance damages heart and blood vessels
- Retinal vascular changes are monitored to assess therapy and disease progression

Chronic hypertension often leads to end-stage renal disease
- Result of progressive sclerosis of renal vessels

Treatment

Medications
- ACE (angiotensin-converting enzyme) inhibitor
- Alpha-adrenergic or beta-adrenergic receptor blocker
- Diuretic
- Calcium channel blocker

Lifestyle changes

Hypotension

Abnormally Low Blood Pressure

Types

Orthostatic (postural) hypotension
- Fall in both systolic and diastolic arterial blood pressure on standing
- Associated with
  - Dizziness
  - Blurred vision
  - Fainting (syncope)

- Caused by insufficient oxygenated blood flow through brain
- Can be acute (temporary) or chronic

Chronic orthostatic hypotension—types
- Primary of unknown cause
- Secondary to certain disease processes
  - Such as:
  - Endocrine
  - Metabolic
  - Central nervous system disorders
- Treatment for secondary hypotension is correction of underlying disease

Aneurysm

Dilation of an arterial blood vessel wall or cardiac chamber
- Danger is rupture of aneurysm

Atherosclerosis is common cause

Arteriosclerosis and hypertension also common in persons with aneurysms

True Aneurysm

Involves all three layers of arterial wall

Causes weakening and ballooning of arterial wall

False or Pseudoaneurysm

Usually result of trauma

Also known as saccular

Separation of arterial wall layers (dissecting) in artery wall (crisis situation—a medical emergency)

Bleeds into dissected space and is contained by arterial connective tissue wall

Thrombus

Blood clot that remains attached to vessel wall and occludes vessel

Dislodged thrombus is a thromboembolus

Causes

Trauma

Interior wall lining irritation/roughening

Infection

Inflammation

Low blood pressure/blood stagnation

Obstruction

Atherosclerosis

Risks Related to Thrombus

Dislodges and moves to lungs, brain, heart

Grows to occlude blood flow

Treatment

Pharmacologic, anticoagulants

Heparin

Warfarin derivatives

Noninvasive Intervention

Balloon-tipped catheter to remove or compress thrombus

Thrombophlebitis Caused by Inflammation (Phlebitis)

Causes

Trauma

Infection

Immobility

Commonly Associated With

Endocarditis

Rheumatic heart disease

Embolism

Mass that is present and circulating in blood

Common Types

Air bubble

Fat

Bacterial mass

Cancer cells

Foreign substances

Dislodged thrombus

Amniotic fluid

Obstructs Vessel

Pulmonary emboli travel through venous side or right side of the heart to the pulmonary artery

Systemic or arterial emboli originate in left side of the heart

Associated with
- Myocardial infarction
- Left-sided heart failure
- Endocarditis
- Valvular conditions
- Dysrhythmias

Peripheral Arterial Disease

Thromboangiitis Obliterans (Buerger's Disease)

Occurs most often in young men who are heavy smokers

Inflammatory disease of peripheral arteries creating thombi and vasospasms

Involves small or medium arteries of feet and often hands
- May necessitate amputation

Raynaud's Disease

Vasospasms and constriction of small arterioles of fingers and toes

Affects young women as a secondary condition

Triggered by cold temperatures, emotional stress, cigarette smoking

Fingertips thicken and nails become brittle

Raynaud's phenomenon is secondary to primary disease, such as
- Scleroderma
- Pulmonary hypertension

Treatment of Underlying Condition

No known origin or treatment

Varicose Veins

Blood pools in veins, distending them
- Tends to be progressive/vein valve failure
- Occurs most commonly in saphenous veins
- Hemorrhoids are varicose veins of anus

Leads to
Swelling and discomfort
Fatigue when in legs
Possible ulcerations

Heart Disorders

Congestive Heart Failure (CHF)—Heart Cannot Pump Required Amounts of Blood

Can be left-sided or right-sided heart failure
Left-sided heart failure (systolic); cannot generate adequate output, causing pulmonary edema
Common causes:
- Myocardial infarction
- Myocarditis
- Cardiomyopathies leading to ischemia

Symptoms of left-sided congestive heart failure include:
- Shortness of breath
- Fatigue
- Exercise intolerance

Right-sided heart failure (diastolic) results in right ventricle stasis, inadequate pulmonary circulation, and peripheral edema/hepatosplenomegaly

Abnormal Heart Rhythms (Conduction Irregularities)

Bradycardia and heart block (atrioventricular block)
- Inadequate conduction impulses from SA node though AV node to AV bundle
- Treatment
  - Cardiac pacemaker to maintain proper heart rate

Flutter—rapid regular contractions (most commonly of atria)
- Symptoms—palpitations
- Treatment
  - Cardioversion (electronic shock to heart)
  - Ablation (radiofrequency catheter destroying tissue causing arrhythmia)

Fibrillation—rapid, erratic, inefficient contractions of atria and ventricles
- Atrial fibrillation—most common (electrical impulses move randomly in atria)
  - Symptoms—palpitation, risk of stroke due to clot formations from poor atrial outputs
- Treatment
  - Cardioversion
  - Ablation

Ventricular fibrillation—life-threatening, random electrical impulses throughout ventricles
- Symptoms—cardiac death or arrest without immediate treatment

Treatment
- Cardioversion
- Digoxin—drug used to slow heart rate
- Implantable defibrillator
- Emergency treatment—automatic external defibrillators (AEDs)
- Radiofrequency catheter ablation (RFA) is a minimally invasive technique used to treat cardiac arrhythmias

Infective Endocarditis

Inflammation of interior-most lining of heart
- Leads to destruction and permanent damage to heart valves
- Caused by
  - Bacteria (most commonly streptococci and staphylococci)
  - Virus
  - Fungi
  - Parasites

Patients with heart defects or damage usually take antibiotics prior to invasive procedures

Pericarditis

Inflammation of pericardium of heart

Common Types
- Acute
- Pericardial effusion
- Constrictive

Rheumatic Fever/Rheumatic Heart Disease

Results in formation of scar tissue of the endocardium and heart valves
- In 10% of cases leads to rheumatic heart disease
- Family tendency to develop
- Begins as carditis (inflammation of all layers of heart wall)
- Long-term effects:
  - Mitral and/or aortic valve disease
  - Stenosis
  - Regurgitation
  - Insufficiency

Tricuspid valve
- Affected in about 10% of cases

Pulmonary valve
- Rarely affected

Valvular Heart Disease

Valves are extensions of endocardial tissue
- Endocardial damage can be congenital or acquired
- Damage leads to stenosis and/or incompetent valve
- Includes
  - Valvular stenosis is narrowing, stiffness, thickening, fusion, or blockage of valve, creating resistance, resulting in increased pressure in cardiac chamber behind valve

- Valvular regurgitation is failure of valve leaflet to close tightly, allowing backflow of blood
- Result of lesions causing valve leaflets to shrink
- Functional valvular regurgitation results in increased chamber size (cardiomegaly)

Stenosis

Aortic Valve Stenosis

Caused by
  Congenital malformation
  Degeneration
  Infection
Results in slowing blood circulatory rate
Symptoms
  Bradycardia
  Faint pulse
  May lead to heart murmur and hypertrophy

Mitral Valve Stenosis

Impaired flow from left atrium to left ventricle
Caused by
  Rheumatic fever
  Bacterial infections
Symptom
  Decreased cardiac output
May lead to
- Pulmonary hypertension
- Right ventricular heart failure
- And/or edema

Valvular Regurgitation

Flow in opposite direction from normal
Mitral regurgitation (MR)
  Backflow of blood from left ventricle into left atrium
Aortic regurgitation (AR)
  Backflow of blood from aorta into left ventricle
Pulmonic regurgitation (PR)
  Backflow of blood from pulmonary artery into right ventricle
Tricuspid regurgitation (TR)
  Backflow of blood from right ventricle into right atrium

Heart Wall Disorders

Acute Pericarditis

Roughening and inflammation of pericardium (sac around heart)

Treatment
  Anti-inflammatory drugs and pain medication

Constrictive Pericarditis (Restrictive Pericarditis)

Forms Fibrous Lesions That Encase Heart

Compresses heart—thickened pericardial sac prevents heart from expanding when blood enters it
  Tamponade occurs when fluid builds up in pericardial space

Pressure stops heart from beating—pericardial effusion or bleeding after heart surgery
Reduces output

Pericardial Effusion

Accumulation of fluid in pericardial cavity
Results in pressure on heart
- Sudden development of pressure on heart is tamponade

Cardiomyopathies

Myocardium: muscular wall (middle layer) of heart musculature
Group of diseases that affect myocardium
Cause
  Idiopathic (most common)
  Underlying condition

Types of Cardiomyopathy

Dilated cardiomyopathy (congestive cardiomyopathy)
- Ventricular distention and impaired systolic function
Hypertrophic cardiomyopathy
- Cause is often hypertensive or valvular heart disease
- Results in thickened interventricular septum (septum between the ventricle chambers)
Restrictive cardiomyopathy
- Myocardium becomes stiffened
- Heart enlarges (cardiomegaly)
- Dysrhythmias common
- Caused by infiltrative diseases such as amyloidosis

Congenital Heart Defects

Coarctation of aorta (CoA)—narrowing of the aorta
- Treatment
  Surgical removal of narrow segment/end-to-end anastomosis
Patent ductus arteriosus (PDA)—opening between aorta and pulmonary artery
- Treatment
  Drugs to close/embolize or plug ductus or tying off surgically
Tetralogy of Fallot—malformation of heart includes four defects
  1. Pulmonary artery stenosis—
     - Narrowing/obstruction
  2. Ventricular septal defect
     - Hole between two bottom chambers (ventricles) of heart
  3. Overriding aorta
     - Shift of aorta to right—aorta overrides the interventricular septum
  4. Hypertrophy of right ventricle
     - Myocardium enlarges to pump blood through narrowed pulmonary artery
     Treatment
     - Open-heart technique with heart-lung machine support to relieve right ventricular outflow tract stenosis and repair of ventriculoseptal defect

Chapter 4: Pathophysiology Quiz

(Quiz Answers Are Located in Appendix B)

1. Lesion of carotid artery may lead to:
   a. heart attack
   b. stroke
   c. peripheral vascular disease
   d. ischemic heart disease
2. This blood pressure is hypertension:
   a. 120/80
   b. 130/70
   c. 140/90
   d. 110/70
3. Infective endocarditis is inflammation of the interior of the lining of the heart, and when caused by streptococci or staphylococci, the infection is:
   a. viral
   b. fungal
   c. bacterial
   d. parasitic
4. Angina pectoris is:
   a. heart block
   b. heart murmur
   c. chest pain
   d. barrel chest
5. In this type of regurgitation, there is a backflow of blood from left ventricle into left atrium:
   a. aortic
   b. pulmonic
   c. tricuspid
   d. mitral
6. In this type of heart wall disorder, fibrous lesions form and encase the heart:
   a. constrictive pericarditis
   b. acute pericarditis
   c. pericardial effusion
   d. cardiomyopathy
7. Which of the following terms means "of unknown cause"?
   a. etiology
   b. manifestation
   c. idiopathic
   d. late effect
8. This condition is also known as congestive cardiomyopathy:
   a. hypertrophic
   b. valvular
   c. dilated
   d. restrictive
9. This peripheral arterial disease most often occurs in young men who are heavy smokers:
   a. Buerger's
   b. Pick's
   c. Addison's
   d. Glasser's
10. This cardiomyopathy results in a thickened interventricular septum:
   a. restrictive
   b. congestive
   c. dilated
   d. hypertrophic

5

Female Genital System and Pregnancy

Terminology

Ovaries (Pair)

Produce ova (single female gamete) and hormones; ova: plural; ovum: singular (Fig. 5.1). Each ovum/gamete contains 23 chromosomes.

Fallopian Tubes (Uterine Tubes or Oviducts)

Ducts from ovary to uterus

Uterus (Womb)

Muscular organ that holds embryo
   Three layers
- Endometrium: inner mucosa
- Myometrium: middle layer/muscle
- Perimetrium/Uterine serosa: outer layer
  - Cervix: lower narrow portion of uterus
  - Fundus: the upper rounded part of the uterus

Vagina

Tube from uterus to outside of body

Vulva

External genitalia
- Clitoris: erectile tissue
- Labia majora: outer lips of vagina
- Labia minora: inner lips of vagina
- Urinary meatus: opening to urethra
- Bartholin's gland: glands on either side of vagina
- Hymen: membrane partially or wholly occludes entrance to vagina

Perineum

Area between anus and vaginal orifice

Accessory Organs (Fig. 5.2)

Breasts

Mammary glands
   Composed of glandular tissue containing milk glands/ lactiferous ducts
   In response to hormones from pituitary gland, milk is produced in acini (also known as alveoli) (lactation)
   Lactiferous ducts transfer milk to nipple
   Nipple, surrounded by areola

Menstruation and Pregnancy

Proliferation Phase

Menstruation (Days 1-5): discharge of blood fluid containing endometrial cells, blood cells, and glandular secretions from endometrium
Endometrium repair (Days 6-12): maturing follicle in ovary produces estrogen (hormone), which causes endometrium to thicken and ovum (egg) to mature in graafian follicle

Secretory Phase

Ovulation (Days 13-14): occurs when graafian follicle ruptures and ovum travels down fallopian tube
   Usually only one graafian follicle develops each month
Premenstruation (Days 15-28): a period of time in which graafian follicle converts to corpus luteum secreting progesterone to stimulate build-up of uterine lining. If after 5 days no fertilization occurs, cycle repeats.

Pregnancy

Prenatal stage of development from fertilization to birth (39 weeks)
   Fertilized ovum or zygote develops in a double cavity: yolk sac (produces blood cells) and amniotic cavity (contains amniotic fluid)

Embryo, stage of development from 4th to 8th week
Fetus, unborn offspring, 9 weeks until birth

Placenta Forms Within Uterine Wall and Produces Hormone—Human Chorionic Gonadotropin (HCG)

HCG is hormone tested in urine pregnancy tests
    HCG stimulates corpus luteum to produce estrogen and progesterone until the third month of pregnancy
    Placenta then produces hormones
    Expelled after delivery (afterbirth)

Gestation, Approximately 266 Days

280 days used when calculating estimated date of delivery (EDD) or time from last menstrual period (LMP)
    Three trimesters

- First   LMP-12 weeks
- Second   13-27 weeks
- Third   28 weeks-EDD

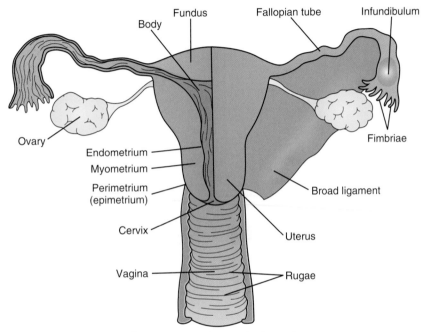

• **Figure 5.1** Female reproductive system.

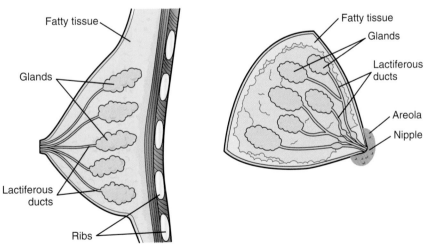

• **Figure 5.2** Breast structure.

TABLE 5-1

Combining Forms

Combining Form	Meaning	Combining Form	Meaning
1. amni/o	amnion	21. metr/o	uterus, measure
2. arche/o	first	22. metr/i	uterus
3. cephal/o	head	23. my/o, muscul/o	muscle
4. cervic/o	cervix	24. nat/a	birth
5. chori/o	chorion	25. nat/i	birth
6. colp/o	vagina	26. obstetr/o	pregnancy/childbirth
7. crypt/o	hidden	27. olig/o	few
8. culd/o	cul-de-sac	28. oo/o	egg
9. episi/o	vulva	29. oophor/o	ovary
10. fet/o	fetus	30. ov/o	egg
11. galact/o	milk	31. ovari/o	ovary
12. gynec/o	female	32. ovul/o	ovulation
13. gyn/o	female	33. perine/o	perineum
14. hymen/o	hymen	34. peritone/o	peritoneum
15. hyster/o	uterus	35. phor/o	to bear
16. lact/o	milk	36. salping/o	uterine tube, fallopian tube
17. lapar/o	abdominal wall	37. top/o	place
18. mamm/o	breast	38. uter/o	uterus
19. mast/o	breast	39. vagin/o	vagina
20. men/o	menstruation, month	40. vulv/o	vulva

TABLE 5-2

Prefixes

Prefix	Meaning
1. ante-	before
2. dys-	painful
3. ecto-	outside
4. endo-	in
5. extra-	outside
6. in-	into
7. intra-	within
8. multi-	many
9. neo-	new
10. nulli-	none
11. nulti-	none
12. post-	after
13. primi-	first
14. pseudo-	false
15. retro-	backwards
16. uni-	one

TABLE 5-3

Suffixes

Suffix	Meaning
1. -arche	beginning
2. -cyesis	pregnancy
3. -gravida	pregnancy
4. -rrhexis	rupture
5. -para	woman who has given birth
6. -parous	to bear
7. -rrhea	discharge
8. -salpinx	uterine tube
9. -tocia	labor
10. -version	turning

TABLE 5-4

Medical Abbreviations

Abbreviation	Meaning	Abbreviation	Meaning
1. AFI	amniotic fluid index	20. EMC	endometrial curettage
2. AGA	appropriate for gestational age	21. ERT	estrogen replacement therapy
3. ARM	artificial rupture of membrane	22. FAS	fetal alcohol syndrome
4. BPD	biparietal diameter	23. FHR	fetal heart rate
5. BPP	biophysical profile	24. FSH	follicle-stimulating hormone
6. BV	bacterial vaginosis	25. HPV	human papillomavirus
7. CHL	crown-to-heel length	26. HSG	hysterosalpingogram
8. CNM	certified nurse midwife	27. HSV	herpes simplex virus
9. CPD	cephalopelvic disproportion	28. IVF	in vitro fertilization
10. CPP	chronic pelvic pain	29. LEEP	loop electrosurgical excision procedure
11. D&C	dilation and curettage	30. LGA	large for gestational age
12. D&E	dilation and evacuation	31. PID	pelvic inflammatory disease
13. DUB	dysfunctional uterine bleeding	32. PROM	premature rupture of membranes
14. ECC	endocervical curettage	33. SHG	sonohysterogram
15. EDC	estimated date of confinement	34. SROM	spontaneous rupture of membranes
16. EDD	estimated date of delivery	35. SUI	stress urinary incontinence
17. EFM	electronic fetal monitoring	36. TAH	total abdominal hysterectomy
18. EFW	estimated fetal weight	37. VBAC	vaginal birth after cesarean
19. EGA	estimated gestational age		

TABLE 5-5

Medical Terms

Term	Meaning	Term	Meaning
Abortion	Termination of pregnancy	Introitus	Opening or entrance to vagina
Amniocentesis	Percutaneous aspiration of amniotic fluid	Ligation	Binding or tying off, as in constricting blood flow of a vessel or binding fallopian tubes for sterilization
Amniotic sac	Sac containing fetus and amniotic fluid		
Antepartum	Before childbirth		
Cesarean	Surgical opening through abdominal wall for delivery	Multipara	More than one pregnancy
		Oophorectomy	Surgical removal of ovary(ies)
Chorionic villus sampling	CVS, biopsy of outermost part of placenta	Perineum	Area between vulva and anus; also known as pelvic floor
Cordocentesis	Procedure to obtain a fetal blood sample; also called a percutaneous umbilical blood sampling	Placenta	A structure that connects fetus and mother during pregnancy
		Postpartum	After childbirth
Curettage	Scraping of a cavity using a spoon-shaped instrument	Primigravida	First pregnancy
		Primipara	First delivered infant/given birth to only one child
Cystocele	Herniation of bladder into vagina		
Delivery	Childbirth	Salpingectomy	Surgical removal of uterine tube
Dilation	Expansion (of cervix)	Salpingostomy	Creation of a fistula into uterine tube
Ectopic	Pregnancy outside uterus (i.e., in fallopian tube)	Tocolysis	Repression of uterine contractions
		Vesicovaginal fistula	Abnormal opening/channel between vagina and bladder
Hysterectomy	Surgical removal of uterus		
Hysterorrhaphy	Suturing of uterus		
Hysteroscopy	Visualization of canal and cavity of uterus using a scope placed through vagina		

Chapter 5: Anatomy and Terminology Quiz

(Quiz Answers Are Located in Appendix B)

1. This is NOT one of the three layers of uterus:
   a. perimetrium
   b. endometrium
   c. myometrium
   d. barametrium
2. Located at the lower end of uterus is the:
   a. cervix
   b. vagina
   c. perineum
   d. labia majora
3. Approximate gestation of a human fetus is:
   a. 266 days
   b. 276 days
   c. 290 days
   d. 292 days
4. LMP is the:
   a. later maternity phase
   b. last menstrual period
   c. low metabolic pregnancy
   d. late menstruation phase
5. Name of stage that describes development of fetus from fertilization to birth is:
   a. postpartum
   b. antepartum
   c. prenatal
   d. natal
6. Which of the following correctly identifies three trimesters of gestation?
   a. LMP to less than 14 weeks 0 days, 14 weeks 0 days to less than 28 weeks 0 days, 28 weeks 0 days until deliver
   b. LMP to less than 16 weeks 0 days, 16 weeks 0 days to less than 28 weeks 0 days, 28 weeks 0 days until deliver
   c. LMP to less than 16 weeks 0 days, 16 weeks 0 days to less than 29 weeks 0 days, 29 weeks 0 days until deliver
   d. LMP to less than 13 weeks 0 days, 13 weeks 0 days to less than 27 weeks 0 days, 27 weeks 0 days until deliver
7. Combining form meaning "few":
   a. oopho/o
   b. olig/o
   c. nati/i
   d. top/o
8. Combining form meaning "hidden":
   a. amni/o
   b. crypt/o
   c. chori/o
   d. fet/o
9. Suffix meaning "beginning":
   a. -cyesis
   b. -rrhea
   c. -arche
   d. -orrhexis
10. Prefix meaning "within":
    a. ante-
    b. dys-
    c. ecto-
    d. endo-

PATHOPHYSIOLOGY

Menstrual and Hormonal Disorders

Dysmenorrhea

Painful menstruation

Common Types
- Primary and secondary

Primary Dysmenorrhea
No underlying condition but begins with commencement of ovulation

Cramping is caused by excess of prostaglandin
- Causes contractions and uterine ischemia
- Develops 24 to 48 hours prior to menstruation

Treatment
- Nonsteroidal anti-inflammatory agents
- Progesterone

Secondary Dysmenorrhea
Caused by an underlying disorder, such as
- Polyps
- Tumors
- Endometriosis
- Pelvic inflammatory disease

Treatment
Directed at underlying disorder

Amenorrhea

Amenorrhea is absence of menstruation

Common Types
- Primary and secondary

Primary Amenorrhea
Menstruation has never occurred
May be genetic disorder
- Turner's syndrome (ovaries do not function)

Secondary Amenorrhea

Cessation of menstruation for 3 cycles or 6 months
- Individual has previously menstruated

Various causes of anovulation/amenorrhea

Examples:
- Tumors
- Stress
- Eating disorders
- Competitive sports participation

Dysfunctional Uterine Bleeding (DUB)

Abnormal bleeding patterns
Occurs when no organic cause can be identified

Abnormal Menstruation Types

Oligomenorrhea: in excess of 6 weeks between periods
    Polymenorrhea: less than 3 weeks between periods
    Metrorrhagia: bleeding between cycles
    Menorrhagia: increase in amount and duration of flow
    Hypomenorrhea: light or spotty flow
    Menometrorrhagia: irregular cycle with varying amounts and duration of flow
    Menorrhea: lengthy menstrual flow
    Dysmenorrhea: painful menstruation

Premenstrual Syndrome (PMS)

Also known as premenstrual tension (PMT)
Occurs before onset of menses (luteal phase) and ends at onset of menses

Cluster of Common Symptoms

Weight gain
Breast tenderness
Sleep disturbances
Headache
Irritability
Cause is unknown

Treatment
- Varies depending on individual symptoms

Endometriosis

Endometrial tissue (uterine lining) develops outside the uterus (on ovaries, fallopian tubes, small intestine, etc.)

Responses to Hormone Cycle

Ectopic (out of place) endometrial tissue degenerates, sheds, and bleeds

Causes
- Irritation
- Inflammation
- Pain
  Continued cycles produce fibrous tissue
- Adhesions and obstructions can then form
- Interferes with normal bodily function

- For example, fallopian tube endometriosis may lead to obstructed tubes
  Primary symptom is dysmenorrhea
- May also cause painful intercourse (dyspareunia)

Risks

Increased risk for cancers
- Breast
- Ovaries
- Non-Hodgkin lymphoma

Treatment Includes

Hormonal suppression

Surgical removal of endometrial tissue
- May require hysterectomy and BSO (bilateral salpingo-oophorectomy)

Infection, Inflammation, and Sexually Transmitted Diseases

Pelvic Inflammatory Disease (PID)

Infection and inflammation of reproductive tract
- Primarily ovaries and fallopian tubes
- Usually originates in cervix or vagina
  - Migrates up through reproductive tract

Types

Acute
Chronic
Commonly forms adhesions and strictures
- May lead to infertility

Candidiasis

Yeast infection
- *Candida albicans (Monilia)*

Not sexually transmitted
Opportunistic infection may follow
- Infection treated with antibiotics
- Period of reduced resistance
- Increased glucose or glycogen levels (often associated with diabetes mellitus)

Affects mucous membranes
- Produces a white, thick, curd-like discharge

Result may be dyspareunia and dysuria

Treatment

Antifungal substances such as nystatin
Identification and treatment of underlying condition

Chlamydia

Most common sexually transmitted disease (STD)

Cause

Bacteria, *Chlamydia trachomatis*

Symptoms
Asymptomatic or mild discharge and dysuria

Treatment
Antimicrobial

Genital Herpes
Cause
Virus, herpes simplex 2 (HSV-2)

Symptoms
Ulcers and vesicles

Treatment
Antiviral, manage outbreaks
There is no cure for genital herpes

Genital Warts
Cause
Virus, human papillomavirus

Symptoms
Polyps or grey lesions

Treatment
Excision

Prevention
Vaccine
There is no cure for genital warts

Gonorrhea
Cause
Bacteria, *Neisseria gonorrhoeae*

Symptoms
Dysuria
Discharge

Treatment
Antibacterial drugs
Some strains are drug-resistant

Syphilis
Cause
Bacteria, *Treponema pallidum*

Symptoms
Primary syphilis
- Ulcer or chancre at site of entry
Secondary syphilis
- Headache
- Fever
- Rash
- Tertiary
- Affects cardiovascular and nervous systems

Treatment
Penicillin

Trichomoniasis
Cause
Protozoan, *Trichomonas vaginalis*

Symptoms
Usually asymptomatic

Treatment
Antimicrobial drugs

Benign Lesions

Leiomyomas—Uterine Fibroids
Well-defined, solid uterine tumor

Also known as
- Uterine fibroids
- Fibromyoma
- Fibroma
- Myoma
- Fibroid
Classification is based on location of tumor within uterine wall
    Submucous: beneath endometrium
    Subserous: beneath serosa
    Intramural: in muscle wall

Symptoms
May be asymptomatic
Abnormal uterine bleeding
Pressure on nearby structures, such as bladder and rectum
Constipation
Pain
Sensation of heaviness

Treatment
Surgical excision of lesions
Hysterectomy may be necessary

Adenomyosis
Within uterine myometrium

Symptoms
Usually asymptomatic
Abnormal menstrual bleeding
Enlarged uterus
    Commonly develops in late reproductive years
    Common in those taking Tamoxifen

Treatment
Symptomatic in mild cases
Surgical in severe cases
- Excision of adenomyosis or hysterectomy

Malignant Lesions

Carcinoma of Breast

Accessory of reproductive system
  Most often develops in upper outer quadrant
  • Due to location, often spreads to lymph nodes
  • May metastasize to lungs, brain, bone, liver, etc.
Majority arise from epithelial cells of ducts and lobules
Second most common cancer of women
Most are adenocarcinoma
  • Invasive ductal carcinoma most common type
  • Invasive lobular carcinoma second most common type
  • Lymph node spread is determined by sentinel node biopsy (SNB)
  • Small primary tumors are excised in a lumpectomy (tumor and immediate surrounding tissue only)
  • Mastectomy is alternative surgical procedure removing entire breast
  • Chemotherapy and radiation may be indicated to prevent recurrence
If neoplasm is responsive to hormone, hormone-blocking agents are administered

Increased Risks
• Heredity
  • Especially history of mother or sister who developed breast cancer
  • Mutated breast cancer gene (BRCA-1)
  • Familial breast cancer syndrome associated with BRCA-2
• Lower socioeconomic status
• Radiation exposure

Carcinoma of Uterus (Endometrial Cancer)

Most frequent pelvic cancer
  Usually postmenopausal
  Associated with higher levels of estrogen

Increases Risk
Obesity (estrogen produced by fat tissue)
Early menarche
Delayed menopause
Hypertension
Diabetes mellitus
Nulliparity (no viable births)
Some types of colorectal cancer
Oral contraceptives (estrogen)
Estrogen-producing tumors

Symptoms
Abnormal, excessive uterine bleeding
Postmenopausal bleeding
No simple screening test available
  • Uterine cells may be aspirated for evaluation

Staging of Endometrial, Cervical, and Ovarian Malignancies
I—Confined to corpus
II—Involves corpus and cervix
III—Extends outside uterus but not outside true pelvis
IV—Extends outside true pelvis or involves rectum or bladder

Treatment
Pharmaceutical
Surgical
Irradiation
Chemotherapy
Combination of above

Carcinoma of Cervix

Routinely found on Papanicolaou (Pap) smear
  Dysplasia is an early change in cervical epithelium

Increases Risks
Herpes simplex virus type 2 (HSV-2)
Human papillomavirus (HPV)
Young age of sexual activity
Smoking
Lower socioeconomic status

Stages of cervical cancer

Stage 1—Carcinoma of cervix
Stage 2—Carcinoma spread from cervix to upper vagina
Stage 3—Carcinoma spread to lower portion of vagina/pelvic wall
Stage 4—Most invasive stage spreading to other body parts

Symptoms
Early stages asymptomatic
Later stages
  • Bleeding
  • Discharge
Biopsy is used to confirm

Treatment
Pharmaceutical
Surgical
Irradiation
Chemotherapy
Combination of above

Carcinoma of Ovary

Cause is unknown—considered silent killer

Increased Risks
Genetic factors (BRCA-1)
Endocrine
  • Nulliparous
  • Early menarche

- Late menopause
- Non–breast feeding
- Late first pregnancy
- Postmenopausal estrogen replacement therapy (ERT)

Tumor Categories

Germ Cell Tumors

Arise from primitive germ cells, usually the testis and ovum

Types

- Germinoma
- Yolk sac
- Endodermal sinus tumor
- Teratoma
- Embryonal carcinoma
- Polyembryoma
- Gonadoblastoma
- Some types of choriocarcinoma

Categories

- Dermoid cysts (benign)
- Malignant tumors
- Primitive malignant
  - Embryonic
  - Extraembryonic cells

Epithelial Tumors

Most common gynecologic cancer

Gonadal Stromal Tumors

Symptoms
Pelvic heaviness
Dysuria
Increased urinary frequency
Sometimes vaginal bleeding

Treatment
Excision
Hysterectomy, including bilateral salpingo-oophorectomy with omentectomy (fold of peritoneum)
Chemotherapy
Radiation therapy
Combination of above

Carcinoma of Fallopian Tubes

Primary Fallopian Tube Tumors

Rare
Must be located within tube to be considered primary
- Adenocarcinoma most common primary tumor
Most tumors are secondary

Symptoms
Often asymptomatic
Bleeding or discharge
Irregular menstruation
Pain

Treatment
Hysterectomy, including bilateral salpingo-oophorectomy with any necessary omentectomy (fold of peritoneum)
Chemotherapy
Radiation therapy
Combination of above

Carcinoma of Vulva

Usually squamous cell carcinoma (90%)
Increased risk with STDs

Symptoms
Can be asymptomatic
Pruritic vulvular lesion

Treatment
Radical vulvectomy with node dissection
Wide local excision

Carcinoma of Vagina

Usually squamous cell carcinoma

Increased Risk
Human papillomavirus (HPV)
Postmenopausal hysterectomy
History of abnormal Pap
History of other carcinomas

Symptoms
Often asymptomatic
Vaginal pain, discharge, or bleeding

Treatment
Squamous cell—radiation
Early tumors may be excised
Vaginectomy
Hysterectomy
Lymph node dissection

Pregnancy

Placenta Previa

Opening of cervix is obstructed by displaced placenta

Types (Fig. 5.3)
Marginal
Partial
Total

Abruptio Placentae (Fig. 5.4)

Premature separation of placenta from uterine wall

Eclampsia

Serious condition of pregnancy characterized by
- Hypertension
- Edema
- Proteinuria

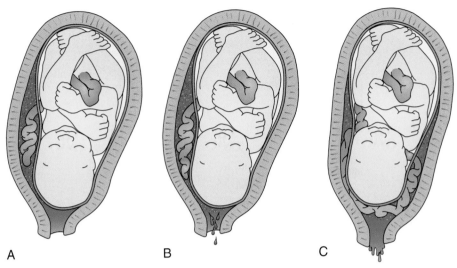

• **Figure 5.3 A.** Marginal placenta previa. **B.** Partial placenta previa. **C.** Total placenta previa.

• **Figure 5.4** Abruptio placentae is classified according to the grade of separation of the placenta from uterine wall. **A.** Mild separation in which hemorrhage is internal. **B.** Moderate separation in which there is external hemorrhage. **C.** Severe separation in which there is external hemorrhage and extreme separation.

Ectopic Pregnancy (Extrauterine)
(Fig. 5.5)

Implantation of fertilized ovum outside uterus
- Often fallopian tubes (tubal pregnancy)

Hydatidiform Mole

Benign tumor of placenta
Secretes hormone (chorionic gonadotropic hormone, CGH)
Indicates positive pregnancy test

Malpositions and Malpresentations

(Fig. 5.6)

Vaginal Delivery

Breech
    Vertex
    Face
    Brow
    Shoulder

Abortion

Types
Spontaneous
- Miscarriage
- Happens naturally
- Uterus completely empties

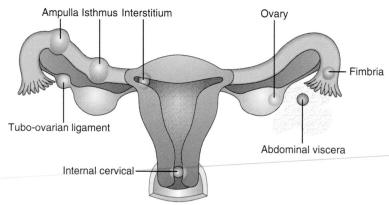

• **Figure 5.5** Ectopic pregnancy most often occurs in fallopian tube. Pregnancy outside the uterus may end in life-threatening rupture.

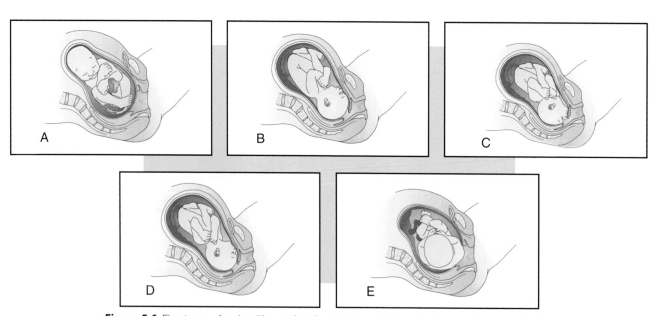

• **Figure 5.6** Five types of malposition and malpresentation of fetus: **A.** Breech. **B.** Vertex. **C.** Face. **D.** Brow. **E.** Shoulder.

Incomplete
- Uterus does not completely empty
- Requires intervention to remove remaining fetal material

Missed
- Fetus dies naturally
- Requires intervention to remove fetal material

Septic
- Similar to missed
- Has added complication of infection
- Requires intervention to remove fetal material
- Vigorous treatment of infection

Methods

D&C
- Dilation and curettage (scraping)

Evacuation (suction)

Intra-amniotic injections
- Saline (salt) solution

Vaginal suppositories
- Such as prostaglandin

Chapter 5: Pathophysiology Quiz

(Quiz Answers Are Located in Appendix B)

1. Most common solution used for intra-amniotic injections is:
   a. prostaglandin
   b. saline
   c. estrogen
   d. chorionic gonadotropic hormone

2. This type of dysmenorrhea is treated with nonsteroidal anti-inflammatory agents and progesterone:
   a. secondary
   b. constrictive
   c. periodic
   d. primary

3. In this type of amenorrhea there is a cessation of menstruation:
   a. secondary
   b. constrictive
   c. periodic
   d. primary

For questions 4 to 6, match the abnormal menstruation type with correct definition from items a-c below.
   a. increased amount and duration of flow
   b. bleeding between cycles
   c. in excess of 6 weeks

4. oligomenorrhea
5. metrorrhagia
6. menorrhagia

7. Increased risks of breast cancer, ovarian cancer, and non-Hodgkin lymphoma exist with this condition:
   a. endometriosis
   b. pelvic inflammatory disease
   c. sexually transmitted disease
   d. dysfunctional uterine bleeding

8. This benign lesion is also known as uterine fibroids:
   a. adenomyosis
   b. squamous cell
   c. leiomyoma
   d. extraembryonic cell primitive

9. Marginal, partial, and total are types of this condition:
   a. abruptio placentae
   b. placenta previa
   c. ectopic pregnancy
   d. hydatidiform mole

10. Which of the following is NOT a malposition of fetus?
   a. breech
   b. shoulder
   c. back
   d. brow

6
Male Genital System

ANATOMY AND TERMINOLOGY

Function, reproduction
> Structure, essential organs, and accessory organs (Fig. 6.1)

Essential Organs

Testes (Gonads)

Produce sperm (male gamete with 23 chromosomes) in seminiferous tubules
> Covered by tunica albuginea, located in scrotum
> Produce testosterone in Leydig cells

Vas Deferens

Is a tube
> End of epididymis

Accessory Organs

Ducts (carry sperm from testes to exterior), sex glands (produce solutions that mix with sperm), and external genitalia

Seminal vesicles produce most seminal fluid
Prostate gland produces some seminal fluid and activates sperm
Bulbourethral gland (Cowper's gland) secretes a very small amount of seminal fluid
External genitalia: penis and scrotum
- Penis contains three columns of erectile tissue: two corpora cavernosa and one spongiosum
- Urethra passes through corpora spongiosum
- Scrotum encloses testes
Passage of sperm from production to exterior

Sperm are produced in seminiferous tubules (testes) and pass into

Epididymis then to vas deferens (within seminal vesicles) to
Ejaculatory duct then through urethra (prostate gland and Cowper's [bulbourethral] gland)
Pass though penis to outside of body

Urinary bladder
Vas deferens
Urethra
Penis
Glans penis
Foreskin
Seminal vesicle
Ejaculatory duct
Prostate gland
Bulbourethral gland
Anus
Epididymis
Testis
Scrotum

• **Figure 6.1** Male reproductive system.

TABLE 6-1

Combining Forms

Combining Form	Meaning
1. andr/o	male
2. balan/o	glans penis
3. cry/o	cold
4. crypt/o	hidden
5. epididym/o	epididymis
6. gon/o	seed
7. hydr/o	water, fluid
8. orch/i	testicle
9. orch/o	testicle
10. orchi/o	testicle
11. orchid/o	testicle
12. prostat/o	prostate gland
13. semin/i	semen
14. sperm/o	sperm
15. spermat/o	sperm
16. test/o	testicle
17. varic/o	varicose veins
18. vas/o	vessel, vas deferens
19. vesicul/o	seminal vesicles

TABLE 6-2

Suffixes

Suffix	Meaning
1. -one	hormone
2. -pexy	fixation
3. -ectomy	removal
4. -stomy	new opening

TABLE 6-3

Medical Abbreviations

Abbreviation	Meaning
1. BPH	benign prostatic hypertrophy
2. PSA	prostate-specific antigen
3. TURBT	transurethral resection of bladder tumor
4. TURP	transurethral resection of prostate

TABLE 6-4

Medical Terms

Term	Meaning
Cavernosa	Connection between cavity of penis and a vein
Cavernosography	Radiographic recording of a cavity, e.g., pulmonary cavity or main part of penis
Cavernosometry	Measurement of pressure in a cavity, e.g., penis
Chordee	Condition resulting in penis being bent downward
Corpora cavernosa	The two cavities of penis
Epididymectomy	Surgical removal of epididymis
Epididymis	Tube located at the top of testes that stores sperm
Epididymovasostomy	Creation of a new connection between vas deferens and epididymis
Meatotomy	Surgical enlargement of opening of urinary meatus
Orchiectomy	Castration, removal of testes
Orchiopexy	Surgical procedure to release undescended testis and fixate within scrotum
Penoscrotal	Referring to penis and scrotum
Plethysmography	Determining changes in volume of an organ part or body
Priapism	Painful condition in which penis is constantly erect
Prostatotomy	Incision into prostate
Transurethral resection, prostate	Procedure performed through urethra by means of a cystoscopy to remove part or all of prostate
Tumescence	State of being swollen
Tunica vaginalis	Covering of testes
Varicocele	Swelling of a scrotal vein
Vas deferens	Tube that carries sperm from epididymis to ejaculatory duct and seminal vesicles
Vasectomy	Removal of segment of vas deferens
Vasogram	Recording of the flow in vas deferens
Vasotomy	Incision in vas deferens
Vasorrhaphy	Suturing of vas deferens
Vasovasostomy	Reversal of a vasectomy
Vesiculectomy	Excision of seminal vesicle
Vesiculotomy	Incision into seminal vesicle

Chapter 6: Anatomy and Terminology Quiz

(Quiz Answers Are Located in Appendix B)

1. This gland activates sperm and produces some seminal fluid:
   a. seminal vesicle
   b. bulbourethral gland
   c. prostate gland
   d. scrotum

2. Carries sperm from testes to ejaculatory duct:
   a. vas deferens
   b. sex gland
   c. tunica
   d. seminal

3. Penis contains these erectile tissues:
   a. one corpora cavernosa and two spongiosa
   b. two corpora cavernosa and two spongiosa
   c. one corpora cavernosa and one spongiosum
   d. two corpora cavernosa and one spongiosum

4. Also known as Cowper's gland:
   a. seminal vesicles
   b. bulbourethral gland
   c. prostate gland
   d. scrotum

5. Which of the following is NOT an accessory organ?
   a. gonads
   b. seminal vesicles
   c. prostate
   d. penis

6. Combining form meaning "male":
   a. andr/o
   b. balan/o
   c. orchi/o
   d. test/o

7. Combining form meaning "glans penis":
   a. balan/o
   b. vas/o
   c. vesicul/o
   d. orch/o

8. Testes are covered by the:
   a. seminal vesicles
   b. androgen
   c. chancre
   d. tunica albuginea

9. This abbreviation describes a surgical resection of prostate that is accomplished by means of an endoscope inserted into the urethra:
   a. TURBT
   b. BPH
   c. UPJ
   d. TURP

10. This abbreviation describes a condition of prostate in which there is an enlargement that is benign:
    a. TURBT
    b. BPH
    c. UPJ
    d. TURP

PATHOPHYSIOLOGY

Male Genital System Disorders

Disorders of Scrotum, Testes, and Epididymis

Cryptorchidism

Undescended testes—condition at birth
- Unilateral or bilateral
- Primarily result from obstruction
- Risk neoplastic processes

Treatment
- May descend spontaneously
- Administration of hormone to stimulate testosterone production
- Surgical intervention (orchiopexy) near age 1 to avoid risk of infertility

Orchitis

Inflammation of testes
Most common cause is virus
- Such as mumps orchitis
- Atrophy with irreversible loss of sperm production at risk

May be associated with
- Mumps or epidemic parotitis
- Gonorrhea
- Syphilis
- Tuberculosis

Symptoms
- Mild to severe pain in testes
- Mild to severe edema
- Feeling of weight in testicular area

Treatment
- Depends on presence of underlying condition

Epididymitis

Inflammation of epididymis
Inflammatory response to trauma or infection
Abscess may form

Types

Sexually transmitted epididymitis
- Gonorrhea
- *T. pallidum*
- *T. vaginalis*

Nonspecific bacterial epididymitis
- *E. coli*
- Streptococci

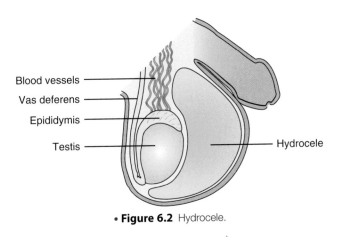

• **Figure 6.2** Hydrocele.

Blood vessels

Vas deferens

Epididymis

Testis

Hydrocele

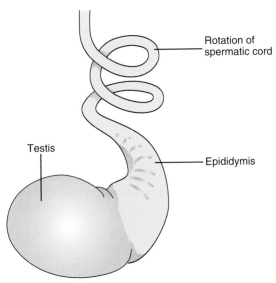

• **Figure 6.3** Torsion of testis.

Rotation of
spermatic cord

Testis

Epididymis

- Staphylococci
- Associated with underlying urological disorder

Symptoms
Scrotal pain
    Swelling
    Erythema
    Perhaps hydrocele formation

Treatment
Antibiotic
    Bed rest
    Ice packs
    Scrotal support
    Analgesics

Hydrocele (Fig. 6.2)
Collection of fluid in membranes of tunica vaginalis
    May be congenital or acquired (response to infection or tumors)
    Congenital hydrocele may reabsorb due to a communication between the scrotal sac and peritoneal cavity and require no intervention

Symptoms
Scrotal enlargement

Usually painless
- Unless infection is present

Varicocele
Abnormal dilation of plexus of veins
Decreases sperm production and motility

Symptoms
Usually painless
    In elderly, may signal renal tumor

Treatment
Surgical intervention

Torsion of Testes (Fig. 6.3)
Twisting of testes
    Congenital abnormal development of tunica vaginalis and spermatic cord
    Trauma may precipitate

Symptoms
Sudden onset of severe pain
    Nausea
    Vomiting
    Scrotal edema and tenderness
    Fever

Treatment
Immediate surgical intervention

Cancer of Testes
Rare form of cancer

Cure rate high (95%)
Cause unknown
Usually occurs in younger men
Two main groups
- Germ cell tumors (GCT)—90% of testicular tumors
- Sex cord–stromal tumors

Cancer of Scrotum
Rare form of cancer
- Squamous cell carcinoma

Symptoms
Asymptomatic in early stages
    Ulcerations in later stages

Treatment
Wide local excision
    Mohs micrographic surgery

- Precise removal of tumor
- Layers are removed until no further microscopic evidence of abnormal cells is seen
  Laser therapy
  Lymph nodes are examined for metastasis

Disorders of Urethra

Epispadias
Congenital anomaly
  Urethral meatus is located on dorsal side of penis
  Usually occurs in conjunction with other abnormalities

Treatment
Surgical reconstruction

Hypospadias
Most common abnormality of penis
Urethral opening on ventral side of penis
Results in curvature of penis
- Due to chordee

Treatment
Surgical reconstruction

Urethritis
Inflammation of urethra

Infectious urethritis can be gonococcal or nongonococcal
Nongonococcal organisms
- C. trachomatis
- *U. urealyticum*

Symptoms
Discharge
Inflammation of meatus
Burning
Itching
Urgent and frequent urination
In nongonococcal, symptoms are fewer

Treatment
Antibiotics based on organism

Disorders of Penis

Balanitis
Inflammation of glans

Causes
Syphilis
  Trichomoniasis
  Gonorrhea
  Candida albicans
  Tinea
  Underlying disease—diabetes mellitus and candidiasis
  No circumcision

Symptoms
Irritation
  Tenderness
  Discharge
  Edema
  Ulceration
  Swelling of lymph nodes

Treatment
Culture of discharge
  Saline irrigation
  Antibiotics

Phimosis and Paraphimosis, Phimosis
Condition in which prepuce (foreskin) is constricted
- Prepuce cannot be retracted over glans penis
  Can occur at any age
  Associated with poor hygiene and chronic infection in uncircumcised males

Symptoms
Erythema
  Edema
  Tenderness
  Purulent discharge

Treatment
Surgical circumcision

Paraphimosis
Condition in which prepuce (foreskin) is constricted
  Prepuce is retracted over glans penis and cannot be moved forward

Symptom
Edema

Treatment
Surgical

Peyronie's Disease
Also known as bent nail syndrome

Fibrotic condition
- Results in lateral curvature of penis during erection
Occurs most often in middle-aged men
Cause is unknown but associated with
- Diabetes
- Keloid development
- Dupuytren's contracture (flexion deformity of toes and fingers)

Treatment
Sometimes spontaneous remission
  Pharmacologic, oxygen-increasing therapies
  Surgical resection of fibrous bands

Cancer of Penis
Rare form of cancer

Occurs most often in men over age 60
Squamous cell carcinoma
Increased risks
- More common in uncircumcised men
- Sexual partner with cervical carcinoma
- Human papillomavirus

Usually begins with small lesion beneath prepuce
Intraepithelial neoplasia is also known as
- Bowen's disease
- Erythroplasia of Queyrat
- Begins as noninvasive

Progresses to invasive if untreated
Metastasis to lymph nodes

Treatment
Excision
    Mohs micrographic surgery
    Radiation therapy
    Laser therapy
    Cryosurgery

Advanced tumors are treated with partial or total penectomy and chemotherapy

Disorders of Prostate Gland

Benign Prostatic Hyperplasia/Hypertrophy (BPH)
Multiple fibroadenomatous nodules; usually located on outside of gland, so easily palpable on digital exam
- Related to aging; common in men over 60 years of age
- Enlarging prostate obstructs bladder neck and urethra
- Decreases urine flow

It is thought that increased levels of estrogen/androgen cause BPH

Symptoms
Increased frequency and urgency of urination
    Nocturia
    Incontinence
    Hesitancy
    Diminished force
    Postvoiding dribble

Screening
Prostate-specific antigen (PSA)
    Digital rectal examination (DRE)

Treatment
Partial prostatectomy
Transurethral resection of prostate (TURP)
Excision of nodules
Hormone therapy
Placement of urethral stents

Pharmaceuticals—those that inhibit production of testosterone and those that relax smooth muscle of gland and neck of bladder

Prostatitis
Inflammation of prostate
- Acute or chronic bacterial prostatitis

Bacterial Causes
Escherichia coli
    Enterococci
    Staphylococci
    Streptococci
    Chlamydia trachomatis
    Ureaplasma urealyticum
    Neisseria gonorrhea

Nonbacterial Causes
Spontaneous
    Prostatodynia

Symptoms
Acute Prostatitis
Fever and chills
    Lower back pain
    Perineal pain
    Dysuria
    Tenderness, suprapubic
    Urinary tract infection

Chronic Prostatitis
Recurring
    Same as acute only with no infection in urinary tract

Treatment
Acute. Antibiotic based on culture
Chronic. No treatment available

Cancer of Prostate
Most common malignancy diagnosed in men, occurring in men over age 60
Indications are that the cause is related to androgens
Predominately adenocarcinoma (95%)
No relationship between BPH and cancer of prostate

Symptoms
Asymptomatic in early stages

Later symptoms include
- Dysuria
- Back pain
- Hematuria
- Frequent urination
- Urinary retention
- Increased incidence of uremia

Stages

Two systems used to stage prostate cancer

- Whitmore-Jewett stages as indicated in Fig. 6.4
- Tumor-node-metastasis (TNM) as indicated in Fig. 6.5

Treatment

Dependent on stage

WHITMORE-JEWETT STAGES:

Stage A is clinically undetectable tumor confined to the gland and is an incidental finding at prostate surgery.
A1: well-differentiated with focal involvement
A2: moderately or poorly differentiated or involves multiple foci in the gland
Stage B is tumor confined to the prostate gland.
B0: nonpalpable, PSA-detected
B1: single nodule in one lobe of the prostate
B2: more extensive involvement of one lobe or involvement of both lobes
Stage C is a tumor clinically localized to the periprostatic area but extending through the prostatic capsule; seminal vesicles may be involved.
C1: clinical extracapsular extension
C2: extracapsular tumor producing bladder outlet or ureteral obstruction
Stage D is metastatic disease.
D0: clinically localized disease (prostate only) but persistently elevated enzymatic serum acid phosphatase
D1: regional lymph nodes only
D2: distant lymph nodes, metastases to bone or visceral organs
D3: D2 prostate cancer patients who relapse after adequate endocrine therapy

- **Figure 6.4** Whitmore-Jewett stages.

TNM STAGES:

Primary Tumor (T)
TX: Primary tumor cannot be assessed
T0: No evidence of primary tumor
T1: Clinically inapparent tumor not palpable or visible by imaging
    T1a: Tumor incidental histologic finding in 5% or less of tissue resected
    T1b: Tumor incidental histologic finding in more than 5% of tissue resected
    T1c: Tumor identified by needle biopsy (e.g., because of elevated PSA)
T2: Tumor confined within the prostate
    T2a: Tumor involves half a lobe or less
    T2b: Tumor involves more than half of a lobe, but not both lobes
    T2c: Tumor involves both lobes; extends through the prostatic capsule
T3a: Unilateral extracapsular extension
T3b: Bilateral extracapsular extension
T3c: Tumor invades the seminal vesicle(s)
T4: Tumor is fixed or invades adjacent structures other than the seminal vesicle(s)
    T4a: Tumor invades any of bladder neck, external sphincter, or rectum
    T4b: Tumor invades levator muscles and/or is fixed to the pelvic wall
Regional lymph nodes (N)
NX: Regional lymph nodes cannot be assessed
N0: No regional lymph node metastasis
N1: Metastasis in a single lymph node, 2 cm or less in greatest dimension
N2: Metastasis in a single lymph node, more than 2 cm but not more than 5 cm in greatest dimension; or multiple lymph node metastases, none more than 5 cm in greatest dimension
N3: Metastasis in a single lymph node more than 5 cm in greatest dimension
Distant metastases (M)
MX: Presence of distant metastasis cannot be assessed
M0: No distant metastasis
M1: Distant metastasis
    M1a: Nonregional lymph node(s)
    M1b: Bone(s)
    M1c: Other site(s)

- **Figure 6.5** TNM stages.

Chapter 6: Pathophysiology Quiz

(Quiz Answers Are Located in Appendix B)

1. What is the condition in which testes do not descend?
   a. cryptorchidism
   b. Bowen's disease
   c. torsion
   d. hypospadias
2. Orchitis is most often caused by a:
   a. bacteria
   b. virus
   c. parasite
   d. fungus
3. A condition that can be either congenital or acquired through trauma and that involves twisting of testes is:
   a. hydrocele
   b. hypospadias
   c. cryptorchidism
   d. torsion

4. Cancer of the _____ is divided into two main groups of germ cell tumors and sex stromal cord tumors.
   a. testes
   b. penis
   c. scrotum
   d. prostate
5. This type of surgical technique involves excision of a lesion in layers until no further evidence of abnormality is seen:
   a. Bowen's
   b. Addison's
   c. Mohs
   d. laser

6. Epispadias is a disorder of the urethra in which urethral meatus is located on the _____ side of penis:
   a. ventral
   b. dorsal
   c. lateral
   d. medial
7. Inflammation of glans is:
   a. phimosis
   b. paraphimosis
   c. urethritis
   d. balanitis
8. This disease is also known as bent nail syndrome:
   a. Bowen's
   b. Peyronie's
   c. Addison's
   d. Whitmore-Jewett

9. Condition in which multiple fibroadenomatous nodules form and lead to decreased urine flow. Condition is thought to be related to increased levels of estrogen/androgen.
   a. BPH
   b. DRE
   c. GCT
   d. TNM
10. Cancer of prostate is predominately this type of cancer:
    a. sex cord
    b. adenocarcinoma
    c. squamous cell
    d. seminoma

7
Urinary System

ANATOMY AND TERMINOLOGY

Removes metabolic waste materials (nitrogenous waste: urea, creatinine, and uric acid)

Conserves nutrients and water
Balances: electrolytes (acids/bases balance)
 Electrolytes are electrically charged molecules required for nerve and muscle function
Assists liver in detoxification

Organs (Fig. 7.1)

Kidneys
 Ureters
 Urinary bladder
 Urethra

Kidneys (Fig. 7.2)

Electrolytes and fluid balance
 Control pH balance (acid/base)
 Secrete renin (which affects blood pressure) and erythropoietin (which stimulates red blood cell production in bone marrow)
 Secrete active vitamin D required for calcium absorption from intestines
 Two organs located behind peritoneum (retroperitoneal space)

Kidney Structure

Cortex (outer layer)
Medulla (inner portion)
Hilum (depression on medial border through which blood vessels and nerves pass)
Pyramids (divisions of medulla)
Papilla (inner part of pyramids)
Pelvis (receptacle for urine within kidney)
Calyces surround top of renal pelvis
Nephrons (3 types) are operational units of kidney

Ureters

Narrow tubes transporting urine from kidneys to bladder

Urinary Bladder
Reservoir for urine

Shaped like an upside-down pear with three surfaces
 • Posterior (base)
 • Anterior (neck)
 • Superior (peritoneum)
Trigone
 • Smooth triangular area inside bladder—size never changes
 • Formed by openings of ureters and urethra

Urethra

Canal from bladder to exterior of body
 Urinary meatus, outside opening of urethra

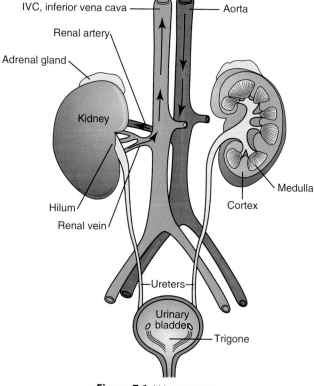

• **Figure 7.1** Urinary system.

TABLE 7-1

Combining Forms

Combining Form	Meaning
1. albumin/o	albumin
2. azot/o	urea
3. bacteri/o	bacteria
4. cali/o	calyx
5. cyst/o	urinary
6. dips/o	thirst
7. glomerul/o	glomerulus
8. glyc/o	sugar
9. glycos/o	sugar
10. hydr/o	water
11. ket/o	ketone bodies/ketoacidosis
12. lith/o	stone
13. meat/o	meatus
14. nephr/o	kidney
15. noct/i	night
16. olig/o	scant, few
17. pyel/o	renal pelvis
18. ren/o	kidney
19. son/o	sound
20. tripsy	to crush
21. tryg/o	trigone region/kidney
22. ur/o	urine
23. ureter/o	ureter
24. urethr/o	urethra
25. uria	urination/urinary condition
26. urin/o	urine
27. vesic/o	bladder

TABLE 7-2

Prefixes

Prefix	Meaning
1. dys-	painful
2. peri-	surrounding
3. poly-	many
4. retro-	behind

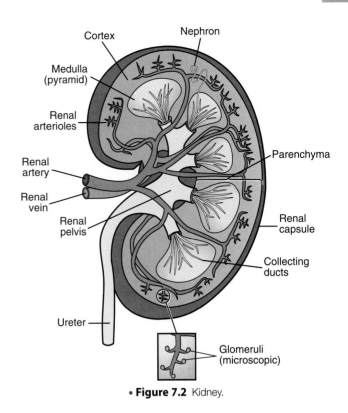

• **Figure 7.2** Kidney.

TABLE 7-3

Suffixes

Suffix	Meaning
1. -eal	pertaining to
2. -lithiasis	condition of stones
3. -lysis	separation
4. -plasty	repair
5. -rrhaphy	suture
6. -tripsy	crush

TABLE 7-4

Medical Abbreviations

Abbreviation	Meaning
1. ARF	acute renal failure
2. BUN	blood urea nitrogen
3. ESRD	end-stage renal disease
4. HD	hemodialysis
5. IVP	intravenous pyelogram
6. KUB	kidney, ureter, bladder
7. pH	symbol for acid/base level
8. PKU	phenylketonuria
9. sp gr	specific gravity
10. UA	urinalysis
11. UPJ	ureteropelvic junction
12. UTI	urinary tract infection

TABLE 7-5

Medical Terms

Term	Meaning	Term	Meaning
Bulbocavernosus	Muscle that constricts vagina in a female and urethra in a male	Nephrocutaneous fistula	An abnormal channel from kidney to skin
Bulbourethral	Gland with duct leading to urethra	Nephrolithotomy	Removal of a kidney stone through an incision made into the kidney
Calculus	Concretion of mineral salts, also called a stone	Nephrorrhaphy	Suturing of kidney
Calycoplasty	Surgical reconstruction of recess of renal pelvis	Nephrostomy	Creation of a channel into renal pelvis of kidney
Calyx	Recess of renal pelvis	Transureteroureterostomy	Surgical connection of one ureter to other ureter
Cystolithectomy	Removal of a calculus (stone) from urinary bladder	Transvesical ureterolithotomy	Removal of a ureter stone (calculus) through bladder
Cystometrogram	CMG, measurement of pressures and capacity of urinary bladder	Ureterectomy	Surgical removal of a ureter, either totally or partially
Cystoplasty	Surgical reconstruction of bladder	Ureterocutaneous fistula	Channel from ureter to exterior skin
Cystorrhaphy	Suture of bladder	Ureteroenterostomy	Creation of a connection between intestine and ureter
Cystoscopy	Use of a scope to view bladder		
Cystostomy	Surgical creation of an opening into bladder	Ureterolithotomy	Removal of a stone from ureter
		Ureterolysis	Freeing of adhesions of ureter
Cystotomy	Incision into bladder	Ureteroneocystostomy	Surgical connection of ureter to a new site on bladder
Cystourethroplasty	Surgical reconstruction of bladder and urethra	Ureteropyelography	Ureter and renal pelvis radiography
Cystourethroscopy	Use of a scope to view bladder and urethra	Ureterotomy	Incision into ureter
Dilation	Stretching or expansion	Urethrocystography	Radiography of bladder and urethra
Dysuria	Painful urination	Urethromeatoplasty	Surgical repair of urethra and meatus
Endopyelotomy	Procedure involving bladder and ureters, including insertion of a stent into renal pelvis	Urethropexy	Fixation of urethra by means of surgery
		Urethroplasty	Surgical repair of urethra
Extracorporeal	Occurring outside of body	Urethrorrhaphy	Suturing of urethra
Fundoplasty	Repair of the bottom of bladder	Urethroscopy	Use of a scope to view urethra
Hydrocele	Sac of fluid	Vesicostomy	Surgical creation of a connection of viscera of bladder to skin
Kock pouch	Surgical creation of a urinary bladder from a segment of the ileum		

Chapter 7: Anatomy and Terminology Quiz

(Quiz Answers Are Located in Appendix B)

1. The outer covering of kidney:
   a. medulla
   b. pyramids
   c. cortex
   d. papilla
2. Which is not a division of kidneys?
   a. pelvis
   b. pyramids
   c. cortex
   d. trigone
3. The inner portion of kidneys:
   a. medulla
   b. pyramids
   c. cortex
   d. papilla
4. The smooth area inside bladder:
   a. pyramids
   b. calyces
   c. trigone
   d. cystocele
5. The narrow tube connecting kidney and bladder:
   a. urethra
   b. ureter
   c. meatus
   d. trigone
6. Which of the following is NOT a surface of urinary bladder?
   a. posterior
   b. anterior
   c. superior
   d. inferior
7. Combining form that means "stone":
   a. azot/o
   b. cyst/o
   c. lith/o
   d. olig/o
8. Term meaning "painful urination":
   a. pyuria
   b. dysuria
   c. diuresis
   d. hyperemia
9. Combining form meaning "scant":
   a. glyc/o
   b. hydr/o
   c. meat/o
   d. olig/o
10. Term that describes renal failure that is acute:
   a. ARF
   b. ESRD
   c. HD
   d. BPH

PATHOPHYSIOLOGY

Renal Failure

Acute Renal Failure

Sudden onset of renal failure

Causes
Extreme hypotension
Trauma
Infection
Inflammation
Toxicity
Obstructed vascular supply

Symptoms
Uremia
Oliguria (decreased output) or anuria (no output)
Hyperkalemia (high potassium in blood)
Pulmonary edema

Types
Prerenal
- Associated with poor systemic perfusion
- Decreased renal blood flow
  - Such as with congestive heart failure

Intrarenal
- Associated with renal parenchyma disease (functional tissue of kidney)
  - Such as acute interstitial nephritis, glomerulopathies, and malignant hypertension

Postrenal
- Resulting from urine flow obstruction outside kidney (ureters or bladder neck)

Treatment
Underlying condition
Dialysis
Monitoring of fluid and electrolyte balance

Chronic Renal Failure

Gradual loss of function
- Progressively more severe renal insufficiency until end stage of
  - Renal disease
  - Irreversible kidney failure

Stages—Based on Level of Creatinine Clearance
Stage 1: Blood flow through kidney increases, kidney enlarges
Stage 2 (mild): Small amounts of blood protein (albumin) leak into urine (microalbuminuria)

Stage 3 (moderate): Albumin and other protein losses increase; patient may develop high blood pressure and kidney loses ability to filter waste

Stage 4 (severe): Large amounts of urine pass through kidney; blood pressure increases

Stage 5: End-stage renal failure. Ability to filter waste nearly stops; dialysis or transplant only option

Causes
Long-term exposure to nephrotoxins
Diabetes
Hypertension

Symptoms
No symptoms until well advanced
Polyuria
Nausea or anorexia
Dehydration
Neurologic manifestations

Stages of Nephron Loss
Decreased reserve
- 60% loss

Renal insufficiency
- 75% loss

End-stage renal failure
- 90% loss

Treatment
No cure
Dialysis
Kidney transplant

Urinary Tract Infections (UTI)

Cystitis—Bacterial
Cause
Bacteria, usually *E. coli*

Symptoms
Lower abdominal pain
Dysuria
Lower back pain
Urinary frequency and urgency
Cloudy, foul-smelling urine

Systemic Signs
Fever
Malaise
Nausea

Treatment
Antibiotics
Increased fluid intake

Cystitis—Noninfectious, Nonbacterial
Cause
Radiation, chemotherapy, autoimmune disorder, etc.
May later produce bacterial infection

Symptoms
Urinary frequency and urgency
Dysuria
Negative urine culture

Treatment
No known treatment

Acute Pyelonephritis (Fig. 7.3)
Bacterial infection with multiple abscesses of renal pelvis and medullary tissue
- May involve one or both kidneys

Causes
E. coli
Proteus
Pseudomonas
Obstruction and reflux of urine from bladder

Symptoms
Fever
Chills
Groin or flank pain
Dysuria
Pyuria
Nocturia

• **Figure 7.3** Acute pyelonephritis. Cortical surface exhibits grayish white areas of inflammation and abscess formation.

Treatment
Antibiotics
Surgical correction of obstruction

Chronic Pyelonephritis

Recurrent infection that causes scarring of kidney
Cause is difficult to determine
- Repeated infections
- Obstructive conditions

Symptoms
Hypertension
Dysuria
Flank pain
Increased frequency of urination

Treatment
Antibiotics for extended periods when reoccurring
Surgical reduction of obstruction

Glomerular Disorders

May be acute or chronic
Function of glomerulus is blood filtration

Glomerulonephritis

Inflammation of glomerulus

Causes
Drugs or toxins
Systemic disorder affecting many organs or idiopathic
May follow acute infections—most commonly streptococcal infections
Vascular pathology
Immune disorders

Treatment
Follows cause

Nephrotic Syndrome (Nephrosis)

Disease of kidneys that includes damage to membrane of the glomerulus causing excessive protein loss to urine

Accompanied by
- Hypoalbuminemia
- Hypercholesterolemia
- Hypercoagulability (excessive clotting)
- Prone to infections
- Edema
- Protein loss of >3.5 g
Damage to glomerulus results from
- Infection
- Immune response
  - Most predominant cause of dysfunction is exposure to toxins

May be a manifestation of an underlying condition, such as diabetes

Symptoms
Edema
Weight gain
Pallor
Proteinuria
Lipiduria

Treatment
Glucocorticoids, such as prednisone
- Reduces inflammation
Sodium- and fat-reduced diet
Protein supplements
Careful monitoring for continued inflammation

Acute Poststreptococcal Glomerulonephritis (APSGN)

Cause
Streptococcus infection
- With certain types of group A beta-hemolytic *Streptococcus* Creates an antigen-antibody complex
- Infiltrates glomerular capillaries
- Results in inflammation in kidneys
- Inflammation interferes with normal kidney function
- Fluid and waste build-up
- Can lead to acute renal failure and scarring Usually occurs in children 3 to 7 years of age
- Most often in boys

Symptoms
Back and flank pain
Cloudy, dark urine
Oliguria (decreased output)
Edema
Elevated blood pressure
Fatigue
Malaise
Headache
Nausea

Treatment
Sodium reduction
Antibiotics
Careful monitoring for continued inflammation

Urinary Tract Obstructions

Interference with urine flow

Causes urine backup behind obstruction of urinary system
Damage occurs to structures behind blockages
Increased urinary tract infection
Obstruction can be

- Functional
- Anatomic
  - Also known as obstructive uropathy

Kidney Stones (Nephrolithiasis—Renal Calculi)

Formed of mineral salts (uric and calcium)

Develop anywhere in urinary tract
Tend to form in presence of excess salt and decreased fluid intake
- Most stones are formed of calcium salts
- Staghorn calculus forms in renal pelvis

Symptoms
Asymptomatic until obstruction occurs

Obstruction results in renal colic
- Extremely intense pain in flank
- Nausea
- Vomiting
- Cold, clammy skin
- Increased pulse rate

Treatment
Stone usually passes spontaneously
May use extracorporeal ultrasound or laser lithotripsy to break up stone (also known as extracorporeal shock wave lithotripsy, or ESWL)
Drugs may be used to dissolve stone
Preventative treatment to adjust pH level
- Increased fluid intake

Bladder Carcinoma

Malignant Tumor
Most common site of malignancy in urinary system
Tumors originate in transitional epithelial lining
Tends to recur
Often metastatic to liver and bone

Tumor Staging for Renal Cancer
Stage 1—Tumor of kidney capsule only
Stage 2—Tumor invading renal capsule/vein but within fascia
Stage 3—Tumor extending to regional lymph nodes/vena cava
Stage 4—Other organ metastasis

Symptoms
Often asymptomatic in early stage
Hematuria
Dysuria
Frequent urination
Infections common

Increased Risks

Cigarette smoking
Males age 50+

Working with industrial chemicals
Analgesics used in large amounts
Recurrent bladder infections

Treatment
Immunotherapy (Bacillus Calmette-Guérin [BCG] vaccine)
Excision
Chemotherapy
Radiation therapy

Hydronephrosis

Distention of kidney with urine
- Due to an obstruction
- Usually as a result of a kidney stone
- May also be due to scarring, tumor, edema from infection, or other obstruction

Symptoms
Usually asymptomatic
Mild flank pain
Infection may develop
May lead to chronic renal failure

Treatment
Treat underlying condition, such as removal of stone or antibiotics for infection
Dilation of stricture

Vascular Disorders

Nephrosclerosis

Excessive hardening and thickening of vascular structure of kidney
- Reduces blood supply
  - Increases blood pressure
  - Results in atrophy and ischemia of structures
  - May lead to chronic renal failure

Symptoms
Asymptomatic in early stages

Treatment
Diuretics
ACE (angiotensin-converting enzyme) inhibitors
Beta blockers that block release of resin
Antihypertensive drugs
Sodium intake reduction

Congenital Disorders

Polycystic Kidney Disease (PKD)

Numerous kidney cysts
Genetic disease

Symptoms
Asymptomatic until 40s
Cysts progressive in development (both kidneys)

Nephromegaly, hematuria, UTI, hypertension, uremia
Develops chronic renal failure
Cysts may spread to other organs, such as liver

Treatment
As for chronic renal failure

Wilms' Tumor—Nephroblastoma
Usually unilateral kidney tumors

Most common tumor in children
Usually advanced at time of diagnosis
- Metastasis to lungs at time of diagnosis is common

Symptoms
Asymptomatic until abdominal mass becomes apparent at
  age 1 to 5

Treatment
Excision
Radiation therapy
Chemotherapy
Usually a combination of above

Chapter 7: Pathophysiology Quiz

(Quiz Answers Are Located in Appendix B)

1. Which of the following is NOT a type of acute renal failure?
   a. prerenal
   b. intrarenal
   c. interrenal
   d. postrenal
2. The loss of nephron function in end-stage renal disease is:
   a. 60%
   b. 70%
   c. 80%
   d. 90%
3. The cause of bacterial cystitis is usually:
   a. Proteus
   b. Pseudomonas
   c. Staphylococcus
   d. *E. coli*
4. The primary treatment for acute pyelonephritis would be:
   a. prednisone
   b. sodium reduction
   c. antibiotics
   d. BCG
5. APSGN stands for:
   a. advanced poststaphylococcal glomerulonephritis
   b. acute poststreptococcal glomerulonephritis
   c. acute poststaphylococcal glomerulonephritis
   d. advanced poststreptococcal glomerulonephritis
6. Obstructive uropathy is also known as:
   a. pyelonephritis
   b. renal failure
   c. urinary tract obstruction
   d. nephrotic syndrome
7. A treatment for kidney stone may be:
   a. ESWL
   b. prednisone
   c. open surgical procedure
   d. diuretics
8. The treatment for hydronephrosis involves:
   a. an open surgical procedure
   b. use of diuretics
   c. treatment of the underlying condition
   d. BCG
9. This is a congenital condition in which numerous cysts form in the kidney:
   a. Wilms' tumor
   b. polycystic kidney
   c. nephrosclerosis
   d. nephrotic syndrome
10. The treatment of Wilms' tumor would NOT include which of the following?
    a. excision
    b. chemotherapy
    c. diuretic
    d. radiation therapy

8
Digestive System

Function: digestion, absorption, and elimination
  Includes gastrointestinal tract (alimentary canal) and accessory organs

Mouth (Fig. 8.1)

Roof: hard palate, soft palate, uvula (projection at back of mouth)
Floor: contains tongue (Fig. 8.2), muscles, taste buds, and lingual frenulum, which anchors tongue to floor of mouth

Teeth

Thirty-two teeth (permanent)

Names of teeth: incisor, cuspid, bicuspid, and tricuspid
Tooth has crown (outer portion), neck (narrow part below gum line), root (end section), and pulp cavity (core)

Salivary Glands (Fig. 8.3)

Surround mouth and produce saliva—1.5 liters daily

Parotid
Submandibular
Sublingual

Pharynx or Throat (Fig. 8.4)

Muscular tube (5 inches long) lined with mucous membrane through which air and food/water travel

Epiglottis covers larynx/esophagus when swallowing

Esophagus

Muscular tube (9-10 inches long) that carries food from pharynx to stomach by means of peristalsis (rhythmic contractions)

Stomach

Sphincter (ring of muscles) at entry into stomach (gastroesophageal or cardiac)

Three parts of stomach:
  Fundus (upper part)
  Body (middle part)
  Antrum/pylorus (lower part)
Lined with rugae (folds of mucosal membrane)
Pyloric sphincter opens to allow chyme (thick liquid) to leave stomach and enter small intestine

Small Intestine

Duodenum (2 inches long): first portion beyond stomach—bile and pancreatic juice delivered here

Jejunum (96 inches long): connects duodenum to ileum
Ileum (132 inches long): attaches to large intestine

Large Intestine

Extends from ileum to anus
Cecum, from which appendix extends, connects ileum and colon
Colon (60 inches long), divided into:
  Ascending
  Transverse
  Descending
  Sigmoid
Sigmoid colon connected to rectum, which terminates at anus

Accessory Organs

Liver produces bile, sent to gallbladder via hepatic duct and cystic duct

Gallbladder stores bile, sent to duodenum from cystic duct into common bile duct
Bile emulsifies fat (breaks up large globules)

A

B

C

• **Figure 8.1** Anatomic structures of the mouth.

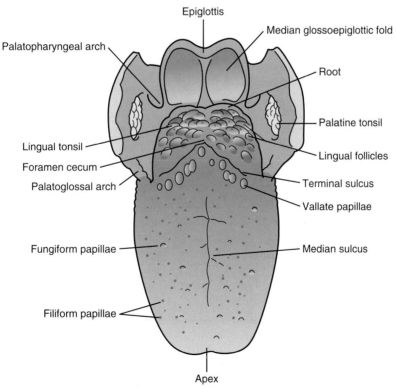

• **Figure 8.2** Dorsum of the tongue.

Pancreas produces enzymes sent through pancreatic duct to hepatopancreatic ampulla (ampulla of Vater) then to duodenum

Pancreatic cells—islets of Langerhans produce insulin and glucagon

Peritoneum

Serous membrane lines abdominal cavity and maintains organs in correct anatomic position

Food passes through digestive tract via:
Mouth—including salivary glands
Pharynx
Esophagus
Stomach
Duodenum—pancreatic enzymes and bile produced in liver and stored in gallbladder enter
Jejunum
Ileum
Cecum
Ascending colon
Transverse colon
Descending colon
Sigmoid colon
Rectum
Anus

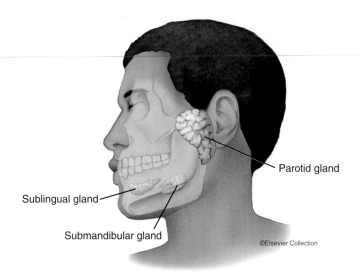

©Elsevier Collection

• **Figure 8.3** Major salivary glands.

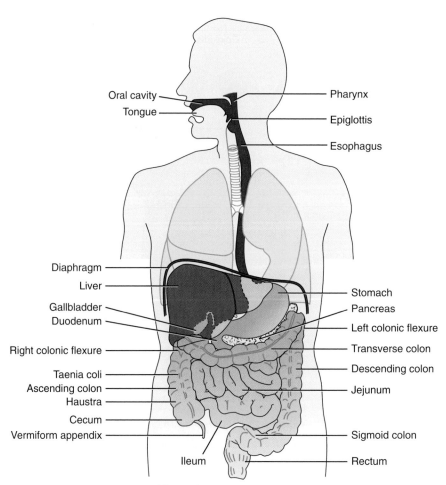

• **Figure 8.4** Digestive system.

TABLE 8-1

Combining Forms

Combining Form	Meaning	Combining Form	Meaning
1. abdomin/o	abdomen	25. herni/o	hernia
2. an/o	anus	26. ile/o	ileum
3. appendic/o	appendix	27. jejun/o	jejunum
4. bil/i	bile	28. labi/o	lip
5. bilirubin/o	bile pigment	29. lapar/o	abdomen
6. bucc/o	cheek	30. lingu/o	tongue
7. cec/o	cecum	31. lip/o	fat
8. celi/o	abdomen	32. lith/o	stone
9. cheil/o	lip	33. or/o	mouth
10. chol/e	gall/bile	34. ordont/o	tooth
11. cholangio/o	bile duct	35. palat/o	palate
12. cholecyst/o	gallbladder	36. pancreat/o	pancreas
13. choledoch/o	common bile duct	37. peritone/o	peritoneum
14. col/o	colon	38. pharyng/o	throat
15. dent/i	tooth	39. polyp/o	polyp
16. diverticul/o	diverticulum	40. proct/o	rectum
17. duoden/o	duodenum	41. pylor/o	pylorus
18. enter/o	small intestine	42. rect/o	rectum
19. esophag/o	esophagus	43. sial/o	saliva
20. faci/o	face	44. sialaden/o	salivary gland
21. gastr/o	stomach	45. sigmoid/o	sigmoid colon
22. gingiv/o	gum	46. steat/o	fat
23. gloss/o	tongue	47. stomat/o	mouth
24. hepat/o	liver	48. uvul/o	uvula

TABLE 8-2

Suffixes

Suffix	Meaning
1. -ase	enzyme
2. -cele	hernia
3. -chezia	defecation
4. -iasis	abnormal condition
5. -phagia	eating
6. -prandial	meal

TABLE 8-3

Medical Abbreviations

Abbreviation	Meaning
1. EGD	esophagogastroduodenoscopy
2. EGJ	esophagogastric junction
3. ERCP	endoscopic retrograde cholangiopancreatography
4. GERD	gastroesophageal reflux disease
5. GI	gastrointestinal
6. HJR	hepatojugular reflux
7. LLQ	left lower quadrant
8. LUQ	left upper quadrant
9. PEG	percutaneous endoscopic gastrostomy
10. RLQ	right lower quadrant
11. RUQ	right upper quadrant

TABLE 8-4

Medical Terms

Term	Meaning	Term	Meaning
Anastomosis	Surgical connection of two tubular structures, such as two pieces of intestine	Hernia	Organ or tissue protruding through wall or cavity that usually contains it
Biliary	Refers to gallbladder, bile, or bile duct	Ileostomy	Artificial opening between ileum and abdominal wall
Cholangiography	Radiographic recording of bile ducts	Imbrication	Overlapping
Cholecystectomy	Surgical removal of gallbladder	Incarcerated	Regarding hernias, a constricted, irreducible hernia that may cause obstruction of an intestine
Cholecystoenterostomy	Creation of a connection between gallbladder and intestine		
Colonoscopy	Fiberscopic examination of entire colon that may include part of terminal ileum	Intussusception	Slipping of one part of intestine into another part
Colostomy	Artificial opening between colon and abdominal wall	Jejunostomy	Artificial opening between jejunum and abdominal wall
Diverticulum	Protrusion in wall of an organ	Laparoscopy	Exploration of the abdomen and pelvic cavities using a scope placed through a small incision in abdominal wall
Dysphagia	Difficulty swallowing		
Enterolysis	Releasing of adhesions of intestine		
Eventration	Protrusion of bowel through an opening in abdomen	Lithotomy	Incision into an organ or a duct for the purpose of removing a stone
Evisceration	Pulling viscera outside of the body through an incision	Lithotripsy	Crushing of a stone by sound wave or force
Exstrophy	Condition in which an organ is turned inside out	Paraesophageal or hiatal hernia	Protrusion of any structure through esophageal hiatus of diaphragm
Fulguration	Use of electric current to destroy tissue		
Gastrointestinal	Pertaining to stomach and intestine	Proctosigmoidoscopy	Fiberscopic examination of sigmoid colon and rectum
Gastroplasty	Operation on stomach for repair or reconfiguration	Sialolithotomy	Surgical removal of a stone of salivary gland or duct
Gastrostomy	Artificial opening between stomach and abdominal wall	Varices	Varicose veins
		Volvulus	Twisted section of intestine

Chapter 8: Anatomy and Terminology Quiz

(Quiz Answers Are Located in Appendix B)

1. This is NOT a part of the small intestine:
   a. ileum
   b. cecum
   c. duodenum
   d. jejunum
2. Term meaning "ring of muscles":
   a. pyloric
   b. parotid
   c. epiglottis
   d. sphincter
3. The throat is also known as the:
   a. larynx
   b. epiglottis
   c. esophagus
   d. pharynx
4. The three parts of the stomach:
   a. pyloric, rugae, fundus
   b. fundus, body, antrum
   c. antrum, pyloric, rugae
   d. ilium, fundus, pyloric
5. The projection at the back of the mouth:
   a. palate
   b. sublingual
   c. uvula
   d. parotid
6. Mucosal membrane that lines the stomach:
   a. cecum
   b. rugae
   c. frenulum
   d. fundus

7. The parts of the colon are:
   a. ascending, transverse, descending, sigmoid
   b. ascending, descending, sigmoid
   c. transverse, descending, sigmoid
   d. descending, sigmoid
8. Combining form meaning "abdomen":
   a. an/o
   b. cec/o
   c. celi/o
   d. col/o
9. Term that means connecting two ends of a tube:
   a. anastomosis
   b. amylase
   c. aphthous stomatitis
   d. atresia
10. Abbreviation that means a scope placed through the esophagus, into the stomach, and to the duodenum:
    a. ERCP
    b. EGD
    c. GERD
    d. PEG

PATHOPHYSIOLOGY

Disorders of Oral Cavity

Cleft Lip and Cleft Palate (Orofacial Cleft) (Fig. 8.5)

Congenital defect
Cleft lip and palate
   Lip and palate do not properly join together
Causes feeding problems
- Infants cannot create sufficient suction for feeding
- Danger of aspirating food
- Results in speech defects

Treatment
Surgical repair of defects

Ulceration

Canker sore—caused by herpes simplex virus
- Ulceration of oral mucosa
  Also known as
- Aphthous ulcer (aphtha: small ulcer)
- Aphthous stomatitis
  Heals spontaneously

Infections

Candidiasis
Candida albicans is naturally found in mouth

Thrush (oral candidiasis) is overarching infection

Causes
Antibiotic regimen
Chemotherapy
Glucocorticoids
Common in patients with diabetes and AIDS patients

Treatment
Nystatin (topical fungal agent)

Herpes Simplex Type 1
Herpetic stomatitis
- Viral cold sores and blisters
- Associated with herpes simplex virus type 1 (HSV-1)

Treatment
No cure
   May be alleviated somewhat by antiviral medications

Cancer of Oral Cavity

Most common type is squamous cell carcinoma
   Kaposi's sarcoma is type seen in AIDS patients
   Increased in smokers
   Lip cancer also increased in smokers, particularly pipe smokers
   Poor prognosis
   Usually asymptomatic until later stages
   Metastasis through lymph nodes

Esophageal Disorders

Scleroderma

Also known as progressive systemic sclerosis

Atrophy of smooth muscles of lower esophagus
Lower esophageal sphincter (LES) does not close properly

• **Figure 8.5** Cleft palate.

- Leads to esophageal reflux
- Strictures form

Symptom

Predominantly dysphagia

Esophagitis

Inflammation of esophagus

Types

Acute

Most common type is that caused by hiatal hernia
Infectious esophagitis is common in patients with AIDS
Ingestion of strong alkaline or acid substances
- Such as those in household cleaners
Inflammation leads to scarring

Chronic

Most common type is that caused by LES reflux

Cancer of Esophagus

Most common type is squamous cell or secondary adenocarcinoma

Usually caused by continued irritation
- Smoking
- Alcohol
- Hiatal hernia
- Chronic esophagitis/GERD
Poor prognosis

Hiatal Hernia (Diaphragmatic Hernia)

Diaphragm goes over stomach
- Esophagus passes through diaphragm at natural opening (hiatus)
- Part of the stomach protrudes (herniates) through opening in diaphragm into thorax

Types (Fig. 8.6)
Sliding
- Stomach and gastroesophageal junction protrude through the hiatus
Paraesophageal/rolling hiatal
- Part of fundus protrudes

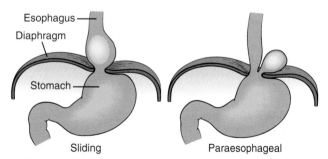

HIATAL HERNIAS

Esophagus

Diaphragm

Stomach

Sliding   Paraesophageal

- **Figure 8.6** Sliding and paraesophageal hernias (hiatal hernias).

Symptoms

Heartburn
Reflux
Belching
Lying down causes discomfort
Dysphagia
Substernal pain after eating

Gastroesophageal Reflux Disease (GERD)

Associated with hiatal hernias
- Reflux of gastric contents
  Lower esophageal sphincter does not constrict properly

Treatment

Reduce irritants, such as
- Smoking
- Spicy foods
- Alcohol
Antacids
Elevate head of bed
Avoid tight clothing

Stomach and Duodenum Disorders

Gastritis

Inflammation of stomach mucosa

Acute Superficial Gastritis

Mild, transient irritation

Causes

Excessive alcohol
  Infection
  Food allergies
  Spicy foods
  Aspirin
  H. pylori (Helicobacter pylori)

Symptoms

Nausea
Vomiting
Anorexia
Bleeding in more severe cases
Epigastric pain

Treatment

Usually spontaneous remission in 2 to 3 days
  Removal of underlying irritation
  Antibiotics for infection

Chronic Atrophic Gastritis

Progressive atrophy of epithelium

Types

Type A, atrophic or fundal
- Involves fundus of stomach
- Autoimmune disease

- Decreases acid secretion
- Results in high gastrin levels

Type B, antral
- Involves antrum region of stomach
- Often associated with elderly
  - May be associated with pernicious anemia
- Low gastrin levels
- Usually caused by infection
- Irritated by alcohol, drugs, and tobacco
  Symptom abatement
- Bland diet
- Alcohol avoidance
- ASA avoidance
- Antibiotics for *H. pylori*

Peptic Ulcers

Erosive area on mucosa
- Extends below epithelium
- Chronic ulcers have scar tissue at base of erosive area
  Ulcers can occur anywhere on gastrointestinal tract but typically are found on the
- Lower esophagus
- Stomach
- Proximal duodenum

Some Causes

Alcohol
Smoking
Aspirin
Severe stress
Bacterial infection caused by *Helicobacter pylori (H. pylori)*, 90% of the time
Genetic factor
Constant use of anti-inflammatory drugs

Symptoms

Epigastric pain when stomach is empty
- Relieved by food or antacid
  Burning
  May include
- Vomiting blood
- Nausea
- Weight loss
- Anorexia
  Severe cases may include
- Obstruction
- Hemorrhage
- Perforation

Treatment

Surgical intervention
  Antacids
  Dietary restrictions
  Rest
  Antibiotics

Gastric Cancer (Malignant Tumor of Stomach)

Most often occurs in men over 40
  Cause is unknown, but often associated with *Helicobacter pylori* (bacterial infection)

Predisposing Factors

Atrophic gastritis
  Pernicious anemia
  History of nonhealing gastric ulcer
  Blood type A
  Geographic factors
  Environmental factors
  Carcinogenic foods
- Smoked meats
- Nitrates
- Pickled foods

Symptoms

Usually asymptomatic in early stages

Treatment

Excision
Chemotherapy
Radiation (poor response)
Prognosis is poor

Pyloric Stenosis

Narrowing of the pyloric sphincter
Signs appear soon after birth
- Failure to thrive
- Projectile vomiting

Treatment

Surgery to relieve stenosis (pyloromyotomy)

Intestinal Disorders

Small Intestine

Malabsorption Conditions

Celiac Disease

Most important malabsorption condition
  Villi atrophy in response to food containing gluten and lose ability to absorb
- Gluten is a protein found in wheat, rye, oats, and barley

Symptoms

Malnutrition
Muscle wasting
Distended abdomen
Diarrhea
Fatigue
Weakness
Steatorrhea (excess fat in feces)

Treatment
Gluten-free diet
Steroids when necessary

Lactase Deficiency

Enzyme deficiency
- Secondary to gastrointestinal damage, such as
  - Regional enteritis
  - Infection
- Common in African Americans, occurring in adulthood

Symptoms
Intolerance to milk
Intestinal cramping
Diarrhea
Flatulence

Treatment
Elimination of milk products

Inflammatory Bowel Disease (IBD)

Affects terminal ileum and colon
For example, Crohn's Disease (Regional Enteritis)

Cause
Unknown

Symptoms
Vary greatly
Inflammatory disease of GI tract
Diarrhea
Gas
Fever
Abdominal pain
Malaise
Anorexia
Weight loss

Treatment
No specific treatment
Palliative medications to control symptoms
Resection of affected section of intestine with anastomosis
Diet modifications

Duodenal Ulcers

Most common ulcer
Develop in younger population
Common in type O blood types

Appendicitis

Inflammation of vermiform appendix that projects from cecum

Obstruction of lumen leads to infection
- Appendix becomes hypoxic (decreased oxygen levels)
- May cause gangrene
- May rupture, causing peritonitis

Symptoms
Periumbilical (around umbilicus) pain, initially
Right lower quadrant (RLQ) pain as inflammation progresses
Nausea
Vomiting
Possible diarrhea

Treatment
Appendectomy
Management of any perforation or abscess

Meckel's Diverticulum

- Appendage of ileum near cecum derived from an unobliterated yolk stalk in fetal development
- Symptoms can mimic appendicitis

Peritonitis

Inflammation of peritoneum (membrane that lines abdominal cavity)
Usually a result of
- Spread of infection from abdominal organ
- Puncture wound to abdomen
- Rupture of gastrointestinal tract—appendicitis or Meckel's diverticulum
Abscesses form, resulting in adhesions
- May result in obstruction

Types
Acute, chronic

Symptoms
Abdominal pain
Vomiting
Rigid abdomen
Fever
Leukocytosis (increased white cells in blood)

Treatment
Antibiotics
Suction of stomach and intestines
If possible, surgical removal of origin of infection, such as appendix
Fluid replacement
Bed rest

Obstruction

Any interference with passage of intestinal contents

May be
- Acute
- Chronic
- Partial
- Total

Types
Nonmechanical

- Paralytic ileus
- Result of trauma or toxin

Mechanical
- Result of tumors, adhesions, hernias
- Simple mechanical obstruction
  - One point of obstruction
- Closed-loop obstruction
  - At least two points of obstruction
- Diverticulosis
- Twisted bowel (volvulus)
- Telescoping bowel (intussusception)

Symptoms
Abdominal distention
Pain
Vomiting
Total constipation

Treatment
Surgical intervention
Symptomatic treatment

Large Intestine
Diverticulosis
Herniation of intestinal mucosa
- Forms sacs in lining, called diverticula

Diverticulitis
Sacs fill and become inflamed
- Common in aged persons

Symptoms
Diarrhea or constipation
Gas
Abdominal discomfort

Complications
Perforation
Bleeding
Peritonitis
Abscess
Obstruction

Treatment
Antimicrobials as necessary
High-fiber diet (greater than 20 g daily)
Stool softeners
Dietary restrictions of solid foods
Surgical intervention if necessary

Ulcerative Colitis (Fig. 8.7)
Inflammation of rectum that progresses to sigmoid colon
    Intermittent exacerbations and remissions
    May develop into toxic megacolon
      - Leads to obstruction and dilation of colon
    Increased risk for colorectal cancer

• **Figure 8.7** Ulcerative colitis.

Symptoms
Diarrhea
- Blood and mucus may be present

Cramping
Fever
Weight loss

Treatment
Remove physical or emotional stressors
    Anti-inflammatory medications
    Antimotility agents
    Nutritional supplementation
    Surgical intervention, if necessary

Colorectal Cancer
Usually develop from polyp
- In those 55 and older

Increased Risks
Genetic factors
    40 years of age and older
    Diets high in
      - Fat
      - Sugar
      - Red meat
    Low-fiber diets

Symptoms
Asymptomatic until advanced
    Some may experience
- Cramping
- Ribbon stools
- Feeling of incomplete evacuation
- Fatigue
- Weight loss
- Change in bowel habits
- Blood in stool

Treatment
Surgical excision

Radiation
Chemotherapy
Combination of above

Disorders of Liver, Gallbladder, and Pancreas

Disorders of Liver
Jaundice (Hyperbilirubinemia)
A sign of biliary disease, not a disease itself
* Results in yellow eyes (sclera) and skin

Types
Prehepatic
* Excess destruction of red blood cells
* Result of hemolytic anemia or reaction to transfusion
Intrahepatic
* Impaired uptake of bilirubin and decreased blending of bilirubin by hepatic cells
* Result of liver disease, such as cirrhosis or hepatitis
Posthepatic
* Excess bile flows into blood
* Result of obstruction
  * Due to conditions such as inflammation of liver, tumors, cholelithiasis

Treatment
Removal of cause

Cancer of Liver
Most commonly a metastasis; primary CA rare
 Risk for primary liver CA
* Hepatitis B, C, and D
* Cirrhosis
* Myotoxins
* Heavy smoking/alcohol use

Treatment
Surgical resection if localized
 Survival typically 3 or 4 months

Viral Hepatitis
Liver cells are damaged
 Results in inflammation and necrosis
 Damage can be mild or severe
 Scar tissue forms in liver
  * Leads to ischemia

Hepatitis A (HAV)
Infectious hepatitis—caused by hepatitis A virus

Transmission
* Most commonly fecal-oral route—contaminated food or water
Does not have a chronic state
Slow onset—complete recovery characteristic

Vaccine available for those who are traveling
Gamma globulin may be administered to those just exposed

Hepatitis B (HBV)
Serum hepatitis

Carrier state is common
Caused by hepatitis B virus
* Asymptomatic but contagious
Long incubation period
Transmission
* Intravenous drug users
* Transfusion
* Exposure to blood and bodily fluids
* Sexual transmission
* Mother-to-fetus transmission
* Immune globulin is temporary prophylactic
* Vaccine is now routine for children and is given to those at risk
Severe forms cause liver cell destruction, cirrhosis, death

Hepatitis C (HCV)
Transmission of virus
* Most commonly by transfusion
* IV drug users
 Half of cases develop into chronic hepatitis
 Increases risk of hepatocellular cancer
 Carrier state may develop

Hepatitis D (HDV)
Transmission of hepatitis D virus
* Blood
* Intravenous drug users
 Hepatitis B is present for this type to develop

Hepatitis E (HEV)
Transmission of hepatitis E virus
* Fecal-oral route
 Does not develop into chronic or carrier

Hepatitis G
Transmission of hepatitis G virus
* IV drug use
* Sexual transmission

Symptoms of Hepatitis
Stages
Preicteric
* Anorexia
* Nausea and vomiting
Liver enzymes may be elevated—indication of liver cell damage
* Fatigue
* Malaise
* Generalized pain with low-grade fever
* Cough

Icteric
- Jaundice
- Hepatomegaly (enlarged liver)
- Biliary obstruction
- Light-colored stools and dark urine
- Pruritus
- Abdominal pain

Posticteric (recovery)
- Reduction of symptoms

Treatment
None
    In early stages gamma globulins may be used
    Interferon may be used for cases of chronic hepatitis B
      and C

Nonviral Hepatitis
Hepatitis that results from hepatotoxins

Symptoms
- Similar to viral hepatitis

Treatment
- Removal of hepatotoxin

Cirrhosis
Profuse liver damage
- Extensive fibrosis
  - Results in inflammation
    Progressive disorder
    Leads to liver failure

Types
Alcoholic liver
- Known as Laënnec's cirrhosis or portal cirrhosis
- Largest group
  Biliary
- Associated with immune disorders
- Obstructions (intrahepatic or extrahepatic blood vessels) occur and disrupt normal function
  Postnecrotic
- Associated with chronic hepatitis (A or C) and exposure to toxins

Symptoms
Asymptomatic in early stages
    Nausea
    Vomiting
    Fatigue
    Weight loss
    Pruritus
    Jaundice
    Edema

Treatment
Symptomatic
    Dietary restrictions
- Reduced protein and sodium

• **Figure 8.8** Resected gallbladder containing mixed gallstones.

- Increased vitamins and carbohydrates
Diuretics
Antibiotics
Liver transplant

Disorders of Gallbladder
Cholecystitis
Inflammation of gallbladder and cystic duct

Cholangitis
Inflammation of bile duct

Cholelithiasis
Formation of gallstones (Fig. 8.8)
- Consists of cholesterol or bilirubin
- Occurs most often in those with high levels of cholesterol, calcium, or bile salts
  Stones cause irritation and inflammation
- May lead to infection
- Obstruction
  - May result in pancreatitis
  - Rupture is possible

Symptoms
Often asymptomatic
    Dietary intolerance particularly to fat
    Right upper quadrant (RUQ) pain
    Pain in back and/or shoulder
    Epigastric discomfort
    Bloating heartburn, flatulence

Treatment
Surgical intervention (laparoscopic cholecystectomy)
    Lithotripsy
    Medical management by use of drugs that break down
      stone

Disorders of Pancreas
Pancreatitis
Inflammation of pancreas resulting from digestive enzyme attack to pancreas

Acute and chronic forms

Commonly associated with alcoholism, biliary tract obstruction, drug toxicity, gallstone obstruction of common bile duct, and viral infections

Symptoms
Severe pain
Fever
Acute form is a medical emergency
Neurogenic shock
Septicemia
General sepsis

Complications
Adult respiratory distress syndrome (ARDS)

Renal failure

Treatment
No oral intake
- IV fluids given and carefully monitored

Analgesics
Stop process of autodigestion
Prevent systemic shutdown

Pancreatic Cancer
Increased Risk
Cigarette smoking
    Diet high in fat and protein

Symptoms
Weight loss
    Jaundice
    Anorexia
    Most types of pancreatic cancer are asymptomatic until well advanced

Treatment
Surgery
    Chemotherapy and radiation therapy

Chapter 8: Pathophysiology Quiz

(Quiz Answers Are Located in Appendix B)

1. This type of hyperbilirubinemia is characterized by excess bile flow into the blood:
   a. intrahepatic
   b. prehepatic
   c. posthepatic
   d. jaundice

2. This type of hepatitis is transmitted by the fecal-oral route:
   a. A
   b. B
   c. C
   d. D

3. Which of the following is the recovery stage of hepatitis?
   a. prehepatic
   b. posthepatic
   c. preicteric
   d. posticteric

4. This type of cirrhosis is also known as portal cirrhosis:
   a. biliary
   b. alcoholic liver
   c. postnecrotic
   d. traumatic

5. This condition is the inflammation of the bile ducts:
   a. cholangitis
   b. cholecystitis
   c. cholelithiasis
   d. cholangioma

6. Formation of gallstones most often occurs with high levels of the following:
   a. bile salts and toxins
   b. cholesterol and toxins
   c. cholesterol and bile salts
   d. toxins

7. The primary factor that increases the risk of pancreatic cancer is:
   a. smoking
   b. alcohol
   c. intravenous drug use
   d. hepatitis

8. A potential complication of this condition is ARDS:
   a. hyperbilirubinemia
   b. hepatitis
   c. pancreatitis
   d. pancreatic cancer

9. The primary treatment for jaundice is:
   a. removal of cause
   b. antibiotics
   c. dialysis
   d. vaccine

10. This condition has the largest group of those who abuse alcohol:
    a. cirrhosis
    b. hepatitis
    c. pancreatitis
    d. pancreatic cancer

9

Mediastinum and Diaphragm

ANATOMY AND TERMINOLOGY

Not an organ system

Mediastinum

That area between lungs that a median (partition) divides (Fig. 9.1) into
- Superior
- Anterior
- Posterior
- Middle
    Space that houses heart, thymus gland, trachea, esophagus, nerves, lymph and blood vessels, and major blood vessels
- Aorta
- Inferior vena cava

Diaphragm

A dome-shaped muscular partition that separates abdominal cavity from thoracic cavity
- Assists in breathing

- Expands to assist lungs in exhalation/relaxation of diaphragm
- Flattens out during inspiration/contraction of diaphragm
- Diaphragmatic hernia: esophageal hernia

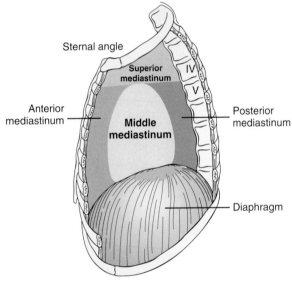

- **Figure 9.1** Mediastinum and diaphragm.

Chapter 9: Anatomy and Terminology Quiz

(Quiz Answers are Located in Appendix B)
1. The mediastinum is NOT an organ system.
    a. true
    b. false
2. The mediastinum is divided into:
    a. superior, anterior, posterior
    b. superior, anterior, posterior, middle
    c. anterior, posterior, middle
    d. middle, anterior, superior
3. During inspiration, the diaphragm:
    a. expands
    b. moves upward
    c. collapses
    d. flattens out
4. Term meaning "partition":
    a. middle
    b. aspect
    c. median
    d. diaphragm

5. The diaphragm is said to be this shape:
   a. square
   b. flat
   c. dome
   d. round
6. This separates the abdominal cavity from the thoracic cavity:
   a. mediastinum
   b. diaphragm
   c. superior
   d. inferior
7. This is the area between the lungs:
   a. mediastinum
   b. diaphragm
   c. superior
   d. inferior
8. This is an esophageal hernia:
   a. mediastinal
   b. diaphragmatic
   c. paraesophageal
   d. hiatal
9. A diaphragmatic hernia is also known as:
   a. esophageal
   b. epiglottis
   c. partitional
   d. medial
10. The diaphragm assists in:
    a. percussion
    b. auscultation
    c. contraction
    d. breathing

10

Hemic and Lymphatic System

ANATOMY AND TERMINOLOGY

Hemic refers to blood

Lymphatic system removes excess tissue fluid
- Lymph tissue is scattered throughout body
- Composed of lymph nodes, vessels, and organs

Lymph

Colorless fluid containing lymphocytes and monocytes
  Originates from blood and after filtering, returns to blood
  Transports interstitial fluids and proteins that have leaked from blood system into venous system
  Absorbs and transports fats from villi of small intestine to venous system
  Assists in immune function

Lymph Vessels

Similar to veins
  Organized circulatory system throughout body

Lymph Organs

Lymph nodes, spleen, bone marrow, thymus, tonsils, and Peyer's patches (lymphoid tissue on mucosa of small intestine)

Lymph nodes, areas of concentrated tissue (Fig. 10.1)
Spleen, located in left upper quadrant (LUQ) of abdomen
- Composed of lymph tissue
  - Function is to filter blood; activates lymphocytes and B cells to filter antigens
  - Stores blood
Thymus secretes thymosin, causing T cells to mature
- Larger in infants and shrinks with age
Tonsils
- Palatine tonsils
- Pharyngeal tonsils/adenoids

Hematopoietic Organ

Bone marrow, contains tissue that produces RBCs, WBCs, and platelets
- Produces stem cells

TABLE 10-1

Combining Forms

Combining Form	Meaning
1. aden/o	gland
2. adenoid/o	adenoids
3. axill/o	armpit
4. cervic/o	neck/cervix
5. immune/o	immune
6. inguin/o	groin
7. lymph/o	lymph
8. lymphaden/o	lymph gland
9. splen/o	spleen
10. thym/o	thymus gland
11. tonsill/o	tonsil
12. tox/o	poison

TABLE 10-2

Prefixes

Prefix	Meaning
1. hyper-	excess
2. inter-	between
3. retro-	behind

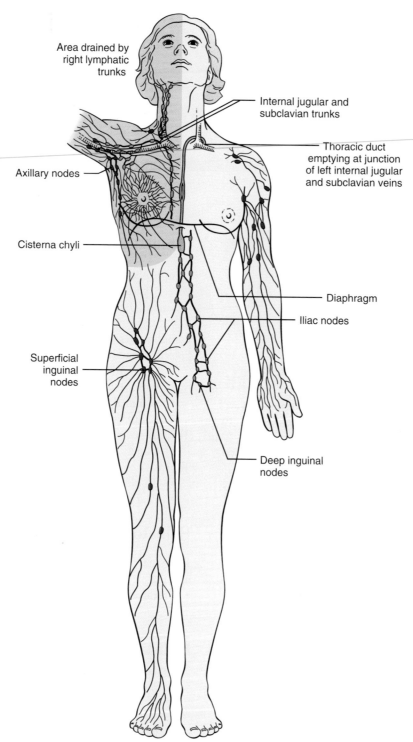

Area drained by
right lymphatic
trunks

Internal jugular and
subclavian trunks

Thoracic duct
emptying at junction
of left internal jugular
and subclavian veins

Axillary nodes

Cisterna chyli

Diaphragm

Iliac nodes

Superficial
inguinal
nodes

Deep inguinal
nodes

• **Figure 10.1** Lymphatic system.

TABLE 10-3

Suffixes

Suffix	Meaning	Suffix	Meaning
1. -ectomy	removal	6. -oma	tumor
2. -edema	swelling	7. -penia	deficient
3. -itis	inflammation	8. -pexy	fixation
4. -megaly	enlargement	9. -phylaxis	protection
5. -oid	resembling	10. -poiesis	production

TABLE 10-4

Medical Terms

Term	Meaning	Term	Meaning
Axillary nodes	Lymph nodes located in armpit	Parathyroid	Produces a hormone to mobilize calcium from bones to blood
Cloquet's node	Also called a gland; it is highest of deep groin lymph nodes	Splenectomy	Excision of spleen
Inguinofemoral	Referring to groin and thigh	Splenography	Radiographic recording of spleen
Jugular nodes	Lymph nodes located next to large vein in neck	Splenoportography	Radiographic procedure to allow visualization of splenic and portal veins of spleen
Lymph node	Station along lymphatic system	Stem cell	Immature blood cell
Lymphadenectomy	Excision of a lymph node or nodes	Thoracic duct	Largest lymph vessel; it collects lymph from portions of body below diaphragm and from left side of body above diaphragm
Lymphadenitis	Inflammation of a lymph node		
Lymphangiography	Radiographic recording of lymphatic vessels and nodes		
Lymphangiotomy	Incision into a lymphatic vessel		
Lymphangitis	Inflammation of lymphatic vessel or vessels	Transplantation	Grafting of tissue from one source to another

Chapter 10: Anatomy and Terminology Quiz

(Quiz Answers Are Located in Appendix B)

1. The spleen is located in this quadrant of the abdomen:
   a. RUQ
   b. LUQ
   c. LLQ
   d. LRQ
2. Produces RBCs and platelets:
   a. thymus
   b. tonsils
   c. lymph node
   d. bone marrow
3. Which of the following is NOT a lymph organ?
   a. adrenal
   b. spleen
   c. thymus
   d. tonsil

4. Lymph transports fluids and _____ that have leaked from the blood system back to veins.
   a. stem cells
   b. lymphocytes
   c. B cells
   d. proteins
5. This is largest in infants and shrinks with age:
   a. tonsils
   b. spleen
   c. thymus
   d. bone marrow
6. Combining form meaning "gland":
   a. axill/o
   b. thym/o
   c. aden/o
   d. tox/o

7. Prefix meaning "excess":
   a. hyper-
   b. hypo-
   c. inter-
   d. retro-
8. Suffix meaning "enlargement":
   a. -edema
   b. -poiesis
   c. -penia
   d. -megaly

9. Lymph node located on neck:
   a. thoracic
   b. jugular
   c. Cloquet's
   d. axillary
10. These cells originate in the bone marrow:
   a. B cells
   b. antigens
   c. erythrocytes
   d. stem cells

PATHOPHYSIOLOGY

Anemia

Reduction in number of erythrocytes or decrease in quality of hemoglobin
- Less oxygen is transported in the blood

Aplastic Anemia

Diverse group of anemias
   Characterized by bone marrow failure with reduced numbers of red and white blood cells and platelets

Causes
Genetic or acquired (primary or secondary)

Toxins/chemical agents
   • Benzene and antibiotics such as chloramphenicol
Irradiation
Immunologic
Idiopathic (unknown)

Treatment
Blood transfusion
Bone marrow transplant

Iron Deficiency Anemia

Characterized by small erythrocytes and a reduced amount of hemoglobin
Caused by low or absent iron stores or serum iron concentrations
   • Blood loss
   • Decreased intake of iron
   • Malabsorption of iron

Symptoms
Pallor
Headache
Stomatitis
Oral lesions
Gastrointestinal complaints
Retinal hemorrhages
Thinning, brittle nails and hair

Treatment
Iron supplement

Pernicious Anemia

Megaloblastic anemia (large stem cells)
Inability to absorb vitamin B_{12} due to a lack of intrinsic factor (found in gastric juices)
Usually in older adults
Caused by impaired intestinal absorption of vitamin B_{12}

Symptoms
Pallor
Weakness
Neurologic manifestations
Gastric discomfort

Treatment
Injections of vitamin B_{12}
Transfusions

Hemolytic Anemia

May be acute or chronic

Shortened survival of mature erythrocytes—excessive destruction of RBCs
   • Inability of bone marrow to compensate for decreased survival of erythrocytes

Treatment
Treat cause

Sickle Cell Anemia

Occurs primarily in those of West African descent
   Abnormal sickle-shaped erythrocytes (sickle cell) caused by an abnormal type of hemoglobin (Hemoglobin S)

Symptoms
Abdominal pain
Arthralgia
Ulceration of lower extremities
Fatigue
Dyspnea
Increased heart rate

Treatment
Symptomatic

Granulocytosis

Increase in granulocytes
- Neutrophils
- Eosinophils
- Basophils

Eosinophilia

Increase in number of eosinophilic granulocytes

Cause
Allergic disorders
Dermatologic disorders
Parasitic invasion
Drugs
Malignancies

Basophilia

Increase in basophilic granulocytes seen in leukemia

Monocytosis

Increased number of monocytes

Cause
Infection
Hematologic factors

Leukocytosis

Increased number of leukocytes

Cause
Acute viral infections, such as hepatitis
Chronic infections, such as syphilis

Leukocytopenia

Decreased number of leukocytes

Cause
Neoplasias
Immune deficiencies
Drugs
Virus
Radiation

Infectious Mononucleosis

Acute Infection of B Cells

Epstein-Barr virus most common cause

Symptoms
Fatigue
Fever
Weakness (asthenia)
Pharyngitis
Atypical lymphocytes in blood
Lymph node enlargement
Splenomegaly
Hepatomegaly

Transmission

Saliva
- Known as kissing disease

Treatment
Rest
Treatment of symptoms

Leukemia

Malignant disorder of blood and blood-forming organs

Leads to dysfunction of cells
- Primarily leads to proliferation of abnormal leukocytes—filling bone marrow and bloodstream

Acute Myelogenous Leukemia (AML)

Rapid onset
Short survival time

Symptoms
Abrupt onset
Fatigue
Lymphadenopathy
Bone pain and tenderness
Anemia
Bleeding
Fever
Infection
Anorexia
Splenomegaly
Hepatomegaly
Headache, vomiting, paralysis

Treatment
Chemotherapy
Bone marrow transplant following high-dose chemotherapy to eradicate leukemic cells

Acute Lymphocytic Leukemia (ALL)

Immature lymphocytes (lymphoblasts)
Most cases occur in children and adolescents
Sudden onset

Treatment
Chemotherapy with drugs that suppress cell division and destroy rapidly dividing cells

Remission
Relapse—leukemia cells in bone marrow and blood requiring treatment

Chronic Myelogenous Leukemia (CML)

Mature and immature granulocytes in bone marrow and blood

Slow, progressive disease (those over 55 years live many years without life threat)
Cells are more differentiated
Gradual onset with milder symptoms
- Majority of cases are in adults

Symptoms
Extreme fatigue
Weight loss
Splenomegaly
Night sweats
Fever
Infections

Treatment
Chemotherapy—target abnormal proteins
Bone marrow transplant following high-dose chemotherapy

Chronic Lymphocytic Leukemia (CLL)

Increased numbers of mature lymphocytes in marrow, lymph nodes, spleen

Most common form seen in elderly
Slowly progressive

Treatment
Chemotherapy

Lymphadenopathy

Lymphadenopathy
Any abnormality of lymph node
Enlargement of lymph node

Lymphangitis
Inflammation of lymphatic vessel

Lymphadenitis
Inflammation of lymph node
Localized inflammation associated with inflamed lesion
Generalized inflammation associated with disease
Inflammation can occur as result of
- Trauma
- Infection
- Drug reaction
- Autoimmune disease
- Immunologic disease

Malignant Lymphoma

Hodgkin Disease
Initial sign is a painless mass commonly located on neck
Giant Reed-Sternberg cells are present in lymphatic tissue

Presentation
Enlarged spleen (splenomegaly)
Abdominal mass
Mediastinal mass
Localized node involvement
- Orderly spreading of node involvement
- Cervical, axillary, inguinal, and retroperitoneal lymph node involvement

Symptoms
Night sweats
Fever
Weight loss
Itching (pruritus)
Anorexia
Weakness

Treatment
If localized: radiation therapy and chemotherapy
If systemic: chemotherapy alone
High probability of cure with new treatments

Non-Hodgkin Lymphoma
No giant Reed-Sternberg cells present
Involves multiple nodes scattered throughout body (follicular lymphoma)
Large cell lymphoma (large lymphocytes in diffuse nodes and lymph tissue)
- Noncontiguous spread of node involvement
- Not localized
Usually begins as a painless enlargement of node

Symptoms
Presents similar to Hodgkin disease

Treatment
Chemotherapy cures or stops disease progression

Burkitt's Lymphoma
Type of non-Hodgkin lymphoma
Usually found in Africa and New Guinea
Characterized by lesions in jaw and face
Epstein-Barr (herpes virus) has been found in Burkitt's lymphoma

Treatment
Radiation and chemotherapy for African type

Myeloma

Multiple Myeloma

B-cell cancer—lymphocytes that produce antibodies destroying bone tissue

- Also known as plasma cell myeloma
  Increased plasma cells replace bone marrow
  Overproduction of immunoglobulins—Bence Jones protein (found in urine)
  Multiple tumor sites cause bone destruction
  Results in weakened bone
  Hypercalcemia
  Anemia
  Renal damage
  Increased susceptibility to infections

Cause
Unknown

Treatment
Chemotherapy
Radiotherapy
Autologous bone marrow transplant (ABMT) prolongs remission—may be a cure
Palliative treatments

Chapter 10: Pathophysiology Quiz

(Quiz Answers Are Located in Appendix B)

1. This condition involves a reduced number of erythrocytes and decreased quality of hemoglobin:
   a. monocytosis
   b. eosinophilia
   c. anemia
   d. leukocytosis
2. This condition is characterized by a shortened survival of mature erythrocytes and inability of bone marrow to compensate for decreased survival:
   a. hemolytic anemia
   b. granulocytosis
   c. eosinophilia
   d. monocytosis
3. The most common cause of this disease is Epstein-Barr virus:
   a. leukocytopenia
   b. infectious mononucleosis
   c. leukocytosis
   d. hemolytic anemia
4. Inflammation of the lymphatic vessels is:
   a. lymphadenitis
   b. lymphoma
   c. lymphadenopathy
   d. lymphangitis
5. What giant cell is present in Hodgkin disease?
   a. B cell
   b. Reed-Sternberg
   c. T cell
   d. C cell
6. This condition increases plasma cells, which replace bone marrow:
   a. Burkitt's lymphoma
   b. multiple myeloma
   c. Hodgkin disease
   d. leukemia
7. Injection of vitamin B may be prescribed for this type of anemia:
   a. pernicious
   b. aplastic
   c. sideroblastic
   d. sickle cell
8. These are large stem cells:
   a. megaloblasts
   b. leukocytes
   c. erythrocytes
   d. granulocytes
9. This is known as the kissing disease:
   a. monocytosis
   b. leukocytopenia
   c. infectious mononucleosis
   d. granulocytosis
10. This lymphoma is usually found in Africa:
    a. multiple
    b. Burkitt's
    c. B-cell
    d. T-cell

11

Endocrine System

ANATOMY AND TERMINOLOGY

Regulates body through hormones (chemical messengers)
   Ductless endocrine glands secrete hormones directly to bloodstream
   Affects growth, development, and metabolism

Endocrine Glands (Fig. 11.1)

Pituitary (Hypophysis): Master Gland

Located at base of brain in a depression in skull (sella turcica)
   Anterior pituitary (adenohypophysis)
   • Adrenocorticotropic hormone (ACTH)—stimulates adrenal cortex and increases production of cortisol
   • Follicle-stimulating hormone (FSH)—males, stimulates sperm and testosterone production; females, with luteinizing hormone (LH) stimulates secretion of estrogen and follicle development and ovulation
   • Growth hormone (GH or somatotropin STH)—stimulates protein processing resulting in growth of bones, muscle, and fat metabolism, and maintains blood glucose levels
   • Luteinizing hormone (LH)—males, stimulates testosterone production; females, stimulates secretion of progesterone and estrogen
   • Melanocyte-stimulating hormone (MSH)—increases skin pigmentation
   • Prolactin (PRL)—secreted by anterior pituitary, stimulates milk production and breast development
   • Thyroid-stimulating hormone (TSH or thyrotropin)—stimulates thyroid gland
   Posterior pituitary (neurohypophysis)—stores and releases hormones
   • Antidiuretic hormone (ADH) or vasopressin—stimulates reabsorption of water by kidney tubules and increases blood pressure by constricting arterioles
   • Oxytocin (OT)—stimulates contractions during childbirth, production and release of milk

Thyroid

Two lobes overlying trachea
   Secretes two hormones that increase cell metabolism—thyroxine (T_4) and triiodothyronine (T_3)—synthesized from iodine
   Secretes one hormone that decreases blood calcium—thyrocalcitonin (nasal spray used to treat osteoporosis)

Parathyroid Glands (4)

Located on posterior side of thyroid
   Secretes PTH (parathyroid hormone) or parathormone
   Promotes calcium homeostasis in bloodstream

Adrenal Gland (Pair)

Located on top of each kidney
   Adrenal cortex—outer region that secretes corticosteroids
   • Cortisol—increases blood glucose
   • Aldosterone—increases reabsorption of sodium (salt)
   • Androgen, estrogen, progestin—sexual characteristics
   Adrenal medulla—inner region that secretes catecholamines (epinephrine to dilate blood vessels to lower blood pressure, increase heart rate, dilate bronchial tubes, and release glycogen for energy and norepinephrine to constrict blood vessels to raise blood pressure)

Pancreas

Located behind stomach
   Contains specialized cells (islets of Langerhans) that produce insulin and glycogen hormones
   Insulin (decreases blood glucose), glucagon (converts glycogen to glucose, raising blood sugar), and somatostatin (regulates other cells of pancreas)

Thymus

Located behind sternum
   Atrophies during adolescence

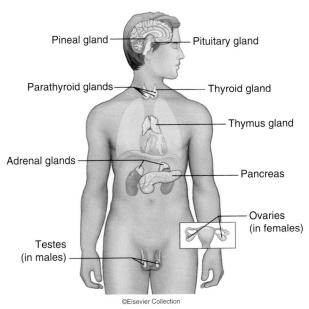

• **Figure 11.1** Endocrine system.

Pineal gland — *Pituitary gland*
Parathyroid glands — *Thyroid gland*
Thymus gland
Adrenal glands — *Pancreas*
Ovaries (in females)
Testes (in males)
©Elsevier Collection

Produces thymosin—stimulates T-lymphocytes, effecting a positive immune response

Hypothalamus (Part of Brain)

Located below thalamus and above pituitary gland
Stimulates anterior pituitary to release hormones and posterior hypothalamus to store and release hormones

Pineal

Located between two cerebral hemispheres and above third ventricle
Secretes melatonin—more so at night, which affects sleep cycle
Also responsible for delaying sexual maturation in children
Also has neurotransmitters such as somatostatin, norepinephrine, serotonin, and histamine

Ovaries (Pair, Females)

Estrogen production stimulates ova production and secondary female sex characteristics
Progesterone—prepares the uterus for and maintains pregnancy

Placenta

Produces HCG (human chorionic gonadotropin) to sustain a pregnancy

Testes (Pair, Males)

Testosterone—male sex characteristics

TABLE 11-1

Combining Forms

Combining Form	Meaning	Combining Form	Meaning
1. aden/o	in relationship to a gland	16. lact/o	milk
2. adren/o	adrenal gland	17. myx/o	mucus
3. adrenal/o	adrenal gland	18. natr/o	sodium
4. andr/o	male	19. pancreat/o	pancreas
5. calc/o, calc/i	calcium	20. parathyroid/o	parathyroid gland
6. cortic/o	cortex	21. phys/o	growing
7. crin/o	secrete	22. pituitar/o	pituitary gland
8. dips/o	thirst	23. somat/o	body
9. estr/o	female	24. ster/o, stere/o	solid, having three dimensions
10. gluc/o	sugar	25. thry/o	thyroid gland
11. glyc/o	sugar	26. thyroid/o	thyroid gland
12. gonad/o	ovaries and testes	27. toc/o	childbirth
13. home/o	same	28. toxic/o	poison
14. hormon/o	hormone	29. ur/o	urine
15. kal/i	potassium		

TABLE 11-2

Prefixes

Prefix	Meaning
1. eu-	good/normal
2. oxy-	sharp, oxygen
3. pan-	all
4. tetra-	four
5. tri-	three
6. tropin-	act upon

TABLE 11-3

Suffixes

Suffix	Meaning
1. -agon	assemble
2. -drome	run, relationship to conducting, to speed
3. -emia	blood condition
4. -in	a substance
5. -ine	a substance
6. -tropin	act upon
7. -uria	urine

TABLE 11-4

Medical Terms

Term	Meaning
Adrenals	Glands, located at top of kidneys, that produce steroid hormones (cortex) and catecholamines (medulla)
Contralateral	Opposite side
Hormone	Chemical substance produced by body's endocrine glands
Isthmus	Connection of two regions or structures
Isthmus, thyroid	Tissue connection between right and left thyroid lobes
Isthmusectomy	Surgical removal of isthmus
Lobectomy	Removal of a lobe
Thymectomy	Surgical removal of thymus
Thymus	Gland that produces hormones important to immune response
Thyroglossal duct	A duct in embryo between thyroid and posterior tongue that occasionally persists into adult life and causes cysts, fistulas, or sinuses
Thyroid	Part of endocrine system that produces hormones that regulate metabolism
Thyroidectomy	Surgical removal of thyroid

Chapter 11: Anatomy and Terminology Quiz

(Quiz Answers Are Located in Appendix B)

1. Which of the following is NOT affected by the endocrine system?
   a. digestion
   b. development
   c. progesterone
   d. metabolism
2. Gland that overlies the trachea:
   a. parathyroid
   b. adrenal
   c. pancreas
   d. thyroid
3. Gland that is located on the top of each kidney:
   a. parathyroid
   b. adrenal
   c. pancreas
   d. thyroid
4. The outer region of the adrenal gland that secretes corticosteroids:
   a. cortex
   b. medulla
   c. sternum
   d. medullary

5. Located on the thyroid:
   a. hypophysis
   b. thymus
   c. pineal
   d. parathyroid
6. Located at the base of the brain in a depression in the skull:
   a. pituitary
   b. thymus
   c. adrenal
   d. pineal
7. Stimulates contractions during childbirth:
   a. cortisol
   b. PTH
   c. ADH
   d. oxytocin
8. Produced only during pregnancy by the placenta:
   a. estrogen and progesterone
   b. melatonin
   c. thymosin
   d. adrenocorticotropic hormone

9. Combining form meaning "secrete":
   a. dips/o
   b. crin/o
   c. gluc/o
   d. kal/i

10. Prefix meaning "good":
   a. tri-
   b. tropin-
   c. pan-
   d. eu-

PATHOPHYSIOLOGY

Diabetes Mellitus

Caused by a deficiency in insulin production or poor use of insulin by body cells
   Islets of Langerhans (pancreatic cells) secrete glucagon and insulin to regulate fat, carbohydrate, and protein metabolism

Types of Diabetes Mellitus

Type 1, IDDM (Insulin-Dependent Diabetes Mellitus), Immune Mediated

Onset before age 30—peak onset age 12
   Includes beta islet cell destruction, insulin deficiency
   Acute onset
   Positive family history
   Requires insulin
   Ketoacidosis (fats improperly burned leads to ketones and acids circulating)

Type 2, NIDDM (Non–Insulin-Dependent Diabetes Mellitus)

Adult onset, after age 30, but it is now occurring earlier
   Insidious onset/asymptomatic
   Positive in immediate family
   Dietary management and/or oral hypoglycemics and/or insulin
   Most common type—85% are obese at onset
   Insulin is present
   Ketoacidosis does not occur

Symptoms

Polyuria
   Polydipsia
   Glycosuria
   Hyperglycemia
   Polyphagia
   Unexplained weight loss

Acute Complications

Hypoglycemia
   Hyperglycemia with coma
   Diabetic ketoacidosis

Chronic Complications

Diabetic neuropathy (Fig. 11.2)
   Retinopathy
   Coronary artery disease (atherosclerosis)

• **Figure 11.2** Patient with diabetes mellitus and neuropathy had severe claw toes, and shear forces across plantar surface of first metatarsal head caused recurrent ulceration.

Stroke
Peripheral vascular disease
Infection

Gestational Diabetes Mellitus—Predisposition to Diabetes

Most often recognized in second trimester
   Glucose intolerance may be temporary, occurring only during pregnancy
   Many will develop diabetes mellitus within 15 years

Pituitary Disorders

Tumors
   Most common cause of pituitary disorders
   May secrete hormone
      Such as prolactin or ACTH

Anterior Pituitary

Dwarfism (Hypopituitarism)

Can be caused by deficiency of somatotropin (growth hormone)

Gigantism (Fig. 11.3) (Hyperpituitarism)

Can be caused by excess of somatotrophin (growth hormone) in childhood

Treatment

Resection of tumor or irradiation of pituitary

• **Figure 11.3** Gigantism. A pituitary giant and dwarf contrasted with normal-size men.

Acromegaly (Hyperpituitarism)

Increased GH in adulthood
Enlargement of facial bones, feet, and hands

Treatment

Pituitary adenoma is irradiated or removed

Posterior Pituitary

Diabetes Insipidus

Insufficient antidiuretic hormone—kidney tubules fail to retain needed water and salts
Causes polyuria, polydipsia, and dehydration
ADH or SIADH—syndrome of inadequate antidiuretic hormone
Excessive secretion of antidiuretic hormone
Causes excessive water retention

Treatment

Some types have no treatment
Others can be controlled with vasopressin (drug)

Thyroid Disorders

Goiter (Fig. 11.4)

Enlargement of thyroid gland in the neck

Cause

Hypothyroid disorders
Hyperthyroid disorders

• **Figure 11.4** Goiter is an enlargement of thyroid gland.

Hyperthyroidism—Thyrotoxicosis

Excessive thyroid hormone production
Most common form: Graves' disease (familial)—results of autoimmune process

Characterized by

Goiter
Tachycardia
Atrial fibrillation
Dyspnea
Palpitations
Fatigue
Tremor
Nervousness
Weight loss
Exophthalmos (protruding eyes)
• Decreased blinking

Treatment

Medication (antithyroid drugs)
Radioactive iodine
Surgical excision

Thyrotoxicosis Storm/Crisis

Thyroid storm/crisis is an acute, life-threatening hypermetabolic state induced by excessive release of thyroid hormones
• Most extreme state of thyrotoxicosis

Hypothyroidism

Primary: inadequate thyroid hormone production
Resulting in increasing levels of thyroid-stimulating hormone (TSH) production
Secondary: inadequate amounts of thyroid-stimulating hormone synthesized

Types

Cretinism
• Congenital
• Occurs in children

- If not treated, it will cause a severe delay in physical and mental development

Myxedema
- Severe form
- Occurs in adults
  - Atherosclerosis
- Symptoms
  - Cold intolerance
  - Weight gain
    - Mental sluggishness
    - Fatigue

Hashimoto's thyroiditis
- Autoimmune disorder

Treatment

Medication (levothyroxine synthetic hormone replacement)

Parathyroid Disorders

Hyperparathyroidism—Excessive Parathyroid Hormone (PTH)

Leads to hypercalcemia
- Affects heart and bones and damages kidneys

Symptoms

Brittle bones
    Kidney stones
    Cardiac disturbances

Treatment

Surgical excision

Hypoparathyroidism—Abnormally Low PTH

Leads to hypocalcemia

Symptoms

Nerve irritability—twitching or spasms
    Muscle cramps
    Tingling and burning (paresthesias) of fingertips, toes, and lips
    Anxiety, nervousness
    Tetany (constant muscle contraction)

Treatment

Calcium and vitamin D

Adrenal Gland Disorders

Cushing Syndrome—Hypercortisolism

Excess levels of adrenocorticotropic hormone (ACTH)

Cause

Hyperfunction of adrenal cortex
    Long-term use of steroid medications

Symptoms

Weight gain

- Fat deposits on face (moonface) and trunk (buffalo hump)

Glucose intolerance
- Diabetes may develop (20%)

Hypernatremia
Hypokalemia
Virilization
Hypertension
Muscle wasting
Osteoporosis
Change in mental status
Delayed healing

Treatment

Medication
    Radiation therapy
    Surgical intervention

Addison's Disease—Primary Adrenal Insufficiency

Deficiency of Adrenocortical Hormones Resulting From Destruction of Adrenal Glands

- Glucocorticoids
- Mineralocorticoids

Cause

Tumors
    Autoimmune disorders
    Viral
    Tuberculosis
    Infection

Symptoms

Decreased blood glucose levels
    Elevated serum ACTH
    Fatigue
    Lack of ability to handle stress
    Weight loss
    Infections
    Hypotension
    Decreased body hair
    Hyperpigmentation

Treatment

Hormone (glucocorticoid) replacement

Hyperaldosteronism

Excess aldosterone secreted by adrenal cortex

Types

Primary hyperaldosteronism (Conn's syndrome)
- Caused by an abnormality of adrenal cortex
  - Usually an adrenal adenoma

Secondary hyperaldosteronism
- Caused by other than adrenal stimuli

Symptoms

Hypertension

Hypokalemia
Neuromuscular disorders

Treatment

Treat the underlying condition that caused hyperaldosteronism
• Such as adrenal adenoma

Adrenal Medulla

Hypersecretion
Pheochromocytoma—benign tumor of medulla
Excessive production of epinephrine and norepinephrine

Symptoms

Severe headaches
Sweating
Flushing
Hypertension
Muscle spasms

Treatment

Antihypertensive drugs
Remove tumor

Androgen and Estrogen Hypersecretion

Androgen, male characteristic hormone
• Virilization, development of male characteristics
Hypersecretion of estrogen, female characteristic hormone
• Feminization

Cause

Underlying condition
• Adrenal tumor
• Cushing syndrome
• Adenomas or carcinomas
• Defects in steroid metabolism

Treatment

Surgical intervention for tumor
Underlying condition

Chapter 11: Pathophysiology Quiz

(Quiz Answers Are Located in Appendix B)

1. This type of diabetes typically occurs before age 30:
   a. type 1
   b. type 2
2. The acronym that indicates that insulin is not required is:
   a. IDDM
   b. NIDDM
   c. PIDDM
   d. NDDMI
3. The most common cause of pituitary disorders is:
   a. hypersecretion
   b. hyposecretion
   c. tumor
   d. infection
4. In excess, this hormone can cause gigantism:
   a. somatotrophin
   b. thyroid
   c. mineralocorticoids
   d. adrenocortical
5. Goiter can be caused by which of the following:
   a. hypothyroidism
   b. parathyroidism
   c. hyperthyroidism
   d. both a and c
6. This type of hypothyroidism is an autoimmune disorder:
   a. myxedema
   b. Hashimoto's
   c. cretinism
   d. hypokalemia
7. Tetany can be caused by:
   a. hypoparathyroidism
   b. hyperthyroidism
   c. hyperparathyroidism
   d. hyperaldosteronism
8. Conn's syndrome is also known as:
   a. primary hypoparathyroidism
   b. primary hyperthyroidism
   c. primary hyperparathyroidism
   d. primary hyperaldosteronism
9. Development of male characteristics is known as:
   a. virilization
   b. feminization
   c. hypertrophy
   d. hyperaldosteronism
10. The treatment for Addison's disease is often:
    a. chemotherapy
    b. radiation
    c. hormone replacement
    d. all of the above

12

Nervous System

ANATOMY AND TERMINOLOGY

Controlling, regulating, and communicating system

Organization
- Central nervous system (CNS), brain and spinal cord
- Peripheral nervous system (PNS), cranial and spinal nerves
  - Autonomic nervous system—motor and sensory nerves of viscera (involuntary)
  - Somatic nervous system—motor and sensory nerves of skeletal muscles

Cells of the Nervous System (Fig. 12.1)

Neurons—Primary Cells of Nervous System

Classified according to function (afferent [sensory], efferent [motor], interneurons [associational])
- Dendrites (receive signals)
- Cell body (nucleus, within cell body)
- Axon (carries signals from cell body)
- Myelin sheath (insulation around axon)

Glia

Astrocytes
    Star shaped—transport water and salts between capillaries and neurons
Microglia
    Multiple branching processes—protect neurons from inflammation
Oligodendrocytes
    Form myelin sheath
Ependymal
    Lining membrane of brain and spinal cord where central spinal fluid circulates

Divisions of Central Nervous System (CNS) (Fig. 12.2)

Brain—Housed in Cranium (Box Comprised of 8 Bones)—Functioning to Enclose and Protect

Listing from inferior to superior

Brainstem
Medulla oblongata—crossover area left to right and center of respiratory and cardiovascular systems
    Pons—connection of nerves (face and eyes)
    Midbrain

Diencephalon
Hypothalamus controls autonomic nervous system, body temperature, sleep, appetite, and control of pituitary
    Thalamus relays impulses to cerebral cortex for sensory system (pain)

Cerebellum
Controls voluntary movement and balance

Cerebrum
Largest part of brain

Functions
Mental processes, personality, sensory interpretation, movements, and memory

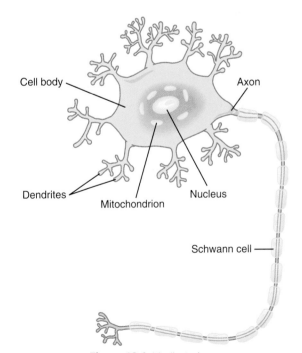

• **Figure 12.1** Myelinated axon.

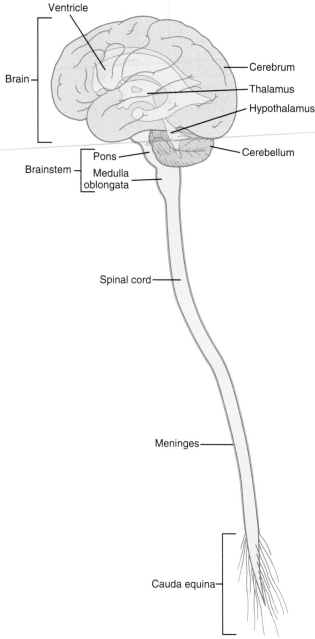

Ventricle

Brain

Cerebrum

Thalamus

Hypothalamus

Cerebellum

Pons

Brainstem

Medulla oblongata

Spinal cord

Meninges

Cauda equina

• **Figure 12.2** Brain and spinal cord.

Two Hemispheres

Right controls left side of body
　Left controls right side of body

Divided Into Five Lobes

- Frontal
- Parietal
- Temporal
- Occipital
- Insula

Vertebral Column—33 Vertebrae

7 cervical
12 thoracic
5 lumbar

5 sacrum (fused)
4 coccygeal (fused)—tailbone

Spinal Cord—Housed Within Vertebrae From Medulla Oblongata to Second Lumbar

Spinal and brain meninges (coverings—dura mater [external], arachnoid, pia mater [internal])
　Spine and brain spaces bathed by cerebrospinal fluid (CSF) (subarachnoid space)
　Cavities within brain contain cerebrospinal fluid (ventricles)

Peripheral Nervous System (PNS)

Cranial nerves, 12 pairs
　Spinal nerves, 31 pairs

Autonomic Nervous System (ANS)—Housed Within Both PNS and CNS

Two divisions
- Sympathetic system—functions in fight and flight (stress)
- Parasympathetic system—functions to restore and conserve energy

TABLE 12-1	
Combining Forms	
Combining Form	**Meaning**
1. cephal/o	head
2. cerebell/o	cerebellum
3. cerebr/o	cerebrum
4. crani/o	cranium
5. dur/o	dura mater
6. encephal/o	brain
7. gangli/o	ganglion
8. ganglion/o	ganglion
9. gli/o	glial cells
10. lept/o	slender
11. mening/o	meninges
12. meningi/o	meninges
13. ment/o	mind
14. mon/o	one
15. myel/o	bone marrow, spinal cord
16. neur/o	nerve
17. phas/o	speech
18. phren/o	mind
19. poli/o	gray matter
20. pont/o	pons
21. psych/o	mind
22. quadr/i	four
23. radic/o	nerve root
24. radicul/o	nerve root
25. rhiz/o	nerve root
26. vag/o	vagus nerve

TABLE 12-2
Prefixes

Prefix	Meaning
1. hemi-	half
2. per-	through
3. quadri-	four
4. tetra-	four

TABLE 12-3
Suffixes

Suffix	Meaning
1. -algesia	pain sensation
2. -algia	pain
3. -cele	hernia
4. -esthesia	feeling
5. -iatry	medical treatment
6. -ictal	pertaining to
7. -kines/o	movement
8. -paresis	incomplete paralysis
9. -plegia	paralysis

TABLE 12-4
Medical Abbreviations

Abbreviation	Meaning
1. ANS	autonomic nervous system
2. CNS	central nervous system
3. CSF	cerebrospinal fluid
4. CVA	stroke/cerebrovascular accident
5. EEG	electroencephalogram
6. LP	lumbar puncture
7. PNS	peripheral nervous system
8. TENS	transcutaneous electrical nerve stimulation
9. TIA	transient ischemic attack

TABLE 12-5
Medical Terms

Term	Meaning	Term	Meaning
Burr	Drill used to create an entry into the cranium	Shunt	An artificial passage
Central nervous system	Brain and spinal cord	Skull	Entire skeletal framework of the head
Craniectomy	Permanent, partial removal of skull	Somatic nerve	Sensory or motor nerve
Craniotomy	Opening of the skull	Stereotaxis	Method of identifying a specific area or point in the brain
Cranium	That part of the skeleton that encloses the brain	Sympathetic nerve	Part of the peripheral nervous system that controls automatic body function and sympathetic nerves activated under stress
Discectomy	Removal of a vertebral disc		
Electroencephalography	Recording of the electric currents of the brain by means of electrodes attached to the scalp		
Laminectomy	Surgical excision of posterior arch of vertebra—includes spinal process	Trephination	Surgical removal of a disk of bone
Peripheral nerves	12 pairs of cranial nerves, 31 pairs of spinal nerves, and autonomic nervous system; connects peripheral receptors to the brain and spinal cord	Vertebrectomy	Removal of vertebra

Chapter 12: Anatomy and Terminology Quiz

(Quiz Answers Are Located in Appendix B)

1. Portion of nervous system that contains cranial and spinal nerves:
   a. central
   b. peripheral
   c. autonomic
   d. parasympathetic

2. Part of neuron that receives signals:
   a. dendrites
   b. cell body
   c. axon
   d. myelin sheath

3. NOT associated with glia:
   a. monocytes
   b. astrocytes
   c. microglia
   d. oligodendrocytes

4. Largest part of brain:
   a. cerebellum
   b. cerebrum
   c. cortex
   d. pons

5. Divided into two hemispheres:
   a. cerebellum
   b. cerebrum
   c. cortex
   d. pons

6. Number of pairs of cranial nerves:
   a. 10
   b. 11
   c. 12
   d. 13

7. Controls right side of body:
   a. left cerebrum
   b. right cerebrum
   c. right cortex
   d. left cortex

8. Combining form that means "brain":
   a. mening/o
   b. mon/o
   c. esthesi/o
   d. encephal/o

9. Prefix that means "four":
   a. per-
   b. tetra-
   c. para-
   d. bi-

10. Combining form that means "speech":
    a. phas/o
    b. rhiz/o
    c. poli/o
    d. myel/o

PATHOPHYSIOLOGY

Dementias—Classified by Causative Factor

Cognitive deficiencies

Causes

Alzheimer's disease
   Vascular disease
   Head trauma
   Tumors
   Infection
   Toxins
   Substance abuse
   AIDS

Alzheimer's Disease

Most common type of dementia
   Progressive intellectual impairment
   • Results in damage to neurons (neurofibrillary tangles)
   • Fatal within 3 to 20 years

Causes

Mostly unknown
   Perhaps genetic defect, autoimmune reaction, or virus

Symptoms

Behavior change
   Memory loss
   Confusion
   Disorientation
   Restlessness
   Speech disturbances
   Personality change—anxiety, depression
   Irritability
   Inability to complete activities of daily living

Treatment

• No cure
• Aricept (drug has modest effect in early stages)
• Symptomatic treatment
• Support for family

Vascular Dementia

Result of brain infarctions (vascular occlusion resulting in loss of brain function)

Nutritional Degenerative Disease

Deficiency
   • B vitamins
   • Niacin
   • Pantothenic acid
Associated with alcoholism

Amyotrophic Lateral Sclerosis (ALS)

Motor neuron disease (MND)
  Also known as Lou Gehrig's disease
    • Baseball player who died of ALS
  Deterioration of neurons of spinal cord and brain
  Results in atrophy of muscles and loss of fine motor skills
  Difficulty walking, talking, and breathing
  Mental functioning remains normal
  Survival is 2 to 5 years after diagnosis
  Genetic cause—familial chromosome 21 aberration
    • Death usually results from respiratory failure

Treatment

Symptomatic only
  Emotional support
  No cure

Huntington's Disease—Chorea

Inherited progressive atrophy of cerebrum

Symptoms

Restlessness
  Rapid, jerky movements in arms and face (uncontrollable jerking and facial grimacing)
  Rigidity
  Intellectual impairment, bradyphrenia, apathy

Treatment

Genetic defect of chromosome 4
  No cure
  Symptomatic

Parkinson's Disease (Parkinsonism)

Decreased secretion of dopamine
  Typically occurs after age 40
  Cause unknown

Symptoms

Muscle rigidity and weakness
  Bradykinesia—slow voluntary movements
  Postural instability, stooped
  Shuffling gait
  Tremors at rest
  Masklike facial appearance
  Depression

Treatment

Medications to reduce symptoms
  Dopamine replacement

Multiple Sclerosis (MS)

Common neurologic condition
  • Demyelination of central nervous system—replaced by sclerotic tissue
Diagnosed in young adults 20–40 years old

Results in myelin destruction and gliosis of white matter of central nervous system
Speculation that it is an autoimmune condition or result of a virus
Exacerbations and remission patterns

Symptoms

Precipitated by "an event," e.g., infection, pregnancy, stress
  Loss of feeling (paresthesias)
  Vision problems
  Bladder disorder
  Mood disorders
  Weakness of limbs—unsteady gait and paralysis

Treatment

Symptomatic
  Management of relapses
  Reducing relapses and disease progression—disease-modifying drugs (DMDs)

Myasthenia Gravis (MG)

Means grave muscle weakness
  Autoimmune neuromuscular condition—antibodies block neurotransmission to muscle cells
  Most have pathologic changes of thymus

Symptoms

Insidious
  Muscle weakness and fatigability
  May be localized or generalized
  Often affects
    • Swallowing
    • Breathing
    • Compromised swallowing and breathing may lead to crisis

Treatment

Anticholinesterase drugs
  • Restores normal muscle strength and recoverability after fatigue
Corticosteroids (prednisone) and immunosuppressive drugs
Thymectomy

Tourette Syndrome

Symptoms

Spasmodic, twitching movements, uncontrollable vocal sounds, inappropriate words
  Begins with twitching eyelids and facial muscles (tics)
  Verbal outbursts

Causes

Unknown
  Excess dopamine or hypersensitivity to dopamine

Treatment

Antipsychotic drugs

Antidepressant drugs
Mood-elevating drugs

Poliomyelitis

Contagious viral disease
Affects motor neurons
Causes paralysis and respiratory failure
Prevent with vaccination

Postpolio Syndrome (PPS)

Also known as postpoliomyelitis neuromuscular atrophy
Progressive muscle weakness
- Past history of paralytic polio

Symptoms

Muscle weakness and fatigability
- May include atrophy and muscle twitching

Treatment

Symptomatic
Maintenance of respiratory function

Guillain-Barré Syndrome

Also known as
- Idiopathic polyneuritis
- Acute inflammatory polyneuropathy
- Landry's ascending paralysis
Demyelination of peripheral nerves—acquired disease

Symptoms

Primary ascending motor paralysis
Variable sensory disturbances

Treatment

Supportive

Congenital Neurologic Disorders

Hydrocephalus

Excessive amounts of circulating cerebrospinal fluid in ventricles of brain
Circulation is impaired in brain or spinal cord
Compresses brain

Treatment

Surgical placement of a shunt

Spina Bifida (Fig. 12.3)

Developmental birth defect that causes incomplete development of spinal cord and its coverings
Vertebrae overlying open portions of spinal cord do not fully form and remain unfused and open
- Spina bifida occulta—may not be noticed, no protrusion through defect
- Spina bifida manifesta, which includes:

- Myelomeningocele (spina bifida cystica)
  - Meninges and spinal cord protrude through defect
- Meningocele
  - Meninges herniated through defect
Results in neurologic deficiencies

Treatment

Surgical repair

Mental Disorders

Schizophrenia

Variety of syndromes
Results in changes in brain
Hereditary factors are considered a cause
- Also, fetal brain damage caused by viral infections, complications of pregnancy, nutritional deficiencies
Stress usually precipitates onset

Symptoms

Delusions of persecution and/or grandeur
Disorganized thought
Repetitive behaviors
Behavior issues
Decreased speech
Decreased ability to solve problems
Loss of emotions/flat affect
Hallucinations
Types are based on characteristics

Treatment

Antipsychotic drugs
Drugs have very unpleasant side effects, such as tardive dyskinesia, with symptoms as follows:
- Excessive movement
- Grimacing
- Jerking
- Tremors
- Shuffling gait
- Dry mouth
- Blurred vision

Depression

Mood (sustained emotional state) disorder
Exact cause is unknown

Symptoms

Sadness
Hopelessness
Lethargy
Insomnia
Anorexia

Treatment

Antidepressant drugs
Electroconvulsive therapy

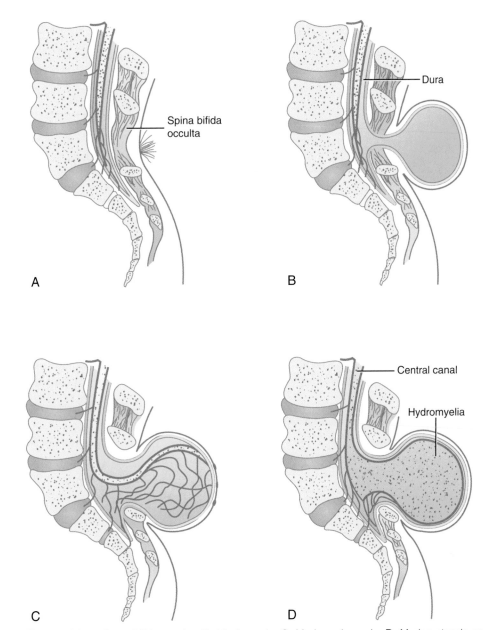

• **Figure 12.3 A.** Spina bifida occulta. **B.** Meningocele. **C.** Myelomeningocele. **D.** Myelocystocele or hydromyelia.

Central Nervous System (CNS) Disorders

Vascular Disorder

Transient Ischemic Attack (TIA)

Temporary reduction of blood flow to brain that produces strokelike symptoms but no lasting damage
    Often a warning sign before cerebrovascular accident

Symptoms
Depend on location of ischemia
• Usual recovery within 24 hours
No loss of consciousness
Slurred, indiscernible speech
May display muscle weakness in legs/arms
Paresthesia (numbness) of face
Mental confusion may be present
Repeated attacks common in the presence of atherosclerotic disease

Cerebrovascular Accident (CVA) or Stroke

Infarction of brain due to lack of blood/oxygen flow
    Necrosis of tissue with total occlusion of vessel

Causes
Atherosclerotic disease—thrombus formation
    Embolus
        Hemorrhage—arterial aneurysm

Symptoms

Depend on location of obstruction
- Thrombus
  - Gradual onset
  - Often occurs at rest
  - Intracranial pressure (ICP) minimal
  - Localized damage
- Embolus
  - Sudden onset
  - Occurs anytime
  - ICP minimal
  - Localized damage unless multiple emboli
- Hemorrhage
  - Sudden onset
  - Occurs most often with activity
  - ICP high
  - Widespread damage
  - May be fatal

Treatment

Anticoagulant drugs (clot dissolving) if caused by thrombus or embolus—tissue plasminogen activator (tPA)
Carotid endarterectomy (removes artherosclerotic plaque)
Oxygen treatment
Underlying condition treated, such as
- Hypertension
- Atherosclerosis
- Thrombus

Aneurysm—Cerebral

Dilation of artery
- May be localized or multiple
Rupture possible, often on exertion
- Fatal if rupture is massive

Symptoms

May display visual effects, such as
- Loss of visual fields
- Photophobia
- Diplopia
- Headache
- Confusion
- Slurred speech
- Weakness
- Stiff neck (nuchal rigidity)

Treatment

Dependent on diagnosis prior to rupture
Surgical intervention

Encephalitis

Infection of parenchymal tissue of brain or spinal cord
- Often viral
Accompanying inflammation
Usually results in some permanent damage

Symptoms

Stiff neck
Headaches
Vomiting
Fever
May have seizure
Lethargy

Some Types of Encephalitis

Herpes simplex
Lyme disease
West Nile fever
Western equine

Treatment

Symptomatic
Supportive

Reye's Syndrome

Associated with viral infection
- Especially when aspirin has been administered
  Changes occur in brain and liver
- Leads to increased intracranial pressure

Symptoms

Headaches
Vomiting
Lethargy
Seizures

Treatment

Symptomatic treatment

Brain Abscess

Localized infection
Necrosis of tissue
Usually spread from infection elsewhere, such as ears or sinus

Symptoms

Neurologic deficiencies
Increased intracranial pressure

Treatment

Antibiotics for bacterial infections
Surgical drainage

Epilepsies

Chronic seizure disorder

Types

Partial Seizures (Focal)

State of altered focus but conscious—simple
Impaired consciousness—complex
Specialized epileptic seizures
Aura
- Auditory or visual sign that precedes a seizure

Generalized Seizures

Absence seizures—petit mal
- Brief loss of awareness
- Most common in children (febrile causation)

Tonic-clonic—grand mal or ictal event
- Loss of consciousness
- Alternate contraction and relaxation
- Incontinence
- No memory of seizure

Causes

Tumor
> Hemorrhage
> Trauma
> Edema
> Infection
> Excessive cerebrospinal fluid
> High fever

Treatment

Correct cause
> Anticonvulsant drugs
> Neurosurgery
> Postictal event—after seizure—neurologic symptoms (weakness, etc.)

Trauma

Head Injury—Traumatic Brain Injury (TBI)

Concussion

Mild blow to head
> Temporary axonal disturbances
> Grade 1: temporary confusion and amnesia (brief)
> Grade 2: memory loss for very recent events and confusion
> Grade 3: amnesia for recent events and disorientation (longer duration)
> Results in reversible interference with brain function
> - Recovery within 24 hours with no residual damage

Contusion

Bruising of brain
> Force of blow determines outcome

Hematomas—Blood Accumulation (Clot)

Compresses surrounding structures

Classified based on location
- Epidural
  - Develops between dura and skull
- Subdural
  - Develops between dura and arachnoid
    - Development within 24 hours is acute
    - Development within a week is subacute
  - ICP increases with enlargement of hematoma
- Subarachnoid
  - Develops between pia and arachnoid
  - Blood mixes with cerebrospinal fluid
    - No localized hematoma forms

- Intracerebral
  - As a result of a contusion

Symptoms

Increased ICP
> Others dependent on location and severity of injury

Treatment

Identification of the location of hematoma
> Medications to decrease edema
> Antibiotics
> Surgical intervention—burr hole if necessary to decrease the ICP

Spinal Cord Injury

Result of trauma to vertebra, cord, ligaments, intervertebral disc

Vertebral Injuries Classified As
- Simple—affects spinous or transverse process
- Compression—anterior fracture of vertebrae
- Comminuted—vertebral body is shattered
- Dislocation—vertebrae are out of alignment
- Flexion injury in which hyperflexion compresses vertebra
  Dislocation
  Rotation

Symptoms

Depend on vertebral level and severity
> Paralysis
> Loss of sensation
> Drop in blood pressure
> Loss of bladder and rectal control
> Decreased venous circulation

Treatment

Identification of area of injury
> Immobilization
> Corticosteroids to decrease edema
> Bladder and bowel management
> Rehabilitation

Tumors of Brain and Spinal Cord

Increases ICP
> Life threatening
> Rarely metastasize outside of central nervous system
> Secondary brain tumors are common
> Metastasis from lung or breast

Gliomas Common Type

Primary malignant tumor—encapsulated and invasive
> Types based on cell from which tumor arises and location of tumor

Glioblastoma

Located in cerebral hemispheres (deep in white matter)
> Highly aggressive

Oligodendrocytoma
Usually located in frontal lobes
  Oligodendroblastoma, more aggressive form

Ependymoma
Located in ventricles
  Most often occurs in children
  Ependymoblastoma, more aggressive form

Astrocytoma
Located anywhere in brain and spinal cord
  Invasive but slow growing

Pineal Region
Germ Cell Tumors
Usually in adolescents
  Rare
  Variable growth rate

Several Other Pineal Tumors
Pineocytoma
  Teratoma
  Germinoma

Blood Vessel
Angioma
Usually located in posterior cerebral hemispheres
  Slow growing

Hemangioblastoma
Located in cerebellum
  Slow growing

Medulloblastoma
Aggressive tumor
  Located in posterior cerebellar vermis (fourth ventricle)

Meningioma
Originates in arachnoid
  Slow growing

Pituitary Tumor
Related to aging
  Slow growing
    • Such as macroadenomas

Cranial Nerve Tumors
Neurilemmomas most common location: cranial nerve VIII
  Slow growing
  Metastatic

Spinal Cord Tumors
Symptoms are based on location of spinal compression
Intramedullary
  • Originates in neural tissue
Extramedullary
  • Originates outside the spinal cord
Metastatic tumors of spinal cord are more common
  • Myeloma—marrow
  • Lymphoma—lymph
  • Carcinomas—lung, breast, prostate
Most common type of primary extramedullary tumor
  • Meningiomas—anyplace in spine
  • Neurofibromas—common in thoracic and lumbar
    regions

Chapter 12: Pathophysiology Quiz

(Quiz Answers Are Located in Appendix B)

1. Most common dementia is:
   a. Alzheimer's disease
   b. secondary
   c. nutritional degenerative disease
   d. Lou Gehrig's disease
2. MND stands for:
   a. maximal neuron disorder
   b. migrating niacin disorder
   c. motor neuron disease
   d. motor neuropathic disorder
3. Dopamine replacement is useful in treating:
   a. multiple sclerosis
   b. Parkinson's disease
   c. Huntington's disease
   d. CVA
4. Condition in which primary symptoms are muscle weakness and fatigability:
   a. amyotrophic lateral sclerosis
   b. multiple sclerosis
   c. dyskinesis
   d. myasthenia gravis
5. Another name for idiopathic polyneuritis is:
   a. Guillain-Barré syndrome
   b. multiple sclerosis
   c. amyotrophic lateral sclerosis
   d. postpolio syndrome
6. This condition is thought to be caused by genetic factors and, possibly, fetal brain damage:
   a. Parkinson's
   b. schizophrenia
   c. spina bifida
   d. Guillain-Barré syndrome

7. This condition is associated with viral infection, especially when aspirin has been administered:
   a. Reye's syndrome
   b. Guillain-Barré syndrome
   c. Lou Gehrig's disease
   d. Conn's syndrome
8. Concussion is a mild blow to the head in which recovery is expected within _____.
   a. 12 hours
   b. 24 hours
   c. 48 hours
   d. 1 week

9. ICP means:
   a. intercranial pressure
   b. intracranial pressure
   c. interior cranial pressure
   d. intensive cranial pressure
10. In this type of hematoma, blood mixes with cerebrospinal fluid:
    a. epidural
    b. subdural
    c. subarachnoid
    d. intracerebral

13

Senses

ANATOMY AND TERMINOLOGY

Sight	Eyes
Hearing	Ears
Smell	Nose
Taste	Tongue
Touch	Skin

Sight: Three Layers of Eye (Fig. 13.1)

Cornea (Outer Layer)

Fibrous, transparent layer that extends over dome of eye
  Refracts (bends) light to focus on receptor cells (posterior eye)
  Avascular (nourished by aqueous humor and tears)

Sclera (Extension of Outer Layer)

White of eye

Extends from edge of cornea (anterior surface) to optic nerve (posterior surface)
  • Lies over choroid

Choroid (Middle Layer)

Vascular layer between sclera and retina
  • Supplies nutrients

Retina (Inner Layer)

Contains rods and cones
  • Rods provide night and peripheral vision
  • Cones provide day and color vision and are stimulated by primary colors of red, green, and blue

Conjunctiva

Covers anterior sclera and lines eyelid (contiguous layer)

Lens

Behind pupil
  Lens is connected by zonules to ciliary body
  Ciliary body muscles cause lens to change shape to refract light rays (accommodation)

Fluids

Aqueous humor (front of lens)—watery substance secreted by ciliary body

Maintains shape of front portion of eye
Refracts light
Nourishes cornea

  Vitreous humor (behind lens)—gel-like substance (not readily re-formed) filling large space behind lens

Maintains shape of eyeball
Refracts light

Optic Nerve

Light rays from rods and cones travel from eye to brain via optic nerve

Optic nerve meets retina in optic disc (no light receptors)—blind spot
Pathway of light ray
  Cornea—refraction site
  Anterior chamber (aqueous humor)—refraction site
  Pupil
  Lens—refraction site
  Posterior chamber (vitreous humor)—refraction site
  Retina (rods and cones)
  Optic nerve fibers—nerve cells act as a cable connecting the eye with the brain
  Optic chiasm
  Thalamus
  Cerebral cortex (occipital lobe)—light is interpreted

Hearing, Three Divisions of Ear

External Ear

Auricle (pinna)—sound waves enter ear
  External auditory canal—tunnel from auricle to middle ear

Middle Ear

Begins with tympanic membrane (eardrum)

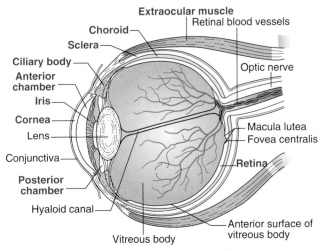

Extraocular muscle
Choroid
Sclera
Ciliary body
Anterior chamber
Iris
Cornea
Lens
Conjunctiva
Posterior chamber
Hyaloid canal
Vitreous body
Retinal blood vessels
Optic nerve
Macula lutea
Fovea centralis
Retina
Anterior surface of vitreous body

• **Figure 13.1** Eye and ocular adnexa.

Ossicles—small bones conducting sound waves from middle to inner ear
- Malleus
- Incus
- Stapes
Eustachian tube—leads to pharynx

Inner Ear (Labyrinth)

Vestibule

Semicircular canals/vestibular apparatus
Cochlea contains perilymph and endolymph (liquids through which sound waves are conducted)
- Organ of Corti—auditory receptor area
Auditory nerve—electrical impulse is conducted to cerebral cortex for interpretation (hearing)

Pathway of sound vibration (exterior to brain)
Pinna
External auditory canal
Tympanic membrane
Malleus
Incus
Stapes

Oval window
Cochlea
Auditory fluid/receptors in organ of Corti
Auditory nerve
Cerebral cortex

Smell

Olfactory Sense Receptors

Located in nasal cavity

Closely related to sense of taste
Cranial nerve I

Taste

Gustatory sense—sweet, salty, and sour differentiated
Taste buds located on anterior portion of tongue
Cranial nerves VII and IX

Touch

Mechanoreceptors

Widely distributed throughout body

React to touch and pressure
- Meissner corpuscles (touch)
- Pacinian corpuscles (pressure)

Proprioceptors

Position and orientation

Dysfunctions
- Vestibular nystagmus—involuntary movement of eyes
- Vertigo—sense of spinning/dizziness

Thermoreceptors

Under skin
Sense temperature changes

Nociceptors

Pain sensors
In skin and internal organs

TABLE 13-1
Combining Forms

Combining Form	Meaning	Combining Form	Meaning
1. ambly/o	dim, dullness	20. opt/o	eye, vision
2. aque/o	water	21. optic/o	eye
3. audi/o	hearing	22. ot/o	ear
4. blephar/o	eyelid	23. palpebr/o	eyelid
5. conjunctiv/o	conjunctiva	24. papill/o	optic nerve
6. cor/o, core/o	pupil	25. phac/o	eye lens
7. corne/o	cornea	26. phak/o	eye lens
8. cycl/o	ciliary body	27. phot/o	light
9. dacry/o	tear	28. presby/o	old age
10. essi/o, esthesi/o	sensation	29. pupill/o	pupil
11. glauc/o	gray	30. retin/o	retina
12. ir/o	iris	31. scler/o	sclera
13. irid/o	iris	32. scot/o	darkness
14. kerat/o	cornea	33. staped/o	stapes
15. lacrim/o	tear	34. tympan/o	eardrum
16. mi/o	smaller	35. uve/o	uvea
17. myring/o	eardrum	36. vitre/o	glassy
18. ocul/o	eye	37. xer/o	dry
19. ophthalm/o	eye		

TABLE 13-2
Prefixes

Prefix	Meaning
1. audi-	hearing
2. eso-	inward
3. exo-	outward

TABLE 13-3
Suffixes

Suffix	Meaning
1. -opia	vision
2. -omia	smell
3. -tropia	to turn

TABLE 13-4
Medical Abbreviations

Abbreviation	Meaning
1. AD	right ear
2. AS	left ear
3. AU	both ears
4. H or E	hemorrhage or exudate
5. IO	intraocular
6. IOL	intraocular lens
7. OD	right eye
8. OS	left eye
9. OU	each eye
10. PERL	pupils equal and reactive to light
11. PERRL	pupils equal, round, and reactive to light
12. PERRLA	pupils equal, round, and reactive to light and accommodation
13. REM	rapid eye movement
14. TM	tympanic membrane

TABLE 13-5

Medical Terms

Term	Meaning	Term	Meaning
Anterior segment	Those parts of eye in the front of and including lens (cornea, iris, ciliary body, aqueous humor)	Labyrinth	Inner connecting cavities, such as internal ear
Apicectomy	Excision of a portion of temporal bone	Labyrinthitis	Inner ear inflammation
Astigmatism	Condition in which refractive surfaces of eye are unequal	Lacrimal	Related to tears
		Mastoidectomy	Removal of mastoid bone
Aural atresia	Congenital absence of external auditory canal	Ménière's disease	Condition that causes dizziness, ringing in ears, and deafness
Blepharitis	Inflammation of eyelid	Myopia	Nearsightedness, eyeball too long from front to back
Cataract	Opaque covering on or in lens	Myringotomy	Incision into tympanic membrane
Chalazion	Granuloma around sebaceous gland	Ocular adnexa	Orbit, extraocular muscles, and eyelid
Cholesteatoma	Tumor that forms in middle ear	Ophthalmoscopy	Examination of the interior of eye by means of a scope, also known as fundoscopy
Conjunctiva	The lining of eyelids and covering of anterior sclera		
Dacryocystitis	Blocked, inflamed infection of nasolacrimal duct	Otitis media	Noninfectious inflammation of middle ear; serous otitis media produces liquid drainage (not purulent), and suppurative otitis media produces purulent (pus) matter
Dacryostenosis	Narrowing of lacrimal duct		
Ectropion	Eversion (outward sagging) of eyelid		
Entropion	Inversion of eyelid (lashes rubbing cornea)	Otoscope	Instrument used to examine ear
Enucleation	Removal of an organ or organs from a body cavity	Papilledema	Swelling of optic disc (papilla)
		Posterior segment	Those parts of eye behind lens
Episclera	Connective covering of sclera	Ptosis	Drooping of upper eyelid
Exenteration	Removal of an organ all in one piece, commonly used to describe radical excision	Sclera	Outer covering of eye
		Strabismus	Extraocular muscle deviation resulting in unequal visual axes
Exophthalmos	Protrusion of eyeball	Tarsorrhaphy	Suturing together of eyelids
Exostosis	Bony growth	Tinnitus	Ringing in the ears
Fenestration	Creation of a new opening in inner wall of middle ear	Transmastoid	Creates an opening in mastoid for drainage antrostomy
Glaucoma	Eye diseases that are characterized by an increase of intraocular pressure	Tympanolysis	Freeing of adhesions of the tympanic membrane
		Tympanometry	Test of the inner ear using air pressure
Hordeolum	Stye—infection of sebaceous gland (nodule on lid margin)	Tympanostomy	Insertion of ventilation tube into tympanum
Hyperopia	Farsightedness, eyeball is too short from front to back	Uveal	Vascular tissue of the choroid, ciliary body, and iris
Keratomalacia	Softening of cornea associated with a deficiency of vitamin A	Vertigo	Dizziness
Keratoplasty	Surgical repair of the cornea	Xanthelasma	Yellow plaque on eyelid (lipid disorder)

Chapter 13: Anatomy and Terminology Quiz

(Quiz Answers Are Located in Appendix B)

1. The middle layer of the eye:
   a. sclera
   b. retina
   c. episclera
   d. choroid
2. The covering of the anterior sclera and lining of eyelid:
   a. aqueous humor
   b. ossicles
   c. vitreous
   d. conjunctiva
3. Which of the following is NOT a bone of the middle ear?
   a. cochlea
   b. stapes
   c. malleus
   d. incus
4. This cranial nerve controls the sense of smell:
   a. I
   b. II
   c. III
   d. IV
5. Which of the following is NOT part of the inner ear?
   a. pinna
   b. vestibule
   c. semicircular canals
   d. cochlea
6. These receptors react to touch:
   a. nociceptors
   b. mechanoreceptors
   c. proprioceptors
   d. thermoreceptors
7. These receptors react to position and orientation:
   a. nociceptors
   b. mechanoreceptors
   c. proprioceptors
   d. thermoreceptors
8. Combining form meaning "eyelid":
   a. aque/o
   b. blephar/o
   c. optic/o
   d. uve/o
9. Combining form meaning "eye lens":
   a. cor/o
   b. irid/o
   c. ocul/o
   d. phak/o
10. Abbreviation meaning the pupils are equal, round, and reactive to light and accommodation:
    a. PERRLA
    b. PERRL
    c. PERL
    d. PURL

PATHOPHYSIOLOGY

Eye

Visual Disturbances

Astigmatism

Irregular curvature of refractive surfaces (cornea or lens) of eye
   Can be congenital or acquired (as a result of disease or trauma)
   Image is distorted

Treatment

Corrected with cylindrical lens

Diplopia

Double vision

Amblyopia

Dimness of vision—impairment of vision without detectable organic lesion of eye

Hyperopia

Farsightedness

Shortened eyeball
   • Can see objects in distance, not close up

Treatment

Corrected with convex lens

Presbyopia

Age-related farsightedness

Treatment

Magnification (reading glasses or bifocals)

Myopia

Nearsightedness

Elongated eyeball
   • Can see objects up close, not in distance

Treatment

Corrected with concave lens thicker at periphery

Nystagmus—Unilateral or Bilateral

Rapid, involuntary eye movements

Movements can be
- Vertical
- Horizontal
- Rotational
- Combination of above

Cause

Brain tumor or inner ear disease
Normal in newborns
Due to underlying condition or adverse effect of drug
Various types, such as
- Vestibular nystagmus
- Rhythmic eye movements

Strabismus

Cross-eyed

Due to muscle weakness or neurologic defect
Forms of strabismus
- Hypotropia (downward deviation of one eye)
- Hypertropia (upward deviation of one eye)
- Estropia (one eye turns inward)
- Exotropia (one eye turns outward)

Treatment
- Eye exercises/patching of normal eye
- Surgery to establish muscle balance

Infections

Conjunctivitis (Pink Eye)

Inflammation of conjunctival lining of eyelid or covering of sclera

Due to
- Infection
- Allergy
- Irritation

Treatment
- Varies with cause
- Antibiotic eye drops

Hordeolum (Stye)

Bacterial infection of eyelid hair follicle
- Usually Staphylococcus
- Results in mass on eyelid

Treatment
- Antibiotics
- Incision and drainage may be necessary

Keratitis

Corneal inflammation

May be caused by herpes simplex virus, contact lens issue, or exposure
Causes tearing and photophobia, pain

Macular Degeneration

Destruction of fovea centralis
- Fovea centralis is small pit in center of retina (fovea centralis retinae)
  Usually age related—leading cause of blindness in elderly
  Results from exposure to ultraviolet rays or drugs
- Also may have a genetic component
  Central vision is lost
  Two types of macular degeneration
- Wet—development of new vascularization and leaking blood vessels near macula
- Dry (85% of cases)—atrophy and degeneration of retinal cells and deposits of drusen (clumps of extracellular waste)

Treatment

None for "dry" macular degeneration

Surgical intervention with laser for "net" macular degeneration to coagulate leaking vessels; success is limited
Medications

Detached Retina

Retinal tear—two layers of retina separate from each other
- Vitreous humor then leaks behind retina
- Retina then pulls away from choroid
  Results in increasing blind spot in visual field
  Condition is painless
  Pressure continues to build if left unattended
  Final result is blindness

Treatment

Surgical intervention with laser to repair tear (emergency/urgency)—photocoagulation for small tears
Scleral buckle for large retinal detachments
Pneumatic retinopexy for medium to large retinal detachment. Gas bubble is injected into vitreous cavity; pressure to tear resulting in retinal reattachment.

Cataracts

Lens becomes opaque with protein aggregates

Classified by Morphology

Size
Shape
Location
Also may be classified by etiology (cause) or time cataract occurs

Examples of Classification

Congenital cataract
- Bilateral opacity present at birth
- Also known as developmental cataract

Heat cataract
- Also known as glassblowers' cataract
- Caused by exposure to radiation

• **Figure 13.2** A concussive injury that resulted in a traumatic cataract.

Traumatic cataract (Fig. 13.2)
• Result of injury to eye
Senile cataract
• Age related
• Usually forms on anterior lens

Symptoms
Blurring of vision
Halos around lights

Treatment
Removal of cataract with intraocular lens implantation
If no intraocular lens implant, then glasses or contact lenses for refraction

Glaucoma
Excess accumulation of intraocular aqueous humor
• High pressure results in decreased blood flow and edema
• Damages retinal cells and optic nerve

Stages of Glaucoma
Mild, moderate, severe
• Based on visual field loss caused by disease

Narrow-Angle Glaucoma
Acute type of glaucoma

Rapid onset is painful

Chronic Glaucoma
Also known as
• Wide-angle glaucoma
• Open-angle glaucoma
  Asymptomatic
  Diagnosed in eye examination using tonometry to test anterior chamber pressure and visual field exams

Treatment
Medications that decrease output of aqueous humor and decrease intraocular pressure (IOP)
Laser treatment to provide drainage

Ear

Infections

Otitis Media
Infection or inflammation of middle ear cavity

Chronic infection produces adhesions
Results in loss of hearing
Often occurs in children in combination with URI (upper respiratory infection)
Causes severe ear pain (otalgia)

Treatment
Antibiotics
Surgical intervention with placement of tubes to allow for drainage
• Useful in patients with recurrent infection

Otitis Externa
Also known as swimmer's ear

Infection of external auditory canal and pinna (exterior ear)
Caused by bacteria or fungus
Results in pain and discharge

Treatment
Antibiotic
Encouraged to keep ear dry

Hearing Loss
Conductive Hearing Loss
Due to a defect of sound-conducting apparatus
• Accumulation of wax
• Scar tissue on tympanic membrane
  Also known as:
• Transmission hearing loss
• Conduction deafness

Treatment
• Hearing aids

Sensorineural
Due to a lesion of cochlea or central neural pathways

Also known as
• Perceptive deafness
May be divided into
• Cochlear hearing loss
  • Due to a defect in receptor or transducing mechanisms of cochlea
• Retrocochlear hearing loss
  • Due to defect located proximal to cochlea (vestibulocochlear nerve or auditory area of brain)
Presbycusis is age-related sensorineural hearing loss

Treatment
- Medication, implant, surgery

Ototoxic Hearing Loss

Caused by ingestion of toxic substance
Also known as toxic deafness

Ménière's Disease

Inner ear disturbance
Also known as idiopathic endolymphatic hydrops
Cause unknown
Common cause of vertigo (dizziness)
Other symptoms include hearing loss and tinnitus

Chapter 13: Pathophysiology Quiz

(Quiz Answers Are Located in Appendix B)

1. This condition can be acquired or congenital and results in an irregular curvature of the refractive surfaces of the eye:
   a. diplopia
   b. hyperopia
   c. nystagmus
   d. astigmatism
2. In this condition, the eyeball is shorter than normal and results in being able to see objects in the distance but not close up:
   a. diplopia
   b. hyperopia
   c. nystagmus
   d. astigmatism
3. Rapid, involuntary eye movement is the predominant symptom of this condition:
   a. diplopia
   b. hyperopia
   c. nystagmus
   d. astigmatism
4. Age-related farsightedness is:
   a. presbyopia
   b. hyperopia
   c. diplopia
   d. myopia
5. Another name for a stye is:
   a. keratitis
   b. hordeolum
   c. hyperopia
   d. strabismus
6. An inflammation of the cornea that is caused by herpes simplex virus is:
   a. keratitis
   b. hordeolum
   c. hyperopia
   d. strabismus
7. In this condition there is destruction of the fovea centralis:
   a. macular degeneration
   b. detached retina
   c. glaucoma
   d. cataract
8. This is an infection that occurs in the middle ear cavity:
   a. otitis media
   b. otitis externa
   c. ototoxic hearing loss
   d. retrocochlear hearing loss
9. The hearing loss that can be due to a lesion on the cochlea is:
   a. conductive
   b. sensorineural
   c. ototoxic
   d. transmission
10. This condition is also known as perceptive deafness:
    a. conductive
    b. sensorineural
    c. otitis media
    d. transmission

PART 2

Reimbursement Issues

14

Reimbursement Issues

Your Responsibility

Ensure accurate coding based upon services provided and documented

Obtain correct reimbursement for services rendered

Recognize upcoding (maximizing) or downcoding is never appropriate

Stay abreast of current and changing
- Reimbursement policies
- Coding guidelines

Health **I**nsurance **P**ortability and **A**ccountability **A**ct of 1996 (HIPAA)
- HIPAA changes are based on various resources such as
  - Centers for Medicare and Medicaid Policy Manuals
  - National Correct Coding Guidelines

Population Changing = Reimbursement Change

According to the Justification of Estimates for Appropriations Committees, FY 2018 report (https://www.acl.gov/sites/default/files/about-acl/2017-05/FY%202018%20ACL%20Budget%20Congressional%20Justification%20v2.pdf):
- The population over age 60 is projected to reach 77.6 million by 2020
  - Increase of 16% between 2015 and 2020
  - Seniors age 65 and older with severe disabilities projected to increase 18%
  Medicare primarily for elderly

Medicare

Those Covered

Originally established for those 65 and older; implemented in 1966

Disabled and permanent renal disease (end-stage renal disease or transplant) patients added in 1972

Persons covered are called "beneficiaries"

Basic Structure

Medicare program established in 1965

Part A: Hospital and Institutional Care Coverage
- This is the part that most inpatient coders will work with

Part B: Supplemental—nonhospital

Example: Physician services and medical equipment
- This is the part that most outpatient coders will work with

Part C: Medicare Advantage Organizations (MAO) plans—combines parts A and B; added in 1997 through Balanced Budget Act

Plans include

  Medicare Health Maintenance Organization (HMO)
  Medicare Preferred Provider Organizations (PPO)
  Medicare Private Fee-for-Service (PFFS)
  Medicare Special Needs Plans (SNPs)
  Medicare Medical Savings Account (MSA)
  HMO Point of Service (HMOPOS)

Part D: Prescription Drug Plan (PDP) (added January 1, 2006)

Plans include
- Medicare Advantage Prescription Drug Plan (MA-PD)
- Private prescription drug plans (PDPs)
- Premium paid by beneficiary

Officiating Office

Department of Health and Human Services (DHHS) (www.hhs.gov)

  Delegated to Centers for Medicare and Medicaid Services (CMS) (formerly HCFA)
- CMS runs Medicare and Medicaid
- CMS delegates daily operation to Medicare Administrative Contractors (MACs)
- MACs are usually insurance companies
- The Medicare Prescription Drug Improvement and Modernization Act of 2003 allowed CMS to reduce the 48 Fiscal Intermediaries to 15 Medicare Administrative Contractors (MACs)
  - By 2014, CMS further reduced the total number of jurisdictions to 12, with no plans for further reductions

Funding for Medicare

Social Security taxes
> Equal match from government
> CMS sends money to MACs
> MACs handle paperwork and pay claims

Medicare Covers

Medical Necessity and Frequency Limitations

Defined in
- LCDs (Local Coverage Determinations)
- NCDs (National Coverage Determinations)

Beneficiary Pays

20% of Medicare-approved amount after deductible is met
> Part A and B annual deductible

Medicare Pays

Part A all covered costs except deductible
Part B 80% of Medicare-allowed amount of covered services after deductible is met
Preventive Services
- Annual Wellness Visit (AWV) co-pay and deductible waived in all POS (G0438—first visit; G0439—subsequent visit)
- Initial Preventative Physical Examination (IPPE) (G0402)—no deductible
- Ultrasound Screening for Abdominal Aortic Aneurysm (AAA) (G0389)—no deductible
- Cardiovascular Disease Screenings (80061)—Lipid Panel; 82465—Cholesterol; 83718—Lipoprotein; 84478—Triglycerides—no copayment/coinsurance, no deductible
- Diabetes Screening Tests (82947)—Glucose, quantitative, blood (except reagent strip)
- 82950—Glucose, post-glucose dose (includes glucose); 82951—Glucose Tolerance Test (GTT), three specimens (includes glucose)—no copayment/coinsurance, no deductible
- Screening PAP—no deductible
- Screening pelvic exam—no deductible
- Screening mammogram—no deductible

Participating Providers

Signed Quality Improvement Organization (QIO) agreement with MACs to accept assignment on Medicare claims

Provider agrees to accept the Medicare Fee Schedule amount as payment in full
- Accepting assignment
Block 27 CMS-1500 (Fig. 14.1)

National Provider Identification (NPI)

10-digit number assigned to all covered health care providers
- Designed to provide one unique identifier for all providers as part of HIPAA

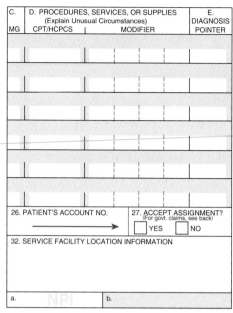

- **Figure 14.1** Block 27, Accept Assignment on the CMS-1500 (02/02), Health Insurance Claim Form.

- Eliminates the need for additional numbers by other carriers

Good Reasons to Participate

- Significant decrease in reimbursement amount for non-participating providers
  Participating providers receive approximately 5% more from Medicare than non-PAR providers
  Check sent directly from MACs to QIO providers
  Faster claims processing
  Provider names listed in QIO directory
- Sent to all beneficiaries

Part A, Hospital Inpatient

Hospitals submit charges electronically or, if an exempt facility, on CMS-1450 (UB-04) form
> MS-DRG basis for payment for Medicare patients
- Using principal diagnosis or principal procedure

Covered In-Hospital Expenses

Semiprivate room
> Meals and special diets in hospital
> All medically necessary services

Noncovered in-Hospital Expenses

Personal convenience items

Example: Slippers, TV
Any service or procedure determined to be "not medically necessary"

Types of Covered Expenses

Rehabilitation

Skilled nursing

Some personal convenience items for long-term illness or disabilities

Home health visits

Hospice care

Not automatically covered
- Must meet certain criteria

Part B, Supplemental

Part B pays services and supplies not covered under Part A

Not automatic

Beneficiaries purchase
- Pay monthly premiums

Types of Items Covered in Part B

Physician services

Outpatient hospital services

Ambulatory surgical services

Home health care

Medically necessary supplies and equipment

Coding for Medicare Part B Services

Three coding systems used to report Part B
- CPT (procedures and service)
- HCPCS (drugs, supplies, equipment, and special services)
- ICD-10-CM (diagnosis codes)

Electronic Transactions

HIPAA
- Created to govern health care portability
- Electronic data interchange (EDI)
  Transactions
- Activities involving transfer of health care information
  Transmission
- Movement of electronic data between two entities
  Today 99% Part A and 95% Part B claims filed electronically
- Using Electronic Remittance Advice (ERA)
  The software that supports electronic transmissions
- 5010 version

National Correct Coding Initiative (NCCI)

Developed by the Centers for Medicare and Medicaid Services to
- Promote national correct coding methods
- Control improper coding that results in inappropriate payment of Part B claims (physician) and hospital outpatient claims
- Complete list may be found at www.cms.gov/National CorrectCodInitEd/

Unbundling

CMS defines unbundling as

- Billing multiple procedure codes for a group of procedures that are covered by a single comprehensive code
  Example: Dividing one service into parts and coding for each part separately, such as:
  - Reporting bilateral procedures unilaterally
  Reporting 31231, bilateral or unilateral diagnostic nasal endoscopy, with modifier -50 (bilateral procedure), rather than correctly as 31231, no modifier
  - Downcoding to use an additional code
  Reporting one of two lacerations of the same complexity and site with a lesser code to enable reporting two separate repairs
  - Separating the surgical approach from the major surgical service
  Coding separately for a thoracic approach during an anterior spine procedure

Federal Register

Government publishes updates, revisions (changes), deletions in laws (Fig. 14.2) (http://www.gpo.gov/fdsys/browse/collection.action?collectionCode=FR)

November and December issues contain major outpatient facility updates

Quality Improvement Organizations (QIO)

Part of U.S. Department of Health and Human Services (HHS) strategy for "providing better care and better health at a lower cost"

Core functions:
- To ensure quality of patient care
- Protect beneficiaries by addressing complaints and appeals
- Ensure Medicare pays only for reasonable and necessary services

Two Types of QIOs

Beneficiary and Family Centered Care (BFCC)

- Assists beneficiaries directly
  - Quality of care reviews
  - Filing complaints or appeals

Quality Innovation Network (QIN)

- Organizes beneficiaries, providers, and community members for improvement initiatives
  - Data-driven approach
  - Focus on safety, health quality, and care coordination

Resource-Based Relative Value Scale (RBRVS)

Physician payment reform implemented in 1992
  Prior to reform, physicians were paid lowest of
- Physician's charge for service
- Physician's customary charge
- Prevailing charge in locality

• Figure 14.2 Example of page from the *Federal Register*.

National Fee Schedule (NFS)

RBRVS payment method
  Termed Medicare Fee Schedule (MFS)
  Payment 80% of MFS, after patient deductible
  Used for physicians and suppliers

Relative Value Units (RVUs)

Assigns national unit values to each CPT code
  Local adjustments made
- Work and skill required
- Overhead costs

- Malpractice costs
  Often referred to as fee schedule
  Annually, CMS updates RVU based on national and local factors

Medicare Fraud and Abuse

Program established by Medicare
- To decrease and eliminate fraud and abuse
  Beneficiary signatures on file
- Service, charges submitted without need for patient signature
  Presents opportunity for fraud

Fraud

Intentional deception to benefit

Example: Submitting for services not provided
Anyone who submits for Medicare services can be violator
- Physicians
- Hospitals
- Laboratories
- Billing services
- YOU

Fraud Can Be

Billing for services not provided
  Misrepresenting diagnosis or CPT/HCPCS codes
  Kickbacks
  Unbundling services
  Falsifying medical necessity
  Systematic waiver of copayment or deductible

Office of the Inspector General (OIG)

Develops and publishes Work Plan annually
  Outlines Medicare monitoring program
  MACs monitor those areas identified in plan

Complaints of Fraud or Abuse

Submitted orally or in writing to MACs or OIG

Allegations made by anyone against anyone
Allegations followed up by MACs or OIG http://oig.hhs.gov/reports-and-publications/archives/workplan/2016/oig-work-plan-2016.pdf

Abuse

Generally involves
- Impropriety
- Lack of medical necessity for services reported
Review takes place after claim submitted
- MACs do historical review of claims

Kickbacks

Bribe or rebate for referring patient for any service covered by Medicare

Any personal-gain kickback
A felony
- $25,000 fine or
- 5 years in jail or
- Both

Protect Yourself

Use your common sense

Submit only truthful and accurate claims
- Stay current with all coding changes
If you are unsure about charges, services, or procedures
- Check with physician or supervisor

Managed Health Care

Network health care providers that offer health care services under one organization

Group hospitals, physicians, or other providers
Majority of people with health care coverage are covered by a Managed Health Care Organization (e.g., HMO, PPO, POS)

Managed Care Organizations

Responsible for health care services to an enrolled group or person
  Coordinate various health care services
  Negotiate with providers and groups

Preferred Provider Organization (PPO)

Providers form network to offer health care services as group
  Enrollees who seek health care outside PPO pay more

Point of Service (POS)

In-network or out-of-network providers may be used
  Benefits are paid at a higher rate to in-network providers
  Subscribers are not limited to providers, but to amount covered by plan

Health Maintenance Organization (HMO)

Total package health care
  Out-of-pocket expenses minimal
  Assigned physician acts as gatekeeper to refer patient to outside organization

TABLE 14-1

Reimbursement Terminology

Term	Meaning	Term	Meaning
Advance Beneficiary Notice	ABN, notification in advance of services that Medicare probably will not pay for and the estimated cost to patient (Fig. 14.3) (formerly WOL, waiver of liability)	Coordination of Benefits	COB, management of multiple third-party payments to ensure overpayment does not occur
		Co-payment	Cost-sharing between beneficiary and payer
Ancillary Service	A service that is supportive of care of a patient, such as laboratory services	Deductible	That portion of covered services paid by the beneficiary before third-party payment begins
Assignment	A legal agreement that allows the provider to receive direct payment from a payer and the provider to accept payment as payment in full for covered services	Denial	Statement from a payer that coverage is denied
		Documentation	Detailed chronology of facts and observations, procedures, services, and diagnoses relative to the patient's health
Attending Physician	The physician legally responsible for oversight of an inpatient's care (in residency programs, the teaching physician that monitors the resident's work)	Durable Medical Equipment	DME, medically related equipment that is not disposable, such as wheelchairs, crutches, and vaporizers
Beneficiary	The person who benefits from insurance coverage; also known as subscriber, dependent, enrollee, member, or participant	Electronic Data Interchange	EDI, computerized submission of health care insurance information exchange
Birthday Rule	When both parents have insurance coverage, the parent with the birthday earlier in the year carries the primary coverage for a dependent	Employer Identification Number	EIN, Internal Revenue Service (IRS)–issued identification number used on tax documents
Certified Registered Nurse Anesthetist	CRNA, an individual with specialized training and certification in nursing and anesthesia administration	Encounter Form Superbill	Medical document that contains information regarding a patient visit for health care services, can serve as a billing and/or coding document
"Clean Claim"	A properly completed claim submitted to a payer with all data fields containing current and accurate information and submitted within the timely filing period required by the insurer	Explanation of Benefits	EOB or EOMB, written, detailed listing of medical service payments by third-party payer to inform beneficiary and provider of payment
Coinsurance	Cost-sharing of covered services	Fee Schedule	List of established payment for medical services arranged by CPT and HCPCS codes
Compliance Plan	Written strategy developed by medical facilities to ensure appropriate, consistent documentation within the medical record and ensure compliance with third-party payer guidelines and the Office of the Inspector General (OIG) Workplan guidelines	Follow-up Days	FUD, established by third-party payers and listing the number of days after a procedure for which a provider must provide services to a patient for no fee. Also known as *global days*, *global package,* and *global period*
Concurrent Care	More than one physician providing care to a patient at the same time	Group Provider Number	GPN, a numeric designation for a group of providers that is used instead of the individual provider number

TABLE 14-1

Reimbursement Terminology—cont'd

Term	Meaning	Term	Meaning
HMO	Health Maintenance Organization	Provider Identification Number	PIN, a number assigned by a third-party payer to providers to be used for identification purposes when submitting claims
Invalid Claim	Claim that is missing necessary information and cannot be processed or paid	Reimbursement	Payment from a third-party payer for services rendered to a patient covered by the payer's health care plan
Medical Record	Documentation about the health care of a patient to include diagnoses, services, and procedures rendered	Rejection/Denial	A claim that did not pass the edits and is returned to the provider as rejected
National Provider Identifier	NPI, 10-digit number assigned to provider by CMS and National Plan and Provider Enumeration System (NPPES) and used for identification purposes when submitting services to third-party payers	Resource-Based Relative Value Scale	RBRVS, a list of physician services with assigned units of monetary value
Noncovered Services	Any service not included by a third-party payer in the list of services for which payment is made	State License Number	Identification number issued by a state to a physician who has been granted the right to practice in that state
Point of Service	POS, a plan in which either an in-network or out-of-network provider may be used with a higher rate paid to in-network providers	UPIN	Unique provider identification number was replaced by the NPI
Preferred Provider Organization	PPO, providers form a network to offer health care services to a group	Usual, Customary, and Reasonable	UCR, used by some third-party payers to establish a payment rate for a service in an area with the usual (standard fee in area), customary (standard fee by the physician), and reasonable (as determined by payer) fee amounts
Prior Authorization	Also known as preauthorization, which is a requirement by the payer to receive written permission prior to patient services in order to be considered for payment by the payer		

A. Notifier:

B. Patient Name: C. Identification Number:

Advance Beneficiary Notice of Noncoverage (ABN)

NOTE: If Medicare doesn't pay for **D.** _____ below, you may have to pay.
Medicare does not pay for everything, even some care that you or your health care provider have
good reason to think you need. We expect Medicare may not pay for the **D.** _____ below.

D.	E. Reason Medicare May Not Pay:	F. Estimated Cost

WHAT YOU NEED TO DO NOW:
- Read this notice, so you can make an informed decision about your care.
- Ask us any questions that you may have after you finish reading.
- Choose an option below about whether to receive the **D.** _____ listed above.
  Note: If you choose Option 1 or 2, we may help you to use any other insurance
  that you might have, but Medicare cannot require us to do this.

G. OPTIONS: Check only one box. We cannot choose a box for you.

☐ **OPTION 1.** I want the **D.** _____ listed above. You may ask to be paid now, but I
also want Medicare billed for an official decision on payment, which is sent to me on a Medicare
Summary Notice (MSN). I understand that if Medicare doesn't pay, I am responsible for
payment, but **I can appeal to Medicare** by following the directions on the MSN. If Medicare
does pay, you will refund any payments I made to you, less co-pays or deductibles.

☐ **OPTION 2.** I want the **D.** _____ listed above, but do not bill Medicare. You may
ask to be paid now as I am responsible for payment. **I cannot appeal if Medicare is not billed.**

☐ **OPTION 3.** I don't want the **D.** _____ listed above. I understand with this choice I
am **not** responsible for payment, and **I cannot appeal to see if Medicare would pay.**

H. Additional Information:

This notice gives our opinion, not an official Medicare decision. If you have other questions on
this notice or Medicare billing, call **1-800-MEDICARE** (1-800-633-4227/**TTY**: 1-877-486-2048).
Signing below means that you have received and understand this notice. You also receive a copy.

I. Signature:	J. Date:

According to the Paperwork Reduction Act of 1995, no persons are required to respond to a collection of information unless it displays a valid OMB control number.
The valid OMB control number for this information collection is 0938-0566. The time required to complete this information collection is estimated to average 7
minutes per response, including the time to review instructions, search existing data resources, gather the data needed, and complete and review the information
collection. If you have comments concerning the accuracy of the time estimate or suggestions for improving this form, please write to: CMS, 7500 Security
Boulevard, Attn: PRA Reports Clearance Officer, Baltimore, Maryland 21244-1850.

Form CMS-R-131 (03/11)   Form Approved OMB No. 0938-0566

• **Figure 14.3** Centers for Medicare and Medicaid Services Advance Beneficiary Notice (ABN).

Chapter 14: Reimbursement Quiz

(Quiz Answers Are Located in Appendix B)

1. Any person who is identified as receiving life or medical benefits:
   a. primary
   b. beneficiary
   c. participant
   d. recipient

2. According to the Birthday Rule, if both parents are covered by an employer-provided health policy, the insurance policy that would be primary for reporting their child's health services is:
   a. parent with the birthday earlier in the year
   b. parent with the birthday later in the year
   c. either parent
   d. parent whose birthday is closer to the child's

3. Abbreviation for durable medical equipment is:
   a. DRG
   b. CRN
   c. DME
   d. DIM

4. Management of multiple third-party payments to ensure that overpayment does not occur:
   a. PRO
   b. COB
   c. DME
   d. FUD

5. CMS delegates the daily operation of the Medicare program to:
   a. DHHS
   b. QIO
   c. RVU
   d. MACs

6. A QIO provider is one who:
   a. ensures quality of patient care
   b. submits charges directly to CMS
   c. receives 5% less than some other physicians
   d. can bill the patient the total remaining balance after payment from Medicare

7. This part of Medicare covers the inpatient portion of covered costs after the deductible has been paid:
   a. Part A
   b. Part B
   c. Part C
   d. Part D

8. This issue of the *Federal Register* contains outpatient major facility changes for CMS programs for the coming year:
   a. October/November
   b. November/December
   c. December/October
   d. November/August

9. This is the RBRVS payment method:
   a. RAI
   b. OPPS
   c. APC
   d. NFS

10. Entity responsible for development of the plan that outlines monitoring of the Medicare program:
   a. MACs
   b. OIG
   c. DHSS
   d. HEW

PART 3

CPT and HCPCS Coding

15
Introduction to CPT

Introduction to Medical Coding

Translates services/procedures/supplies/drugs into CPT/HCPCS codes
    Translates diagnosis(es) into ICD-10-CM codes

Two Levels of Service Codes

1. Level I CPT
2. Level II HCPCS, National Codes

Diagnosis Codes, ICD-10-CM

ICD-10-CM, International Classification of Diseases, 10th Revision, Clinical Modification
- Classification system
- Translates diagnosis(es) (dx) into standardized codes that explain why service was provided
- Very specific in nature
- May be up to seven characters
- Example: Diabetes becomes E11.9

CPT

Developed by the AMA in 1966
    Five-digit codes to report services provided to patients
    Updated each November for use January 1
- Historically in numerical order
- Not the case for more than 100 codes
- Pound symbol (#) appears before the resequenced codes

Example: In the 51725-51798 range, code 51797 follows 51729 (in numeric order). Code 51797 also appears in correct numeric order in the CPT, but next to the code a note states "Code is out of numerical sequence. See 51725-51798."
See Appendix N of the CPT for a complete list of the resequenced codes.

Types of CPT Codes

- Medical
- Surgical
- Diagnostic services
- Anesthesia
- Evaluation and Management

CPT Codes

Allow communication that is both effective and efficient
    Inform third-party payers of services/procedures provided
    Used as a basis of payment

Incorrect Coding

Results in providers being paid inappropriately (either overpayment or underpayment)

Outpatient Physician (Non-Hospital) Services

Reported on standardized insurance form
    CMS-1500 example (Fig. 15.1)

CPT Format

Symbols

Used to convey information
- Bullet = New code symbol
- ▲ Triangle = Revised code
- ▶◀ Right and left triangles = Beginning and ending of text change
- + Plus = Add-on code
  - Full list in Appendix D of CPT
- ⊘ Circle with line = Modifier -51 exempt code
  - Modifier -51 cannot be used with these codes
  - Full list in Appendix E of CPT
- ★ Star = Telemedicine Services
  - Such as 97802, medical nutrition therapy
  - Full list in Appendix P of CPT
- ⚡ Lightning bolt symbol = Codes for which the FDA status is pending
  - Full list in Appendix K of CPT
- \# Number sign = Resequenced CPT codes
  - Such as 21552, excision of tumor, 3 cm or greater, resequenced code in 2010
  - Full list in Appendix N
- ○ Circle = Recycled/reinstated code

HEALTH INSURANCE CLAIM FORM

APPROVED BY NATIONAL UNIFORM CLAIM COMMITTEE (NUCC) 02/12

CARRIER

PICA [ ][ ]   PICA [ ][ ]

1. MEDICARE [ ] (Medicare#)   MEDICAID [ ] (Medicaid#)   TRICARE [ ] (ID#DoD#)   CHAMPVA [ ] (Member ID#)   GROUP HEALTH PLAN [ ] (ID#)   FECA BLK LUNG [ ] (ID#)   OTHER [ ] (ID#)   1a. INSURED'S I.D. NUMBER   (For Program in Item 1)

2. PATIENT'S NAME (Last Name, First Name, Middle Initial)

3. PATIENT'S BIRTH DATE MM | DD | YY   SEX   M [ ]   F [ ]

4. INSURED'S NAME (Last Name, First Name, Middle Initial)

5. PATIENT'S ADDRESS (No., Street)

6. PATIENT RELATIONSHIP TO INSURED   Self [ ]   Spouse [ ]   Child [ ]   Other [ ]

7. INSURED'S ADDRESS (No., Street)

CITY   STATE

8. RESERVED FOR NUCC USE

CITY   STATE

ZIP CODE   TELEPHONE (Include Area Code)   ( )

ZIP CODE   TELEPHONE (Include Area Code)   ( )

9. OTHER INSURED'S NAME (Last Name, First Name, Middle Initial)

10. IS PATIENT'S CONDITION RELATED TO:

11. INSURED'S POLICY GROUP OR FECA NUMBER

a. OTHER INSURED'S POLICY OR GROUP NUMBER

a. EMPLOYMENT? (Current or Previous)   YES [ ]   NO [ ]

a. INSURED'S DATE OF BIRTH MM | DD | YY   SEX   M [ ]   F [ ]

b. RESERVED FOR NUCC USE

b. AUTO ACCIDENT?   YES [ ]   NO [ ]   PLACE (State)

b. OTHER CLAIM ID (Designated by NUCC)

c. RESERVED FOR NUCC USE

c. OTHER ACCIDENT?   YES [ ]   NO [ ]

c. INSURANCE PLAN NAME OR PROGRAM NAME

d. INSURANCE PLAN NAME OR PROGRAM NAME

10d. CLAIM CODES (Designated by NUCC)

d. IS THERE ANOTHER HEALTH BENEFIT PLAN?   YES [ ]   NO [ ]   *If yes,* complete items 9, 9a, and 9d.

READ BACK OF FORM BEFORE COMPLETING & SIGNING THIS FORM.

12. PATIENT'S OR AUTHORIZED PERSON'S SIGNATURE I authorize the release of any medical or other information necessary to process this claim. I also request payment of government benefits either to myself or to the party who accepts assignment below.

SIGNED _____ DATE _____

13. INSURED'S OR AUTHORIZED PERSON'S SIGNATURE I authorize payment of medical benefits to the undersigned physician or supplier for services described below.

SIGNED _____

PATIENT AND INSURED INFORMATION

14. DATE OF CURRENT ILLNESS, INJURY, or PREGNANCY(LMP) MM | DD | YY   QUAL.

15. OTHER DATE QUAL.   MM | DD | YY

16. DATES PATIENT UNABLE TO WORK IN CURRENT OCCUPATION MM | DD | YY   FROM   TO   MM | DD | YY

17. NAME OF REFERRING PROVIDER OR OTHER SOURCE   17a.   17b. NPI

18. HOSPITALIZATION DATES RELATED TO CURRENT SERVICES MM | DD | YY   FROM   TO   MM | DD | YY

19. ADDITIONAL CLAIM INFORMATION (Designated by NUCC)

20. OUTSIDE LAB?   YES [ ]   NO [ ] $ CHARGES

21. DIAGNOSIS OR NATURE OF ILLNESS OR INJURY Relate A-L to service line below (24E)   ICD Ind.

A. | B. | C. | D. |
E. | F. | G. | H. |
I. | J. | K. | L. |

22. RESUBMISSION CODE   ORIGINAL REF. NO.

23. PRIOR AUTHORIZATION NUMBER

24. A. DATE(S) OF SERVICE					B. PLACE OF SERVICE	C. EMG	D. PROCEDURES, SERVICES, OR SUPPLIES (Explain Unusual Circumstances) CPT/HCPCS MODIFIER	E. DIAGNOSIS POINTER	F. $ CHARGES	G. DAYS OR UNITS	H. EPSDT Family Plan	I. ID. QUAL.	J. RENDERING PROVIDER ID. #
From MM	DD	YY	To MM	DD	YY									
1													NPI
2													NPI
3													NPI
4													NPI
5													NPI
6													NPI

25. FEDERAL TAX I.D. NUMBER   SSN [ ] EIN [ ]

26. PATIENT'S ACCOUNT NO.

27. ACCEPT ASSIGNMENT? (For govt. claims, see back)   YES [ ]   NO [ ]

28. TOTAL CHARGE $

29. AMOUNT PAID $

30. Rsvd for NUCC Use $

31. SIGNATURE OF PHYSICIAN OR SUPPLIER INCLUDING DEGREES OR CREDENTIALS (I certify that the statements on the reverse apply to this bill and are made a part thereof.)

SIGNED _____ DATE _____

32. SERVICE FACILITY LOCATION INFORMATION

a. NPI   b.

33. BILLING PROVIDER INFO & PH # ( )

a. NPI   b.

PHYSICIAN OR SUPPLIER INFORMATION

NUCC Instruction Manual available at: www.nucc.org   *PLEASE PRINT OR TYPE*   APPROVED OMB-0938-1197 FORM 1500 (02-12)

• **Figure 15.1** The CMS-1500 Health Insurance Claim Form.

CPT Sections

1. Evaluation & Management (E/M)
2. Anesthesia
3. Surgery
4. Radiology
5. Pathology and Laboratory
6. Medicine

> **NOTE**
>
> During your examination, the front section of the CPT (Introduction and Illustrations) is an excellent resource on the format, definitions of terms, medical terms, and instructions in the CPT. Review these well before the examination to familiarize yourself with where to find the information that is contained in the front section.
>
> Also, flag the different sections of the CPT for easy access during the examination—for example, the list of illustrations section, E/M Guidelines, Appendices, and other major sections of the manual.

Categorized by

Sections
    Subsections
    Subheadings
    Categories
        Anatomy
            Knee or Shoulder
        Procedure
            Incision or Excision
        Condition
            Fracture or Dislocation
        Description
            Cast or Strap
        Surgical approach
            Anterior Cranial Fossa or Middle Cranial Fossa

Guidelines

Section-specific information begins each section
    Provides instruction pertinent to entire section

Notes

Located throughout CPT
    Provides instruction pertinent to specific subsection

Two Types of Code Descriptions

1. **Stand-alone:** Full description
   Example: 10080 Incision and drainage of pilonidal cyst; simple
2. **Indented:** Dependent on preceding stand-alone for meaning
   Example: 10080 Incision and drainage of pilonidal cyst; simple
           10081   complicated

Semicolon

- Description preceding semicolon is the common part of the description and applies to any indented codes under it
- You must return to stand-alone for full description
  Example: 10081 Incision and drainage of pilonidal cyst; complicated

Modifiers Add Information

CPT Modifier

Appended to the end of the CPT/HCPCS code
    Some modifiers are informational; others affect reimbursement
    Example: 43820 gastrojejunostomy
- -62 two primary surgeons
- 43820-62 two surgeons performed a gastrojejunostomy
- Only used if both surgeons submit same CPT code and both surgeons dictate a separate operative report

Level II HCPCS Modifiers

"-AS" physician's assistant
    "-F1" Left hand, second digit
    All modifiers used on CPT or HCPCS codes
    All HCPCS modifiers begin with a letter
    Modifiers are placed in Block D, Modifier (see Fig. 15.1)

Unlisted Services

Codes usually end in "99" = "no specific code" in Category I or Category III
Used when a more specific code cannot be assigned
Written report must accompany claim form indicating
- Nature
- Extent
- Need
- Time
- Effort
- Equipment used

Category II Codes—Supplemental Tracking Codes

Used for performance measurements
- Optional unless practice participating in Quality Payment Program (QPP)
  These codes collect data concerning the quality of care and test results
  Alphanumeric and end in the letter "F" (0005F)
  Located after the Medicine section in CPT
- On CPC exam

Category III Codes—New Technology

Temporary codes—may be included in this section up to 5 years
Identify emerging technology, services, and procedures
Located after Category II codes
Alphanumeric and end in the letter "T" (0055T)

- May or may not receive future Category I code status
- Category I codes (00100-99607)
- Approved by AMA and the Food and Drug Administration (FDA)
- Proven clinical effectiveness (efficacy)
- Category III has not been approved and has no proven clinical effectiveness (efficacy)
- Use Category III code instead of unlisted code if no Category I code appropriate
- Use unlisted code if no Category III code exists
- On CPC exam

The Index

Used to locate service/procedure terms and codes
Speeds up code location
Uses dictionary format

- First entries and last entries on top of page
- Code display in index
  - Single code: 38115
  - Multiple codes: 26645, 26650
  - Range of codes: 22310-22325

Location Methods

Service/procedure: Repair, excision
  Anatomic site: Meniscus, knee
  Condition or disease: Cleft lip, clot
  Synonym: Toe and interphalangeal joint
  Eponym: Jones procedure, Heller operation
  Abbreviation: ECG, PEEP (positive end-expiratory pressure)
"See" in Index
Cross-reference terms: "Look here for code"
Index: Stem, Brain: *See* Brainstem

Appendices of CPT

Appendix A: Modifiers
Appendix B: Summary of Additions, Deletions, and Revisions
Appendix C: Clinical Examples (E/M Codes)
Appendix D: Summary of CPT Add-on Codes
Appendix E: Summary of CPT Codes Exempt from Modifier -51
Appendix F: Summary of CPT Codes Exempt from Modifier -63
Appendix G: Summary of CPT Codes That Include Moderate (Conscious) Sedation (Deleted for 2017)
Appendix H: Alphabetical Clinical Topics Listing (AKA-Alphabetical Listing) (Moved to AMA website)
Appendix I: Genetic Testing Code Modifiers (Deleted for 2013)
Appendix J: Electrodiagnostic Medicine Listing of Sensory, Motor, and Mixed Nerves
Appendix K: Product Pending FDA Approval
Appendix L: Vascular Families
Appendix M: Renumbered CPT Codes—Citations Crosswalk
Appendix N: Summary of Resequenced CPT Codes
Appendix O: Multianalyte Assays with Algorithmic Analyses
Appendix P: CPT Codes That May Be Used For Synchronous Telemedicine Services
Review information in the CPT appendices prior to examination

16

Evaluation and Management (E/M) Section (99201-99499)

Subsections by type of service
Types of service
- Consultation
- Office Services
- Hospital Services, etc.

Integral Factors When Selecting E/M Codes

1. Place of Service

Explains setting of service
- Office
- Emergency Department
- Nursing Home

2. Type of Service

Physicians provide many types of service
- Consultations (not reported for Medicare)
- Admissions
- Office visits

3. Patient Status

The four status types are
1. New patient
2. Established patient
3. Outpatient
4. Inpatient

New Patient

Has not received any professional service in last 3 years from the same physician or another physician of the same specialty and in the same group

New patients are more labor-intensive for physician, medical staff, and clerical staff

Established Patient

Has received professional services in last 3 years from the same physician or another physician of the same specialty in the same group

Medical record available with current, relevant information

Outpatient

One who has not been admitted to a health care facility

Example: Patient receives services at clinic, ED, or same-day surgery center

Inpatient

One who has been formally admitted to a health care facility

Example: Patient admitted to hospital or nursing home
Physician dictates
- Admission orders
- H&P (history and physical)
- Requests for consultations

Levels of E/M Service Based on

Skill required to provide service
Time spent
Level of knowledge necessary to treat the patient
Effort required
Responsibility required/assumed

E/M Levels Divided Based on

Key Components (KC)

- History (Hx)
- Physical examination (PE)
- Medical decision making (MDM)

Contributory Factors (CF)

- Counseling
- Coordination of care
- Nature of presenting problem

Every Encounter Contains Varying Amount of KC and CF

More extensive component/factor
- Higher level of service
  - Less extensive component/factor
- Lower level of service

Key Components

Four Elements of a History

1. Chief Complaint (CC)
2. History of Present Illness (HPI)
3. Review of Systems (ROS)
4. Past, Family, or Social History (PFSH)

Chief Complaint (CC)—Subjective

Reason for encounter or presenting problem: Patient's current complaint in patient's own words
   Documented in medical record for each encounter

History of Present Illness (HPI)—Subjective

Description of development of current illness, e.g., date of onset
   Patient describes HPI
   Provider must personally document

Physician and Patient Dialogue

Development of a CC of Abdominal Pain (HPI):
"Started Thursday night and was mild. During the night, it got worse. Friday morning I went to work but had to leave because the pain got so bad."
   Location. Specific source of pain
      "Pain was in lower left-hand side, a little toward back."
   Quality. Is pain sharp, intermittent, burning?
      "Pain is really sharp and constant."
   Severity. Is pain intense, moderate, mild?
      "Pain is terrible, worst pain I have ever had." (intensity of pain/scale)
   ***Duration.** How long has pain been present?
      "Pain has been going on now for 3 days."
   Timing. Is pain constant or does it come and go?
      "Pain just continues. It just doesn't go away."
   Context. When does it hurt most?
      "Pain is just there, it doesn't matter what I am doing."
   Modifying factors. Does anything make it better or worse?
      "Nothing I do makes it any better or any worse."

---

*Duration is not listed in CPT as HPI element.

Associated signs and symptoms. Does anything else feel different when pain is present?
   "Yes, I have nausea when pain is worst."

Review of Systems (ROS)—Subjective

Questions posed to the patient to identify signs and symptoms that have been or are being experienced relating to the HPI
   Organ systems (OS), e.g., respiratory system, cardiovascular system
   Extent of ROS depends on CC and patient status (new, established, inpatient, outpatient)

ROS Elements

Constitutional—General, fever, weight loss or gain
   Eyes—Organ System (OS)
   Ears, Nose, Mouth, Throat (OS)
   Cardiovascular (OS)
   Respiratory (OS)
   Gastrointestinal (OS)
   Genitourinary (OS)
   Musculoskeletal (OS)
   Integumentary (OS)
   Neurological (OS)
   Psychiatric (OS)
   Endocrine (OS)
   Hematologic/Lymphatic (OS)
   Allergic/Immunologic (OS)

Past, Family, and Social History (PFSH)
Past

Contains relevant information about past illness, injury, or treatment, including
- Major illnesses/injuries
- Operations
- Hospitalizations
- Allergies
- Immunizations
- Dietary status
- Current medications

Family History

Health status or cause of death of family members
- Parents
- Siblings
- Children
Family history items related to CC
- Hereditary diseases

Social History

Review of past and current activities
- Marital status
- Employment
- Occupational history
- Military history
- Use of drugs/alcohol/tobacco

- Educational activities
- Sexual history
- Other relevant or contributory factors

Four History Levels

1. Problem Focused (PF)
2. Expanded Problem Focused (EPF)
3. Detailed (D)
4. Comprehensive (C)

Problem-Focused History

CC
    Brief HPI
    No ROS
    No PFSH

Expanded Problem-Focused History

CC
    Brief HPI
    Problem Focused ROS
    No PFSH

Detailed History

CC
    Extended HPI
    Problem pertinent ROS, extended to include a limited number of additional systems
    Pertinent PFSH directly related to problem

Comprehensive History

CC
    Extended HPI
    Complete ROS directly related to CC, plus review of 10+ systems
    Complete PFSH
    Summary of elements required for each level of history (Fig. 16.1)

History Elements

Chief Complaint (CC)
    Reason for the encounter in the patient's words

History of Present Illness (HPI)
    Location
    Quality
    Severity
    Duration*
    Timing
    Context
    Modifying factors
    Associated signs and symptoms

Review of Systems (ROS)
    Constitutional symptoms (fever, weight loss, etc.)
    Ophthalmologic (eyes)
    Otolaryngologic (ears, nose, mouth, throat)
    Cardiovascular
    Respiratory
    Gastrointestinal
    Genitourinary
    Musculoskeletal
    Integumentary (skin and/or breast)
    Neurologic
    Psychiatric
    Endocrine
    Hematologic/Lymphatic
    Allergic/Immunologic

Past, Family, and/or Social History (PFSH)
    Past major illnesses, operations, injuries, and treatments
    Family medical history for heredity and risk
    Social activities, both past and current

Elements Required for Each Level of History

		Problem Focused	Expanded Problem Focused	Detailed	Comprehensive
History	HPI	Brief 1-3	Brief 1-3	Extended 4+	Extended 4+
	ROS	None	Problem-pertinent 1	Extended 2-9	Complete 10+
	PFSH	None	None	Pertinent 1	Complete 2-3

*Duration is not listed in the CPT E/M Guidelines, but is listed in the DGs.

• **Figure 16.1** History elements required for each level of history.

Four Examination Levels (Objective)

Problem-Focused Examination (1995 Documentation Guidelines [DG])

Limited examination of affected body area or organ system

Expanded Problem-Focused Examination (1995 DG)

Limited examination of affected body area or organ system
  Other related body area(s) or organ system(s)

Detailed Examination (1995 DG)

Extended examination of affected body area(s) and other symptomatic or related organ system(s)

Comprehensive Examination (1995 DG)

Eight or more organ systems
  Summary of elements required for each level of examination (Fig. 16.2)

Medical Decision Making Complexity (MDM)

Management Options

Based on number of possible diagnoses
  Levels: Minimal, limited, multiple, or extensive

Data Reviewed

Laboratory, radiology; any test/procedure results are documented along with the data reviewed and the identity of the reviewer in medical record
- "Hemoglobin within normal limits."
- "Chest x-ray, negative."
  Old medical records (data) from others may be requested and reviewed
  Levels: Minimal, limited, moderate, or extensive

Risks

Risks of morbidity (poor outcome), complications, or mortality (death) associated with problem, diagnostic procedure

Other diseases or factors (co-morbidities)
- Diabetes
- Extreme age
Urgency relates to risks
- Myocardial infarction
- Ruptured appendix
Levels: Minimal, low, moderate, or high
See Fig. 16.3, CMS Table of Risk

Examination Elements

General (OS)
  Constitutional

Body Areas (BA)
  Head (including the face)
  Neck
  Chest (including breasts and axillae)
  Abdomen
  Genitalia, groin, buttocks
  Back
  Each extremity

Organ System (OS)
  Ophthalmologic (eyes)
  Otolaryngologic (ears, nose, mouth, throat)
  Cardiovascular
  Respiratory
  Gastrointestinal
  Genitourinary
  Musculoskeletal
  Integumentary
  Neurologic
  Psychiatric
  Hematologic/Lymphatic/Immunologic

Elements Required for Each Level of Examination

	Problem Focused	Expanded Problem Focused	Detailed	Comprehensive
Examination	Limited to affected BA or OS	Limited to affected BA or OS and other related OS(s)	Extended of affected BA(s) and other related OS(s)	General multi-system (OSs only)

• **Figure 16.2** Examination elements required for each level of examination.

TABLE OF RISK
(Total = highest risk in any one category)

Level of risk	Presenting problem(s)	Diagnostic procedure(s) ordered	Management options selected
Minimal	• One self-limited or minor problem, e.g., cold, insect bite, tinea corpus	• Laboratory tests requiring venipuncture • Chest x-rays • EKG/EEG • Urinalysis • Ultrasound, e.g., echocardiography • KOH prep	• Rest • Gargles • Elastic bandages • Superficial dressings
Low	• Two or more self-limited or minor problems • One stable chronic illness, e.g., well controlled hypertension or non-insulin dependent diabetes, cataract, BPH • Acute uncomplicated illness or injury, e.g., cystitis, allergic rhinitis, simple sprain	• Physiologic tests not under stress, e.g., pulmonary function tests • Non-cardiovascular imaging studies with contrast, e.g., barium enema • Superficial needle biopsies • Clinical laboratory tests requiring arterial puncture • Skin biopsies	• Over-the-counter drugs • Minor surgery with no identified risk factors • Physical therapy • IV fluids without additives
Moderate	• One or more chronic illnesses with mild exacerbation, progression, or side effects of treatment • Two or more stable chronic illnesses • Undiagnosed new problem with uncertain prognosis, e.g., lump in breast • Acute illness with systemic symptoms, e.g., pyelonephritis, pneumonitis, colitis • Acute complicated injury, e.g., head injury with brief loss of consciousness	• Physiologic tests under stress, e.g., cardiac stress test, fetal contraction stress test • Diagnostic endoscopies with no identified risk factors • Deep needle or incisional biopsy • Cardiovascular imaging studies with contrast and no identified risk factors, e.g., arteriogram, cardiac catheterization • Obtain fluid from body cavity, e.g., lumbar puncture, thoracentesis, culdocentesis	• Minor surgery with identified risk factors • Elective major surgery (open, percutaneous, or endoscopic) with no identified risk factors • Prescription drug management • Therapeutic nuclear medicine • IV fluids with additives • Closed treatment of fracture or dislocation without manipulation
High	• One or more chronic illnesses with severe exacerbation, progression, or side effects of treatment • Acute or chronic illnesses or injuries that pose a threat to life or bodily function, e.g., multiple trauma, acute MI, pulmonary embolus, severe respiratory distress, progressive severe rheumatoid arthritis • Psychiatric illness with potential threat to self or others • Peritonitis • Acute renal failure • An abrupt change in neurologic status, e.g., seizure, TIA, weakness, or sensory loss	• Cardiovascular imaging studies with contrast with identified risk factors • Cardiac electrophysiological tests • Diagnostic endoscopies with identified risk factors • Discography	• Elective major surgery (open, percutaneous, or endoscopic) with identified risk factors • Emergency major surgery (open, percutaneous or endoscopic) • Parenteral controlled substances • Drug therapy requiring intensive monitoring for toxicity • Decision not to resuscitate or to de-escalate care because of poor prognosis

• **Figure 16.3** Centers for Medicare and Medicaid Services (CMS) Table of Risk.

Four Levels of MDM Complexity

1. Straightforward MDM

Number of diagnoses or management options: Minimal
   Amount or complexity of data: Minimal/None
   Risk of complications or death: Minimal

2. Low-Complexity MDM

Number of diagnoses or management options: Limited
   Amount or complexity of data: Limited
   Risk of complications or death: Low

3. Moderate-Complexity MDM

Number of diagnoses or management options: Multiple
   Amount or complexity of data: Moderate
   Risk of complications or death: Moderate

4. High-Complexity MDM

Number of diagnoses or management options: Extensive
   Amount or complexity of data: Extensive
   Risk of complications or death: High
   Summary of elements required for each level of MDM
      (Fig. 16.4)
   The diagnosis or management options, amount or complexity of data, and risk are totaled to arrive at the level of MDM

- Only two of three categories must meet or exceed each other in any level to assign the MDM
   Example: Moderate complexity for diagnosis or management options and moderate complexity of amount or complexity of data, but only a low risk would be assigned a moderate level MDM
   Example: Low risk of death, moderate diagnosis or management options, and high amount or complexity of data: Assign the moderate level of MDM

Contributory Factors

Counseling

Provided to patient or family members (synopsis must be stated in medical record)
   Discussion of diagnosis, test results, impressions, recommendations, prognosis, risks/benefits of treatment options or lack thereof, and risk factor reduction

Coordination of Care

Work done on behalf of patient by physician to provide care

Nature of Presenting Problem

Type of problem patient presents to physician with or reason for encounter

---

Medical Decision Making Elements

Number of Diagnoses or Management Options
Minimal
Limited
Multiple
Extensive

Amount or Complexity of Data to Review
Minimal/None
Limited
Moderate
Extensive

Risk of Complications or Death If Condition Goes Untreated
Minimal
Low
Moderate
High

Elements Required for Each Level of Medical Decision Making

	Straightforward	Low	Moderate	High
Number of diagnoses or management options	Minimal	Limited	Multiple	Extensive
Amount or complexity of data to review	Minimal/None	Limited	Moderate	Extensive
Risk	Minimal	Low	Moderate	High

• **Figure 16.4** Elements required for each level of medical decision making.

Levels of Presenting Problem

Minimal Presenting Problem

May not require a physician
Example: A dressing change or removal of an uncomplicated suture

Self-Limiting or Minor Presenting Problem

Self-limiting problems are minor and with a good outcome
and no complications predicted
Example: Sore throat or a slightly irritated skin tag

Low-Severity Presenting Problem

Without treatment, low risk
Example: A middle-aged, healthy male with an upper
respiratory infection

Moderate-Severity Presenting Problem

Without treatment, moderate risk
Example: An elderly male with bacterial pneumonia

High-Severity Presenting Problem

Without treatment, high risk
Example: An elderly male in very poor health with diabetic ketoacidosis

Time

Direct face-to-face: Physician or Other Qualified Health
Care Professional and patient together

Example: Clinic visit or at bedside in hospital
  Calculated for code assignment beginning and ending
    times documented in medical record
  Unit/Floor: Time spent by physician on patient's floor
    or unit, also at patient's bedside
Example: Reviewing patient records or at chart desk and
  then with patient

> **NOTE**
>
> Over 50% of the total time should include counseling and/or
> coordination of care, and the documentation must reflect the
> total time of the visit and the time spent counseling and/or in
> coordination of care to qualify to assign the code based on
> time.

Use of E/M Code

Codes are grouped by type of service and place of service
- Consultation
- Office visit
- Hospital admission
  Different codes are required for various levels of service
assignment
  New patient (99201-99205) services to new patient in
office or other outpatient setting

Selection of Level of E/M Services

For the following categories/subcategories, all three of the
key components must meet or exceed the level stated in the
code description:
- Office or Other Outpatient Services, New Patient
- Hospital Observation Services
- Initial Hospital Care
- Observation of Inpatient Care Services
- Office or Other Outpatient Consultations
- Inpatient Consultations
- Emergency Department Services
- Initial Nursing Facility Care
- Other Nursing Facility Services
- Domiciliary, Rest Home (e.g., Boarding Home), or Cus-
  todial Care Services, New Patient
- Home Services, New Patient
  For the following categories/subcategories, two of the
three key components must meet or exceed the level stated
in the code description:
- Office or Other Outpatient Services, Established
  Patient
- Subsequent Observation Care
- Subsequent Hospital Care
- Subsequent Nursing Facility Care
- Domiciliary, Rest Home (e.g., Boarding Home), Estab-
  lished Patient
- Home Services, Established Patient

New Patient (99201-99205)

All new patients must be seen by physician

Established Patient (99211-99215)

99211 may not require a physician's presence
  No such code in New Patient category; all new patients
are seen by physician

Hospital Observation Status (99217-99220, 99224-99226, 99234-99236)

Not officially admitted to "inpatient status"

Patient not ill enough to admit but is too ill not to be
  monitored or discharged
Read notes at beginning of subsection
Observation services are not codes for "inpatient" services
Observation admission can be reported only for first day of
  service
*When patient admitted on observation status and discharged
  on same day:*
- Assign code from 99234-99236 (Observation or
  Inpatient Care Services category including admission
  and discharge)
  *Patient in hospital overnight for observation but less than
    48 hours:*
  - **First day:** 99218-99220 (Initial Observation
    Care)

- **Second day:** 99217 (Observation Care Discharge Services)

If observation stay longer than 48 hours:
  - **First day:** 99218-99220 (Initial Observation Care)
  - **Second day:** 99224-99226 (Subsequent Observation Care)
  - **Third day:** 99217 (Observation Care Discharge Services)

Initial Observation Care

- Beginning of observation care service
- Does not require a specific hospital unit; can be a regular bed on a floor or in emergency department (ED)
- Status specified as "observation"
  E/M services immediately prior to admission bundled into observation service
  Example: Office visit prior to observation, bundled into observation service

Hospital Inpatient Services (99221-99239)

Officially admitted to a hospital setting
  Total (all day and night)
  Partial (all day and no night, all night and no day, or a variation)
  - Time in and out must be specified in medical record

Types of Physician Status

Attending: Primary or admitting physician
  Consultant: Physician whose opinion and advice requested by attending physician
  Referring: Physician requesting a consultation from another physician regarding a patient's health status

Types of Care

Concurrent care given to patient by more than one physician each of different specialties
  Example: Pulmonologist and cardiologist both treating patient for different conditions at same time

Three Types of Hospital Inpatient Services

Initial Hospital Care (99221-99223)

First service includes admission
  Initial paperwork
  Initial treatment plans and orders
  Used only once for each admission
  - Only one admission by the attending or admitting physician billable per hospitalization

Subsequent Hospital Care (99231-99233)

After initial service
  Physician reviews patient's progress using documentation, information received from nursing staff, examination of patient
  - May be reported by multiple physicians of different specialties managing different conditions

(concurrent care); only one per day per physician per specialty

Hospital Discharge Services (99238, 99239)

Final day of hospital stay when patient in hospital more than 1 day
  Documentation indicates final patient status
  Time based
  - Total time
  - Does not need to be continuous time
  Beginning and ending time or total time spent must be documented to assign the extended discharge code or use lowest level code

Final Status of Patient

Summary of Stay (Discharge)

Condition (final examination)
  Medications
  Plan for return (follow-up care) to physician
  How hospital stay progressed
  Discharged destination (to home, nursing facility, etc.)
  Only attending physician can use discharge code (only one discharge per admission)
  Code based on time spent in service
  Beginning and ending time or total time spent must be documented to assign the extended discharge code or must use lowest level code

Consultation Services (99241-99255)

One physician or appropriate source requests another physician's opinion or advice
  Either inpatient or outpatient; outpatient consultations include those provided in ED
  Outpatient consultations (99241-99245)
  Inpatient consultations (99251-99255)
  Effective January 1, 2010, CMS no longer recognized CPT consultation codes (ranges 99241-99245 and 99251-99255) for inpatient facility and office/outpatient settings.
  Consultation services reported with:
  New patient office/outpatient (99201-99205)
  Established patient office/outpatient (99211-99215)
  Initial hospital codes (99221-99223)

Third-Party-Payer Consultations

Request consult for
- Past medical treatment
- Current condition
- Payers may request prior to approving procedure
- Report services with -32, mandated services

Emergency Department Services (99281-99288)

No distinction between new and established patients
  Must be open 24 hours a day to qualify as ED (ER)
  ED services often require additional codes from Critical Care Services
  - Typically billed by ED physicians

Other Emergency Services (99288), reports two-way communication for emergency care

Critical Care Services (99291, 99292)

Example: Vital organ failure

Critical care services are provided to patients over 71 months of age in life-threatening (critically ill/injured) situations

Time-based codes
- Total time under 30 minutes reported with appropriate E/M code (e.g., ED)

Critical Care Services (99291, 99292)

Time must be documented in medical record to select from this code range; does not need to be continuous
- Over 71 months of age
  99291 and 99292 reports total length of time a physician spends caring for critically ill patient
- 99291: 30-74 minutes
- 99292: Each additional 30 minutes

Nursing Facility Services (99304-99318)

Non-hospital settings with professional staff
- Provide continuous health care services to patients who are not acutely ill

Formerly known as Skilled Nursing Facility (SNF), Intermediate Care Facility (ICF), and Long-Term Care Facility (LTCF)

Various levels of nursing facility services

Initial Nursing Facility Assessment (99304-99306)

Provided at time of patient's initial admission/readmission

Subsequent Nursing Facility Care Codes (99307-99310)

99307 stable, recovering, or improving
99308 not responding or minor complication
99309 significant complication or new problem
99310 significant new problem requiring immediate physician attention

Nursing Facility Discharge Services (99315, 99316)

For final discharge service

Time-based
- Total time, does not need to be continuous
  Other Nursing Facility Services (99318)
- Annual Nursing Facility Assessment

Domiciliary, Rest Home, or Custodial Care Services (99324-99337)

Health care services are not available on site

Types of services provided are lodging, meals, supervision, personal care, leisure activities

Residents cannot live independently

Codes for either new or established patients

Domiciliary, Rest Home, or Home Care Plan Oversight Services (99339, 99340)

Read notes at beginning of subsection

Reports individual physician supervision of patient in home or domiciliary rest home

Services not face-to-face

Time-based
- 99339 15-29 minutes
- 99340 30 minutes or more

Reported once per 30-day period

Home Services (99341-99350)

Care provided in patient's home

Travel time not separately billable
- Not included in determining CPT code

Services based on key components and contributory factors

Codes for new or established patients

Prolonged Services (99354-99360; 99415-99416)

Time codes for direct face-to-face and without direct face-to-face contact

Report time beyond the usual E/M service
- Time must be documented in medical record

Codes for first 30-74 minutes and each additional 30 minutes thereafter

If less than 30 minutes, do not report service as prolonged

Standby Services (99360)

Not caring for other patient(s) to use these codes

Standing by only for that patient, if needed

Standby requested by another physician
- Must be documented in medical record

Report in 30-minute increments

Less than 30 minutes—do not report

Can report for subsequent 30 minutes only if a full 30 minutes

Carriers have strict policies regarding reimbursement for this service

Case Management Services (99366-99368)

Medical Team Conferences (99366-99368)

Codes for with or without face-to-face patient/family contact
- Minimum of three health care professionals, different specialties/disciplines participate in team
- Each member must have performed face-to-face evaluation in past 60 days
- Documentation must reflect member's contribution of information and treatment recommendation
- Not reported for organization or facility contracted services

Time-based

Begins and ends at start and conclusion of review

Care Plan Oversight Services (99374-99380)

Used to report supervision of patient care in home health agency, hospice, domiciliary, or equivalent environment

Patient not present

Codes are time-based

- 15-29 minutes
- 30 minutes or more
- Time must be documented in medical record

Reported once for each 30-day period

Preventive Medicine Services (99381-99429)

Used to report services when patient is not currently ill

Example: Annual checkup

Codes divided by new or established and age

If significant problem is encountered during preventive examination

- E/M code also reported, append modifier -25

Counseling Risk Factor Reduction and Behavior Change Intervention (99401-99429)

Patient is seen specifically to promote health and/or wellness

Example: Diet, exercise program

Patient without symptoms or an established diagnosis to use these codes

Codes based on

- Time, individual or group, and physician review of assessment data

Non-Face-to-Face Services (99441-99449)

Physician E/M services using telephone/online

- 99441-99443 telephone E/M services
  Established patient, family member of the patient, or a guardian
- 99444 online E/M services
  Established patient, family member of the patient, or a guardian
- 99446-99449 report interprofessional telephone/internet consultations
  - Usually provided on urgent/emergency basis
  - No face-to-face, based on total time

Special E/M Services (99450-99456)

- 99450 is reported for services provided for insurance or disability assessments
  Involves no treatment; any treatment provided would be coded separately
  99455-99456 report work related or medical disability evaluation
  Codes divided
- 99455: Assessment by treating physician
- 99456: Assessment by nontreating physician

Newborn Care (99460-99465)

Initial and subsequent care in/other than hospital or birthing center

For normal newborn infant

Per day, for E/M services

99463, initial hospital/birthing center when admission and discharge are same day

Delivery/Birthing Room Attendance and Resuscitation Services (99464-99465)

99464, attendance at delivery

Documented request by attending in medical record

Provides initial stabilization

99465, resuscitation and ventilation

Inpatient Neonatal Intensive Care Services and Pediatric and Neonatal Critical Care Services (99466-99486)

Pediatric Critical Care Patient Transport

99466-99467; 99485-99486

Critically ill or injured patient

24 months or younger

99466, first 30-74 minutes

Each additional 30 minutes, 99467

Reports face-to-face interfacility transport

99485, 99486, supervision by a control physician

First 30 minutes (99485) and each additional 30 minutes (99486)

Inpatient Neonatal and Pediatric Critical Care

99468-99476

Divided by

Initial day

Subsequent day

Divided by age

Neonatal (Age 28 days or younger)

Pediatric (29 days through 24 months)

Pediatric (2 through 5 years)

Initial and Continuing Intensive Care Services

99477-99480

Hospital Care

99477 for neonate 28 days of age or younger

99478-99480 divided by birth weight

very low birth weight (VLBW) ≤1500 grams (≤3.3 pounds)

low birth weight (LBW) 1501-2500 grams (3.3-5.5 pounds)

normal birth weight 2501-5000 grams (5.51-11.01 pounds)

Subdivided on day

Initial

Subsequent

Care Management Services (99487-99490)

Chronic Care Management Services (99490)

- 99490 establishment, implementation, revision, or monitoring of a comprehensive care plan for a patient with 2+ chronic conditions
- Last at least year or result in the death
- At least 20 minutes of physician supervised clinical staff time per month

Complex Chronic Care Management Services (99487, 99489)

- Per month
- At least 60 minutes of physician directed clinical staff time
- Compliance with chronic care criteria
- Substantial revision of a comprehensive care plan

Transitional Care Management Services (99495-99496)

- Patient transition clinical setting to community setting
- MDM is moderate or high with first face-to-face service

Advance Care Planning (99497-99498)

- Face-to-face physician services with a patient/surrogate to counseling and/or develop advance directives
- Time based, first 30 minutes/each additional 30 minutes

Other Evaluation and Management Services (99499)

- 99499 reports unlisted E/M services Accompanied by a special report

---

PRACTICE EXERCISE 16.1   PROGRESS NOTE, ACUTE AND CHRONIC RENAL FAILURE

Progress Note

LOCATION: Inpatient, Hospital
PATIENT: Mike Lumbardi
ATTENDING PHYSICIAN: George Orbitz, MD
  NEPHROLOGY PROGRESS NOTE: Mike had no major events. He tolerated the angiogram very well. He had peripheral vascular disease, but nothing to bypass, unfortunately. The patient denies any chest pain, shortness of breath. He has no nausea or vomiting. He has no leg edema and no GI symptoms.
  PHYSICAL EXAMINATION: His vital signs were stable this morning. Temperature 36.9°C. Blood pressure 165/85. Heart rate 52 per minute. Respirations 16 per minute. Sats were 96% on room air. The patient was not in any respiratory, cardiac, or neurologic distress. He had no increase in jugulovenous pressure; regular rate and rhythm. The lungs were clear bilaterally without any crackles. The abdomen was soft and nontender; no organomegaly. No edema, with decreased pulses bilaterally, with signs of chronic venous and arterial insufficiency.
  Intake/output in the past 8 hours: 1286 in, 1050 out.
  Labs are pending from this morning, but his creatinine yesterday was 1.3.
IMPRESSION
  1. Acute on top of chronic renal failure related to intravascular volume depletion, with creatinine coming down from 1.6 to 1.3.
  2. Peripheral vascular disease.
  3. Hypertension.

RECOMMENDATIONS
  1. Basic metabolic panel is pending today.
  2. If his creatinine goes up over time, he might need to have a renal MRA to look for renal artery stenosis.
  3. Since patient is making urine, I don't think that his creatinine will go up acutely after his angiogram yesterday.
     CPT Code(s): _____

     _____

     ICD-10-CM Code(s): _____

     _____

Abstracting Questions
  1. Are all three key elements (history, examination, and MDM complexity) documented? _____

     _____

  2. How many key elements are required for this type of service? _____

  3. Should both acute and chronic renal failure be reported, and if so, which is reported first? _____

     _____

  4. Is the volume depletion reported? _____

     _____

PRACTICE EXERCISE 16.2 CLINIC VISIT, DIARRHEA

Clinic Note

FOLLOW-UP CLINIC VISIT

SUBJECTIVE: This is a 3½-year-old girl who presents today. Mother states that patient has had diarrhea over the past 3-4 days. Yesterday she had about 4-5 stools. They have been mustard colored, real runny, sometimes in little slivers. No blood has been present. She threw up 3-4 days ago, but this has since ended. Her eating is down, although she is drinking a lot. She will complain of her stomach hurting. Her temperature was as high as 103° F, and that was about 3 days ago. She is taking Motrin.

OBJECTIVE: On general appearance: She is alert and does not appear to be in any acute distress. Temperature is 97.2°F. Weight is 42 pounds. **HEENT:** Eyes are clear. The right TM has some increased erythema present. Landmarks are still seen. The left TM is nice and clear with good landmarks. Oropharynx is unremarkable. Neck is supple. Heart reveals a regular rate and rhythm without murmur. GU: Normal female genitalia.

ASSESSMENT
1. Viral gastroenteritis.
2. Possibly early right otitis media.

PLAN: I did discuss with mother that we could put her daughter on an antibiotic now, but we also could wait to see if she starts complaining of right ear pain or if her fever comes back. If that is the case, I did give mother a prescription for Amoxicillin to have her daughter take 375 mg p.o. t.i.d. × 10 days, and I would want to recheck her ear in 3 weeks. If she does not have any complaints or fever, mother will hold off just so Amoxicillin does not worsen her diarrhea. Mother was in agreement with this plan.

CPT Code(s): _____

_____

ICD-10-CM Code(s): _____

_____

Abstracting Questions

1. What category of E/M codes is used to report this service?

   _____

2. What body system is reviewed in the statement "right TM"?

   _____

PRACTICE EXERCISE 16.3 VOMITING

Dr. Sutton is an employee of the hospital.
LOCATION: Outpatient, Hospital
PATIENT: Penny Karlin
PRIMARY CARE PHYSICIAN: Ronald Green, MD
ED PHYSICIAN: Paul Sutton, MD
SUBJECTIVE: This is a 50-year-old female who is presenting to the emergency department today with a complaint of vomiting.

HISTORY OF PRESENT ILLNESS: This patient has quite significant recent medical history; recently diagnosed with grade IV esophageal cancer. She has been to the Lato Clinic and evaluated there, as well as in Los Angeles with endoscopy, and eventually to the Lato Clinic for further workup. With her workup there they found that she had quite extensive cancer with metastatic disease to the bones as well as to the stomach and thought that palliative oncologic treatment was all that could be offered and she should return to the area for this. She is scheduled to have a central line placed tomorrow and also considerations to nutritional needs. She stated that over the past several days she has had some fundraisers and some events for her and she really wanted to attend even though she was not able to keep foods and fluids down. She has been taking only small sips at a time. It seems like her ability to swallow is getting quite impaired, and as a result she cannot swallow her pain pill, so she is having severe pain in her back, hip, and abdomen. She has had increasing fatigue, has vomited several times, and just is not doing well and comes in for this at this time.

PAST MEDICAL HISTORY: Remarkable for esophageal cancer grade IV adenocarcinoma, noted with pelvic mets.
MEDICATIONS: Oxycodone and promethazine.
ALLERGIES: NKA, other than latex.
SOCIAL HISTORY: No smoking or alcohol.
REVIEW OF SYSTEMS: Negative for fever or chills. No shortness of breath. No headache. Patient's got nausea and abdominal and lower chest pain as positives on her review of systems.

On admission to the emergency department today, the patient's vital signs show a temperature of 36.8, pulse of 99, respiratory rate at 18, and blood pressure 132/84. General: This is a 50-year-old female who is awake, alert, and cooperative. **HEENT:** Head is normocephalic and atraumatic. Pupils are reactive to light. Conjunctivae clear. Nares patent. TMs are clear. Mouth reveals a somewhat dry oropharynx with some chapping of the lips, which appear parched. Neck is supple. Trachea is midline. Examination of lungs reveals clear breath sounds. Cardiovascular: S1 and S2 without murmur, click, or rub. Abdomen is soft. There is mild tenderness to palpation in the epigastric region. No mass, guarding, or rigidity. Extremities are without deformity or edema. Skin exam shows no rash. Cranial nerves 2 through 12 grossly intact. No gross motor or sensory deficits noted at this time.

SUMMARY OF EMERGENCY DEPARTMENT COURSE: The patient is seen and evaluated for the above-mentioned complaint. Orthostatic blood pressures were obtained: lying 112/87 with a pulse of 78, sitting 108/74 with a pulse of 98, and standing 102/80 with a pulse of 116. So she had quite an increase in her heart rate with standing, which I believe is significant. I did start an IV here in the department with normal saline; I gave her a liter of normal saline and 4 mg of morphine for her pain, which did help her pain significantly. It came down from an 8 to a 3. Checked some blood counts and metabolic panel as well as giving her some Phenergan for nausea, and this did help take away the nausea. Her CBC shows a hemoglobin level of 9.1, white count is okay, and her electrolytes are normal. So I think she is on the cusp of dehydration; certainly some anemia present here. I spoke with Dr. Green, who is covering for Dr. White, the patient's oncologist here, and he agreed to come in and evaluate the patient and did admit the patient to his service for further evaluation and treatment.

ASSESSMENT
1. Acute nausea and vomiting and dehydration.
2. Adenocarcinoma of the esophagus with metastatic disease.

PLAN: As above, the patient will be admitted for further evaluation and treatment per Dr. Green, certainly to control her pain, and it looks to me that the patient is going to have to change her pain regimen from oral to either parenteral or transdermal delivery system. She is going to have a line placed tomorrow, and further evaluation and treatment will be based on Dr. Green's plan for the patient. These plans as mentioned above were reviewed with the patient, who was in agreement. She will be admitted in fair condition with poor prognosis.

CPT Code(s): _____

_____

ICD-10-CM Code(s): _____

_____

Abstracting Questions

1. What level of history was documented? _____

_____

2. What level of examination was documented? _____

_____

3. What level of medical decision making was documented?

_____

4. This case began in the emergency department, but what was the ultimate disposition of this patient? _____

_____

5. Why is a neoplasm code not the first-listed diagnosis?

_____

PRACTICE EXERCISE 16.4 WELL-CHILD CHECK

Clinic Note

LOCATION: Outpatient, Hospital
PATIENT: Bradley Wellingstone
PHYSICIAN: Rolando Ortez, MD
    SUBJECTIVE: This is a 3-week-old former 32-week gestational male infant who was in RNICU from birth. He did have some mild respiratory difficulties, oxygen requirements that resolved without further sequelae. He was also there for sepsis and feeding difficulties as well as apnea. He was discharged home on caffeine citrate, home apnea monitoring. He did return 2 days ago to get his first dose of Synagis. He is here for general checkup otherwise.
    OBJECTIVE: He is on 24-calorie Enfamil and is taking that well without difficulty, taking almost 2 ounces at feeding; urinating and stool schedule is normal. No other complaints from his mother.
    ASSESSMENT: On exam, alert, in no distress, and afebrile. His weight is up to 2341 grams, which is up 150 grams. Fontanelle, eyes, ears, nose, and pharynx are clear. Neck is supple. Lungs are clear to auscultation. Heart is regular rate and rhythm without murmur. Abdomen benign. Extremities: Full range of motion. No hip abnormalities. Skin is without rash. Neurologic exam without defect.
    IMPRESSION: Thriving former 32-weeker. Now 3 weeks old.
    PLAN: Anticipatory guidance discussed. We talked about feeding issues, accident prevention, car seat use, sleeping position on the side or the back. We will see them back in 1 month for his next Synagis dose as well as a recheck. We will have him on caffeine citrate 10 mg/day along with home apnea monitoring with plans to stop the caffeine in 1 month. With any problems, they need to give us a call or come back in sooner for re-evaluation.

CPT Code(s): _____

_____

ICD-10-CM Code(s): _____

_____

Abstracting Questions

1. From what CPT section would a code be located to report this? _____

2. From what CPT subcategory would this service be reported? _____

3. Was the patient a new or established patient with the provider? _____

4. Does the age of the patient affect code assignment? _____
_____

5. What type of diagnosis code was reported? _____
_____

PRACTICE EXERCISE 16.5   NICU PROGRESS NOTE, VENTILATOR ASSIST

Dr. Ortez has been following this infant since birth.

LOCATION: Inpatient, Hospital

PATIENT: Loren Black

ATTENDING PHYSICIAN: Rolando Ortez, MD

SUBJECTIVE: Baby is currently 2 days old, slightly under 48 hours.

OBJECTIVE: Weight today is 1716 kg (decreased by 135 grams). He is down 5.1% of his weight since birth. OFC is 30 cm (decreased 0.5 cm). Intake yesterday was 152 cc, 82 cc/kg/day. Output was 170 cc, 3.8 cc/kg/hour. He has had no stools since birth. Vital signs reveal his temperature to be acceptable while on an open, radiant warmer. Heart rate is generally in the 110s-120s. Respiratory rate has generally been equal to the IMV (60). Mean blood pressures have generally been in the 40s-50s. Oxygen saturations have remained in the high 90s.

PHYSICAL EXAMINATION: In general, he is pink, on current ventilator settings. He does have slightly dysmorphic features with wide-set eyes and slightly down-slanting palpebral fissures. Ears are low set and posteriorly rotated. Endotracheal tube was in place. Neck was without masses. Chest reveals symmetric expansion and lungs are clear to auscultation on current ventilator settings. Cardiac Exam: Regular rate without murmur or click. Peripheral pulses are 2+ and symmetric. Abdominal Exam: UAC in place. Liver is palpable 1 cm below the right costal margin. No splenomegaly or masses were noted. Genital Exam: Normal male. Testes are not palpable. Extremity Exam: No fixed decreased range of motion, deformity, or joint abnormality. Neurologic Exam: Mild, diffuse hypotonia. No focal deficits are appreciated.

CURRENT MEDICATIONS

1. Ampicillin 90.4 mg IV q12h.
2. Gentamicin 5.4 mg IV q18h.
3. Morphine sulfate 0.18 mg IV q6h and q1h p.r.n.
4. Dopamine 5 mcg/kg/min.
5. Vecuronium 0.18 mg IV q1-2h p.r.n.

LABORATORY STUDIES: Last arterial blood gas was obtained on ventilator setting of IMV 60, pressures of 24/4, and FIO_2 of 0.5 revealed pH 7.27, PCO_2 51.1, PO_2 66.5, and bicarbonate 22.5. Chemistry panel this morning reveals sodium of 134, potassium of 4.9, chloride of 102, glucose of 111, BUN of 18, creatinine of 1.0, calcium of 7.5, magnesium of 3.8, phosphorus of 7.7, bilirubin of 7.8. CBC reveals a white count of 6190. Platelet count was 98,000. Chest x-ray continues to show significant evidence of hyaline membrane disease. Endotracheal tube is near the carina and has been withdrawn somewhat.

IMPRESSION/RECOMMENDATIONS

1. Two-day-old infant who was born at 30 weeks' gestation. He does have clinical features suggestive of Noonan syndrome.
2. Respiratory: Continues to show evidence of hyaline membrane disease with respiratory failure. He has received three doses of surfactant therapy. He does have echocardiographic evidence of PDA, and we will be treating this at this time. We will attempt to decrease his ventilator settings based on serial clinical examination, pulse oximetry, arterial blood gas determinations, and chest x-ray.
3. Cardiovascular: Status is acceptable at this time while on dopamine at 5 mcg/kg/min. Echocardiogram shows a patent ductus arteriosis. There also appears to be a slight abnormality to the pulmonary valve, which could be associated with his possible Noonan syndrome. He is going to receive indomethacin therapy.
4. Gastrointestinal: Abdominal exam remains benign. He is NPO. He does have mild hyperbilirubinemia. Direct antibody test was negative. We will begin phototherapy at this time.
5. Hematologic: Serial CBCs have been acceptable except for mild thrombocytopenia. We will continue to monitor, especially in light of the indomethacin therapy. He has not required any blood product transfusions since birth.
6. Infectious Disease: Blood culture remains negative at this time. We have discontinued his gentamicin, and he is being placed on cefotaxime because of the indomethacin.
7. Neurologic: Exam remains acceptable given his extreme prematurity. He will require screening intracranial ultrasound and long-term neurodevelopmental follow-up.
8. Renal/Metabolic: Urine output remains adequate and renal function studies are acceptable. Previous metabolic parameters are acceptable. We will repeat in the morning.
9. Fluids/Electrolytes/Nutrition: Weight loss is acceptable and electrolytes are in the more normal range today. We will adjust his TPN accordingly.
10. Apnea/Bradycardia: None since birth.
11. Health Care Maintenance: None yet.

SOCIAL HISTORY: Mom and dad are being kept up to date with regard to the patient's condition. Their questions have been answered, and they are in agreement with the outlined management plan.

CPT Code(s): _____

_____

ICD-10-CM Code(s): _____

_____

Abstracting Questions

1. The surfactant therapy was given for which diagnosis?

_____

2. What does PDA mean? _____

_____

17

Anesthesia Section (00100-01999)

Anesthesiologist

Doctor of medicine specializing in anesthesia

Usually outside practices, e.g., Anesthesia Associates, Inc., or Pain Clinic, Ltd.
Professional services reported separately

CRNA

Certified Registered Nurse Anesthetist

Uses of Anesthesia

Manage unconscious patients, life functions, and resuscitation

Analgesia

Relieve pain

Some Methods of Anesthesia

Endotracheal: Through mouth (general anesthesia)
  Local: Application to area (injection or topical)
  Epidural: Between vertebral spaces—injection into epidural space
  Regional: Field or nerve block
  MAC: Monitored anesthesia care (service provided by an anesthesiologist or CRNA)
  Patient is monitored, and if necessary, sedation (including general anesthesia) may be provided
  Spinal: Anesthesia applied to the spinal cord area, outside the dura mater
  General: State of unconsciousness accomplished through drug administration or by inhalation

Patient-Controlled Analgesia (PCA)

Patient self-administers drug
  Used to relieve chronic pain or temporarily for severe pain following surgery

Moderate (Conscious) Sedation

Codes in Medicine Section of CPT

99151-99153 assigned when sedation is provided by same physician performing procedure
99155-99157 assigned when another physician administers sedation
  • Trained observer must be present
    Decreased level of consciousness
    Codes divided by age (under 5, 5 and over) and time (15 minutes and each additional 15 minutes)

Anesthesia Formula

(B + T + M) × conversion factor = Anesthesia payment

B Is for Base Units

Published in *Relative Value Guide (RVG)* by American Society of Anesthesiologists
  National unit values for anesthesia services based on complexity of service

T Is for Time

Patient record indicates time, e.g., 60 minutes

Usually, 15 minutes = 1 unit
Example: 60 minutes = 4 units
Some payers may indicate 1 unit = 1 minute
Begins: Anesthesiologist begins to prepare patient for induction—preoperative
Continues throughout procedure—intraoperative
Ends: Patient no longer under care of anesthesiologist—postoperative

M Is for Modifying Unit

Additional units based on physical status of patient (see modifiers that follow)

Physical Status Modifiers, P1-P6

Located in Anesthesia Guidelines

Not reported to Medicare
Help to show complexity of service
- P1 Normal healthy
- P2 Mild systemic disease
- P3 Severe systemic disease
- P4 Severe systemic disease is constant threat to life
- P5 Not expected to survive without the operation
- P6 Clinically brain dead

Qualifying Circumstances Codes (99100-99140)

Anesthesia services provided under difficult circumstances

Located in both Anesthesia Guidelines and Medicine section
Listed in addition to primary anesthesia code
More than one may be reported

Summing Up Formula

Base units (from *RVG*) based on CPT codes

Time units (usually 15 min is a unit)
- Total time ÷ 15 = time units

Modifiers [Qualifying Circumstances (99100-99140) and/or Physical Status (P1-P6)]

Conversion Factors

CMS anesthesia conversion factors

Sum of money allocated by payer, per unit for payment of anesthesia services

Anesthesia for Multiple Surgical Procedures

Once anesthetized, length of time, not number of procedures performed during session

Report highest relative value guide (RVG) valued CPT code
Example: Two procedures during same session
- One, 10 base units; the other, 5 base units
- Report only 10 base units and combined time for all procedures

Anesthesia Modifiers

Anesthesia code reported twice
- Once for anesthesiologist
- Once for CRNA
  Each reports service on separate claim form
- One claim for anesthesiologist's service
- One claim for CRNA's service
  Anesthesia modifiers report supervision/direction circumstances
- AA, anesthesia services performed personally by anesthesiologist
- AD, medical supervision >4 concurrent procedures
- QK, medical direction of 2-4 concurrent procedures
- QX, CRNA service with medical direction
- QY, medical direction of 1 CRNA
- QZ, CRNA service without medical
  Anesthesia modifier always precedes the physical status modifier

---

PRACTICE EXERCISE 17.1 PERFORATED APPENDICITIS

Assign anesthesia code(s) and any necessary modifiers. Do not assign surgery codes. Do not assign diagnosis codes. During this procedure the anesthesiologist was medically directing two CRNAs providing anesthesia for concurrent procedures. The patient's physical status is P2.

OPERATIVE REPORT
LOCATION: Inpatient, Hospital
PATIENT: Laurence Hooper
ATTENDING PHYSICIAN: Gary Sanchez, MD
SURGEON: Gary Sanchez, MD
PREOPERATIVE DIAGNOSIS: Perforated appendicitis.
POSTOPERATIVE DIAGNOSIS: Same.
ANESTHESIA: General.
ANESTHESIOLOGIST: Janice E. Larson, MD
  PROCEDURE: The patient was brought to the operating room, placed under general anesthesia, and prepped and draped sterilely. The patient's advanced age is a concern, since he is 92. A right lower quadrant skin incision was made with a #10 blade, and dissection was carried down through the subcutaneous tissue using electrocautery. The anterior sheath of the rectus fascia was opened. The rectus was retracted medially. The posterior sheath and peritoneum were grasped with curved clamps and sharply incised, allowing entry into the peritoneal cavity. There were a few adhesions, which we took down sharply. We then delivered the appendix up and into the wound. We took down the mesoappendix between Kelly clamps and tied the vascular pedicles with 2–0

silk free ties. The base of the appendix was then crushed. It was tied with 0 Vicryl. It was inverted into the base of the cecum with a 3–0 silk pursestring suture. The abdomen was then irrigated with saline until returns were clear. We closed the posterior sheath and peritoneum with running 0 Vicryl, closed the anterior sheath with interrupted 0 Vicryl, and closed the skin with subcuticular 4–0 undyed Vicryl. Steri-Strips and sterile Band-Aids were applied. All sponge and needle counts were correct. Before the patient left the operating room, the wound was anesthetized with a total of 30 cc of 0.50% Sensorcaine with epinephrine solution.

CPT Code(s): _____

_____

Abstracting Questions

1. What is the main term referenced in the index of the CPT to locate the code? _____

_____

2. What was the subterm used in the CPT index to locate the anesthesia code? _____

_____

3. Does the quadrant entered to perform the surgical procedure affect CPT anesthesia code assignment? _____

_____

Continued

PRACTICE EXERCISE 17.1 PERFORATED APPENDICITIS—cont'd

4. Was the procedure at the abdominal wall or intraperitoneal?

_____

5. Were there any Qualifying Circumstances to report?

_____

6. Who decides what Physical Status Modifier should be reported? _____

_____

7. Was the anesthesiologist providing service or medically directing cases? _____

_____

PRACTICE EXERCISE 17.2 LEFT BREAST BIOPSY

Assign anesthesia code(s) only. Do not assign surgery codes. Do not assign diagnosis codes. The patient's physical status is P1.

OPERATIVE REPORT

LOCATION: Outpatient, Hospital

PATIENT: Adrienne Gardener

ATTENDING PHYSICIAN: Gary Sanchez, MD

SURGEON: Gary Sanchez, MD

PREOPERATIVE DIAGNOSIS: Left breast mass.

POSTOPERATIVE DIAGNOSIS: Same.

PROCEDURE PERFORMED: Left breast biopsy.

ANESTHESIA: Local with IV sedation and monitored anesthesia care.

ANESTHESIOLOGIST: Janice E. Larson, MD

   PROCEDURE: The patient was brought to the operating room, given IV sedation, and then anesthetized with a total of 30 cc of 1% Sensorcaine with epinephrine solution. Incision was made over the top of the mass with a #15 blade, and dissection was carried down through subcutaneous tissues sharply. We encountered the mass, which appeared to be a fibroadenoma. We excised this sharply. We got the entire lesion. We controlled bleeding with electrocautery. We then closed the skin with subcuticular 4–0 undyed Vicryl. Steri-Strips and sterile Band-Aids were applied. She tolerated this well and was taken to recovery room in stable condition.

   Pathology Report Later Indicated: Fibroadenoma.

CPT Code(s): _____

_____

Abstracting Questions

1. Do you report the sedation with CPT anesthesia codes or medicine codes? _____

_____

2. Was the procedure superficial (subcutaneous) or deep (internal structures)? _____

_____

PRACTICE EXERCISE 17.3 TAKEDOWN COLOSTOMY AND CHOLECYSTECTOMY

Assign anesthesia code(s) only. Do not assign surgery codes. Do not assign diagnosis codes. The anesthesiologist was supervising two concurrent procedures. The patient's physical status is P2.

OPERATIVE REPORT

LOCATION: Inpatient, Hospital

PATIENT: Simon Sulten

ATTENDING PHYSICIAN: Gary Sanchez, MD

SURGEON: Gary Sanchez, MD

PREOPERATIVE DIAGNOSES

   1. Colostomy for obstructing colon cancer.

   2. Symptomatic cholelithiasis.

POSTOPERATIVE DIAGNOSES: Same.

PROCEDURE PERFORMED

   1. Takedown colostomy with end-to-end colorectostomy.

   2. Open cholecystectomy.

ANESTHESIA: General.

ANESTHESIOLOGIST: Janice E. Larson, MD

   PROCEDURE: The patient was brought to the operating room, placed under general anesthesia, and prepped and draped sterilely. The previous midline was reopened with the #10 blade, and we excised the old scar. We carried out dissection through subcutaneous tissues using electrocautery. Midline fascia was divided sharply. We entered the peritoneal cavity and entered the midline fascia along the length of the incision. We took down numerous filmy adhesions and ran the small bowel from the terminal ileum to the ligament of Treitz, which appeared normal. First, we placed an Omni retractor and exposed the right upper quadrant. We identified the cystic duct and cystic artery and tied them off with 0 silk ties proximally and distally before transecting them. We then shelled the gallbladder from its fossa using electrocautery. We placed a pack up by the liver bed. We then identified the rectal stump and dissected this free. We then made an elliptical incision around the colostomy opening and carried our dissection down to fascia, freed up the stoma, and fired our TLC 75 stapler across the descending colon. We sent the specimen to pathology for permanent. We mobilized the left colon along the avascular line of Toldt up and around the splenic flexure. Once we had adequate length, we placed a Glassman clamp proximally on the rectum and distally on the descending colon. We then performed a two-layer, hand-sewn, end-to-end anastomosis with an outer layer of 3–0 silk Lembert and inner layer of running 3–0 Vicryl. There was a patent anastomosis, and we could easily milk contents through with no evidence of spilling. We then closed the fascia from the colostomy site with interrupted 0 Vicryl and running 0 PDS. We closed the skin with skin clips. All sponge and needle counts were correct. Patient tolerated this well and was taken to recovery in stable condition.

   CPT Code(s): _____

_____

Abstracting Question

1. Was a supervision modifier required? _____

_____

PRACTICE EXERCISE 17.4 INCISION AND DRAINAGE OF PERIRECTAL ABSCESS

Assign anesthesia code(s) only. Do not assign surgery codes. Do not assign diagnosis codes. The patient's physical status is P3.

OPERATIVE REPORT

LOCATION: Outpatient, Hospital

PATIENT: Suzy Tarsinski

ATTENDING PHYSICIAN: Gary Sanchez, MD

SURGEON: Gary Sanchez, MD

PREOPERATIVE DIAGNOSIS: Perirectal abscess.

POSTOPERATIVE DIAGNOSIS: Same.

PROCEDURE PERFORMED: Incision and drainage of perirectal abscess.

ANESTHESIA: Spinal.

ANESTHESIOLOGIST: Janice E. Larson, MD

  PROCEDURE: The patient was brought back to the operating room, and after a spinal anesthetic had been given, the area of the rectum was cleaned and draped in the usual fashion after the patient had been placed in a jackknife position. An incision was made over the top of this abscess with a #10-blade scalpel. We entered the abscessed cavity, which returned large amounts of purulent material. We broke up the loculations, debrided the necrotic tissue with a #10 blade, and irrigated with a liter of saline. We then were able to pack the cavity with sewed Kerlix. The patient tolerated the procedure well, and all sponges and needles were accounted for at the end of the procedure. Soon she could be transferred to the Post Anesthesia Care Unit in stable condition.

CPT Code(s): _____

_____

Abstracting Question

1. For the purpose of locating an anesthesia code in the CPT manual, what was the location of the I&D? _____

_____

PRACTICE EXERCISE 17.5 INTRACEREBRAL HEMATOMA

Assign anesthesia code(s) only. Do not assign surgery codes. Do not assign diagnosis codes. The patient is not expected to survive without this procedure.

OPERATIVE REPORT

LOCATION: Inpatient, Hospital

PATIENT: Suzy Kunklemann

ATTENDING PHYSICIAN: Gary Sanchez, MD

SURGEON: Gary Sanchez, MD

PREOPERATIVE DIAGNOSIS: Intracerebral hematoma, right temporal lobe.

POSTOPERATIVE DIAGNOSIS: Intracerebral hematoma, right temporal lobe.

PROCEDURE PERFORMED: Osteoplastic craniotomy, right temporal area; evacuation of intracerebral hematoma.

ANESTHESIA: General.

  PROCEDURE: This patient is not expected to survive without this procedure, and at this point we have no other choice but to proceed. Under general anesthesia, the patient's head was placed in the Mayfield pins. The right frontal temporoparietal area was prepped and draped in the usual manner. A linear incision was made extending from the midline of the temporal fossa up to the midportion of the scalp. The skin was incised. The temporalis muscle was separated and divided off the bone. I did a craniotomy here the size of a half dollar coin and made a burr hole. I utilized the craniotome to elevate the bone flap, which was a free bone flap. This was then removed. We placed the Weitlaners into the wound and then incised the dura in a cruciate fashion over the temporal lobe. I then entered the middle temple gyrus, irrigated much of the clot from the temporal and posterior parietal areas, and evacuated the clot from the area. This took copious irrigation. We used cotton balls for hemostasis. I did this numerous times until all the bleeders were coagulated. I then lined the cystic cavity with Gelfoam and coagulated the edges of the raw brain. I closed the dura with 4–0 Vicryl. This was closed in a watertight fashion. I used 2–0 Vicryl to elevate the dura to the bone flap with Wurzburg plates, two of them, using plates and screws. I then closed the scalp in one layer using 0 Vicryl on the temporalis muscle and fascia, and the skin was approximated with 2–0 nylon interrupted mattress sutures. Dressing was applied, and the patient was on the ventilator and discharged to the surgical intensive care unit.

CPT Code(s): _____

_____

Abstracting Question

1. Would a physical status modifier be required? _____

_____

18

CPT/HCPCS Level I Modifiers (-22 to -99)

Alters CPT or HCPCS code

Full list, CPT, Appendix A
- Two separate lists
  - One for physician use
  - One for hospital outpatient use

Modifier Functions

Altered (i.e., increased or reduced service)

Bilateral
Multiple
Only portions of service (i.e., professional service only)
More than one surgeon

-22 Increased Procedural Service

Indicates services significantly greater than usual

Accompanied by written report and supportive documentation

-23 Unusual Anesthesia

Use of general anesthesia where local or regional is norm

Example: Highly agitated senile patient
Used only with anesthesia codes
Written report with submission of modifier

-24 Unrelated E/M Services by Same Physician or Other Qualified Health Care Professional During a Postoperative Period

Service not related to surgery
    If E/M provided during postoperative global period, no payment considered without -24

-25 Significant, Separately Identifiable E/M Service, by Same Physician or Other Qualified Health Care Professional on the Same Day of the Procedure or Other Service

Documentation must support service
    Example: Patient seen for sinus congestion, provider performs H&P, prescribes decongestant, notes and removes lesion on back

Code: Procedure + E/M-25

-26 Professional Component

Professional component (physician, -26)
    Technical component (technician + equipment, -TC)

-32 Mandated Service

Mandated by payer, workers' comp, or official body or court of law
    Not request of patient, patient's family, or another physician
    Example: Workers' Compensation requests examination of person currently receiving disability benefits

-33 Preventive Services

Patient Protection and Affordable Care Act (PPACA) requires health insurance coverage of preventive services without cost
    US Preventive Services Task Force (USPSTF) grades preventive services:
- Grade A: High certainty that the net benefit is substantial
- Grade B: High certainty that the net benefit is moderate or there is a moderate certainty that the next benefit is moderate to substantial

Task Force list located at: https://www.uspreventiveservices taskforce.org/Page/Name/uspstf-a-and-b-recommendations/
Example of services:
- Grade A
- Topic: Blood pressure screening
- Description: The USPSTF recommends screening for high blood pressure in adults aged 18 and older.

-47 Anesthesia by Surgeon

Surgeon administers regional or general anesthesia

Physician acts as both surgeon and anesthesiologist
Used only with Surgery codes

-50 Bilateral Procedure

Organs that are bilateral

Example: Procedure on kidneys
Caution: Some codes describe bilateral procedures
Typically not used on Integumentary System codes

-51 Multiple Procedure—Three Types

1. Same procedure, different sites
2. Multiple operation(s), same operative session
3. Procedure performed multiple times
   - List most resource-intense procedure first, then descending order of resource intensity
   - Next, other procedure(s) + -51 (unless code is -51 exempt or add-on code) Usual procedure payment: 1st 100%, 2nd 50%, 3rd 25%-50%, depending on payer

-52 Reduced Services

Service reduced or not performed to the extent described in code description

There is no other code that accurately reflects the service actually provided
Physician directed reduction
Documentation substantiates reduction
Not to be used for patient unable to pay
Submit regular charge amount, payer will adjust

-53 Discontinued Procedure

Surgical/diagnostic procedures

Procedure started then stopped due to patient's condition
Does not apply to presurgical discontinuance
Submit regular charge, payer will adjust
DO NOT USE -53
- When patient cancels scheduled procedure
- With E/M codes
- With time-based code

-54 Surgical Care Only

Physician provides only procedure (intraoperative); other physician performs preoperative and postoperative service

Documented patient transfer must be in record
Some payers require copy of transfer order

-55 Postoperative Management Only

Physician provides only the care after hospital discharge; report surgical code + modifier -55

If transferred while patient hospitalized, report postoperative management with subsequent hospital codes 99231-99233
Documentation of transfer in medical record

-56 Preoperative Management Only

Physician provided only preoperative care; report surgical code + modifier -56

Not acceptable for Medicare
Usual reimbursement for portions, surgical package
- 10% preoperative
- 70% intraoperative
- 20% postoperative
Each payer determines reimbursement for portions

-57 Decision for Surgery

E/M, 99201-99499

Medicine, 92002, 92004, 92012, and 92014 ophthalmologic services
Medicare: Only for preoperative period of major surgery (day before or day of)

-58 Staged/Related Procedure or Service by Same Physician or Other Qualified Health Care Professional During Postoperative Period

Subsequent procedure planned at time of initial surgery
- During postoperative period of previous surgery in series
  Example: Multiple skin grafts completed in several sessions
- Do not use when code describes total sessions
  Example: 67208 destruction of lesion of retina, one or more sessions
- More extensive than original procedure or
- For therapy following diagnostic procedure (e.g., breast biopsy and subsequent mastectomy)

-59 Distinct Procedural Service

Used to report non-E/M services not normally reported together

- Different session or encounter
- Different procedure
- Different site

Separate incision, excision, lesion, injury

Example: Physician removes several lesions from patient's leg; also notes a suspicious lesion on torso and biopsies it

- Excision code for lesion removal + biopsy code for torso lesion with −59
- Indicates biopsy as distinct procedure, not part of lesion removal

CMS established four HCPCS subset modifiers:

- referred to as −X{EPSU} modifiers
- more descriptively define modifier -59
- payer specific

-62 Two Surgeons

Both function as cosurgeons (equals)

Usually of different specialties
Each reports same code + -62
Each dictates operative/procedure note for their portion
Total reimbursement = 125%; each physician = 62.5%

-63 Procedure Performed on Infants Less Than 4 kg

Kilogram = 2.2 pounds (4 kg = 8.8 lb)

Small size increases complexity
Use with all Surgery section codes except Integumentary System or directed otherwise (see parenthetical guideline following 63702)

-66 Surgical Team

Team: Several physicians with various specialties plus technicians and other support personnel

Very complex procedures
Payers may increase payment up to 50%
- Each physician's service must be documented in the medical record

-76 Repeat Procedure/Service by Same Physician or Other Qualified Health Care Professional

Assigned to indicate necessary service

Example: X-rays before and after fracture repair

-77 Repeat Procedure/Service by Another Physician or Other Qualified Health Care Professional

Performed by one physician, repeated by another physician

Submitted with written report to establish medical necessity and identity of performing physician
- Do not append to E/M codes

-78 Unplanned Return to Operating/ Procedure Room by the Same Physician or Other Qualified Health Care Professional Following Initial Procedure for a Related Procedure During Postoperative Period

For complication of first procedure
   Example: Patient had outpatient procedure in morning; was returned to operating room in afternoon with severe hemorrhage
Indicates not typographical error
- Medical record must specifically document need for service provided

-79 Unrelated Procedure or Service by Same Physician or Other Qualified Health Care Professional During Postoperative Period

Example: Several days after discharge for procedure, patient returns for unrelated problem

Diagnosis code would also be different

-80 Assistant Surgeon

Reimbursed at 15% to 30%

Payers identify procedures for which they reimburse assistant at surgery

-81 Minimum Assistant Surgeon

Services at a level less than that described in -80

Reimbursed at 10% if services reported with the modifier are recognized by payer

-82 Assistant Surgeon (When Qualified Resident Surgeon Not Available)

Teaching hospitals
- Have residents who assist as part of education
- Must demonstrate no qualified resident available to use -82
  - Unavailability must be documented in written report

-90 Reference (Outside) Laboratory

Physician has business relationship with outside lab

Physician pays lab
Physician bills payer for lab services

• **Figure 18.1** 3-6 CMS-1500 (02/12) allows for multiple placement of modifiers. (Courtesy U.S. Department of Health and Human Services, Centers for Medicare and Medicaid Services.)

-91 Repeat Clinical Diagnostic Laboratory Test

Repeat same laboratory tests on same day for multiple test results
- e.g., serial troponin levels for acute MI confirmation
  Not tests rerun to confirm or negate original test results
  Not assigned for malfunction of equipment, loss of specimen, or technician error

-92 Alternative Laboratory Platform Testing

Used to report a laboratory test using portable instrument or kit

Usually single use
  86701-86703 HIV testing

-95 Synchronous Telemedicine Services

Used when a provider and patient interact from separate locations

Star (★) symbol appears next to code.
  Reference full list of applicable codes in Appendix P.

-99 Multiple Modifiers

Used when service needs more than one modifier but payer allows for only one modifier with each code

CMS-1500 (Fig. 18.1)

HCPCS Level II Modifiers

Examples of HCPCS Anatomical Modifiers

-LT   Left side
-RT   Right side
-E1   Upper left, eyelid
-E2   Lower left, eyelid
-E3   Upper right, eyelid
-E4   Lower right, eyelid
-FA   Left hand, thumb
-F1   Left hand, second digit
-F2   Left hand, third digit
-F3   Left hand, fourth digit
-F4   Left hand, fifth digit
-F5   Right hand, thumb
-F6   Right hand, second digit
-F7   Right hand, third digit
-F8   Right hand, fourth digit
-F9   Right hand, fifth digit
-TA   Left foot, great toe
-T1   Left foot, second digit
-T2   Left foot, third digit
-T3   Left foot, fourth digit
-T4   Left foot, fifth digit
-T5   Right foot, great toe
-T6   Right foot, second digit
-T7   Right foot, third digit
-T8   Right foot, fourth digit
-T9   Right foot, fifth digit
-LC   Left circumflex coronary artery
-LD   Left anterior descending coronary artery
-RC   Right coronary artery
  Anatomical modifiers are not used with skin procedures
  Example: Removal of skin tags, any area
  Exception is with codes for procedures on sites including sweat glands, eyelids, and breasts

HCPCS Modifiers for Selective Identification of Subsets of Distinct Procedural Services (-59 Modifier)

-XE Separate Encounter

A service that is distinct because it occurred during a separate encounter

-XS Separate Structure

A service that is distinct because it was performed on a separate organ/structure

-XP Separate Practitioner

A service that is distinct because it was performed by a different practitioner

-XU Unusual Non-Overlapping Service

The use of a service that is distinct because it does not overlap usual components of the main service

Example: -XE
- Patient seen in the morning for a cardiovascular stress test and then later in the day patient returns for a rhythm ECG

- Patient is seen in the outpatient infusion center at 8:00 a.m. and seen again in the outpatient infusion center for another treatment at 6:00 p.m.

Example: -XS

- Patient seen for destruction and during procedure unrelated to the destruction the physician obtains tissue for pathologic examination
- Patient under goes a laparoscopy, surgical, ablation of one or more liver tumor(s) and during the surgery, patient has ultrasonic guidance for needle placement

Example: -XP

- Patient undergoes a hernia repair at 7:00 a.m. Later in the day the patient develops acute abdominal pain and returns for another physician to perform a surgical laparoscopic appendectomy

Example: -XU

- Patient seen for two separate lesions; a lipoma is excised on upper thigh region (3 cm), and a separate lipoma excised on the lower leg region (less than 3 cm)

PRACTICE EXERCISE 18.1 MASSIVE DEBRIDEMENT

OPERATIVE REPORT
LOCATION: Inpatient, Hospital
PATIENT: Pam Tieg
ATTENDING PHYSICIAN: Leslie Alanda, MD
SURGEON: Gary Sanchez, MD
PREOPERATIVE DIAGNOSES
1. Massive abdominal wound.
2. Status post multiple small-bowel fistula repair.
POSTOPERATIVE DIAGNOSES
1. Massive abdominal wound.
2. Status post multiple small-bowel fistula repair.
SURGICAL FINDINGS: There was a 28 × 50-cm open wound in the abdomen extending predominantly to the right over past the midline on the left with a more inferior extension near the inguinal ligament. The primary areas of concern were pockets that were at least 8 to 10 cm in diameter in their total dimensions that had undermined in the retroperitoneal space behind the bowel. This contained malodorous fat necrosis and other necrotic tissue, and the odor smelled like Gram-negative organisms. We noted that the bowel was anterior in this space and probably came down on the psoas muscle posteriorly on the right side. Also, there were various areas of fat necrosis overlying the superficial aspect of the wound and fat necrosis along the edges of the wound that was quite malodorous. Multiple cultures and sensitivities were obtained, particularly of the area around the ileostomy site, the large area of fat necrosis in the left side of the abdomen, and the two undermined retroperitoneal areas. There was some extrusion of the mesh with the surrounding coagulative necrosis superiorly.
SURGICAL PROCEDURE: Massive debridement of open abdominal wound and status post multiple enterotomy repairs, small bowel.
ANESTHESIA: General, administered through tracheostomy tube.
ESTIMATED BLOOD LOSS: Approximately 50 cc.
ADDENDUM: Dr. White was called to observe the wound at his request and advised us regarding the dissection retroperitoneally in the proximity of the bowel in the area.
PROCEDURE: The abdomen was prepped as well as possible considering the conditions with Betadine scrub and solution and draped in a routine sterile fashion. A major 3-cm area of fat necrosis was initially debrided, and I debrided multiple sites of fat necrosis over the exposed surface of the wound, and then along the marginal surface there were

multiple sites that were malodorous. Culture and sensitivity were obtained of the original fat necrosis area, the area around the ileostomy, and the more malodorous areas along the skin edges. We then, on the right side, lifted up the abdominal contents and dissected behind this, encountering foul-smelling, anaerobic-smelling collection of tissue, which probably consisted of old blood clot and fat necrosis. This was gently curetted out without entering the bowel. The bowel was in immediate proximity. We came down on what appeared to be the psoas area, which apparently connected with this pocket on the right side. We packed the right side with metronidazole-soaked Kerlix roll and vaginal packing, then also did the same on the left side. We covered the areas of the wound that were most accessible with fine mesh gauze soaked in metronidazole. ABD pads were then applied. The patient tolerated the procedure well and left the area in good condition.

CPT Code(s): _____

_____

ICD-10-CM Code(s): _____

Abstracting Questions

1. Was debridement superficial, deep, or both? _____

2. Was the skin debridement code selection affected by the infection? _____

_____

3. Does the skin debridement code include the retroperitoneal exploration? _____

_____

4. Was there a CPT code for re-exploration of a recent abdominal surgery site? _____

_____

5. Why would code 11008 not be reported? _____

_____

6. Were there different diagnosis codes required to report the necrotic status of abdominal fat, skin, and retroperitoneum?

_____

PRACTICE EXERCISE 18.2   NEVUS EXCISION

OPERATIVE REPORT

One week prior to this report, Dr. Erickson, plastic surgeon, removed a portion of a nevus from the right arm of Leonardo Zapata. Dr. Erickson believed that a further excision was necessary but wanted another opinion. Mr. Zapata was referred to Dr. Matalo to obtain his opinion on the further excision (staged procedure). Dr. Matalo recommended further excision, and today Dr. Erickson performed the other surgery. The follow-up for the first procedure was 10 days.

LOCATION: Outpatient, Hospital

PATIENT: Leonardo Zapata

PRIMARY CARE PHYSICIAN: Ronald Green, MD

SURGEON: Mark Erickson, MD

   INDICATION: This patient had a 1-cm lesion excised from the right arm approximately 1 week ago. There was a question as to whether or not this was a Spitz nevus versus melanoma, and this was referred to Dr. Matalo at the New York Clinic for a second opinion. His opinion was that this was a Spitz nevus, and further conservative excision was recommended if that had not already been done. Since we only took a 5-mm margin, we are going to take about another 1 cm or so off around the previously excised area.

PREOPERATIVE DIAGNOSIS: Spitz nevus, right arm.

POSTOPERATIVE DIAGNOSIS: Spitz nevus, right arm.

SURGICAL FINDINGS: A healed incision of the right arm 2 cm in diameter.

ANESTHESIA: Six cc of 1% Xylocaine with 1:100,000 epinephrine.

   PROCEDURE: The arm was prepped with Betadine solution and draped in the routine sterile fashion. The lesion was anesthetized and excised elliptically. Bleeders were electrocoagulated, and the wound was closed with interrupted subcuticular 3–0 Monocryl sutures and two twists of 4–0 Prolene. Half-inch Steri-Strips were applied. The patient tolerated the procedure well and left the area in good condition. He will use the sling that he used with his previous incision.

   Pathology Report Later Indicated: Nevus, right arm, re-excision. Skin showing biopsy site with fibrosis, granulation tissue, and suture.

CPT Code(s): _____

ICD-10-CM Code(s): _____

_____

Abstracting Questions

1. Is a modifier required to indicate the patient is in the global period from a previous procedure? _____

2. What modifier reports a more extensive procedure than the initial procedure performed during the global period of a previous procedure? _____

_____

_____

3. What was the excised diameter of the initial excision?

_____

4. What is the excised diameter for the re-operation? _____

_____

PRACTICE EXERCISE 18.3   ECHOCARDIOGRAM

Remember to report only the profession portion of the service when the physician is not an employee of the facility in which the service is being provided.

ECHOCARDIOGRAM REPORT

LOCATION: Outpatient, Hospital

PATIENT: Loralee Branigan

ATTENDING/ADMIT PHYSICIAN: James Noonar, MD

RADIOLOGIST: Morton Monson, MD

PERSONAL PHYSICIAN: Ronald Green, MD

INDICATIONS: Valvular heart disease, atrial fibrillation, left ventricular dysfunction.

   The M-Mode echo measurements are listed on the accompanying data sheet. They are essentially within normal limits.

   The two-dimensional echocardiogram clearly demonstrates some thickening and calcification of the mitral valve leaflets as well as thickening of the aortic valve leaflets. The aortic valve opening is normal, and the mitral valve opening is probably normal as well. Left ventricular contractility is definitely diminished. The ejection fraction is in the range of about 20-25% only.

   The Doppler and color Doppler studies do confirm the presence of mild tricuspid insufficiency. The RV systolic pressure is 32 mm Hg, which is consistent with mild pulmonary hypertension.

   CONCLUSION: Depression of left ventricular function, as described above, with mild valvular pathology, as described above.

CPT Code(s): _____

ICD-10-CM Code(s): _____

Abstracting Questions

1. What approach was used for the cardiac echocardiogram?

_____

2. Is the Doppler study also reported? _____

_____

3. Is the Doppler color flow study reported? _____

_____

4. What modifier is required on the CPT code? _____

_____

PRACTICE EXERCISE 18.4 CERVICAL CERCLAGE PREOPERATIVE EXAMINATION

LOCATION: Outpatient, Clinic
PATIENT: Chandelle Jackson
ATTENDING PHYSICIAN: Andy Martinez, MD
SURGEON: Andy Martinez, MD
ADMITTING DIAGNOSIS: Decreased cervical length with suspected incompetent cervix.
PROCEDURE PLANNED: Cervical cerclage.

HISTORY OF PRESENT ILLNESS: The patient is a 26-year-old woman, gravida 5, para 2, whose last menstrual period was August 12 of this year, giving her an estimated date of confinement of May 17 of next year. This presently places her at 19 weeks and 3 days gestation. Her due date has been confirmed by pelvic ultrasound, the earliest of which was at 15 weeks gestation. We suspect possible incompetent cervix. The patient does have a history of two preterm deliveries, the first was 3 years ago in March when she delivered at 32 weeks after a 7-hour labor. Her previous obstetrician had therefore discussed with her that perhaps a cervical cerclage would be appropriate. Her history did not seem overly convincing for incompetent cervix. She had had LEEP procedure about 5 years ago. She then had a miscarriage the following year, for which she had a D&C, and then had a therapeutic abortion 2 years later. I have been following cervical length on this pregnancy. On initial scan at 15 weeks' gestation, cervical length was not performed but a week later was found to be 2.7 cm. Follow-up ultrasound done at 17 weeks' gestation showed cervical length to be 3.1 cm. The most recent ultrasound from 19 weeks' gestation showed cervical length decreased to 2.5 cm, and with the patient's questionable history the decision has been made to proceed with cervical cerclage.

OBSTETRIC AND GYNECOLOGIC HISTORY: As noted above.

PAST MEDICAL AND SURGICAL HISTORY: The patient had a tonsillectomy at age 14 and a hallux vagus correction at age 20.

MEDICATIONS: Prenatal vitamins.
PHYSICAL EXAMINATION: Blood pressure: 108/60. Height: 5'6". Weight: 132 lb. Lungs: Clear to auscultation bilaterally. Heart: Sounds normal. Abdomen: Gravid with uterus palpable at the level of the umbilicus. Fetal heart rate is in the 140s. Bimanual examination was carried out, and the cervix is long, soft, and closed.

ASSESSMENT AND PLAN: The patient has had two previous preterm deliveries with history questionable for incompetent cervix, and now has decreased cervical length of 2.5 cm on ultrasound at 19 weeks' gestation. After discussing risks and alternatives, the patient has consented to proceed with cervical cerclage. She is aware of the risks, such as general anesthetic, hemorrhage, infection, ruptured membranes, and ultimately loss of the pregnancy. She does, however, consent to proceed, and the surgery has been scheduled for tomorrow.

CPT Code(s): _____

_____

ICD-10-CM Code(s): _____

_____

Abstracting Questions

1. What section of the CPT would be referenced to locate a code to report the service provided in this report? _____

_____

2. Was the patient admitted to the hospital after the clinic examination? _____

_____

PRACTICE EXERCISE 18.5 ETHMOIDECTOMY, SPHENOIDOTOMY, AND SEPTOPLASTY

Ready for a challenge? This case will give your coding skills an excellent workout. There will be five service codes and five diagnosis codes. The most extensive procedure is the septoplasty, and that code will be sequenced first.
LOCATION: Outpatient, Hospital
PATIENT: Russell Price
ATTENDING PHYSICIAN: Jeff King, MD
SURGEON: Jeff King, MD
PREOPERATIVE DIAGNOSES
  1. Septal deviation.
  2. Bilateral sinonasal polyposis.
  3. Pansinusitis.
  4. Bilateral inferior turbinate hypertrophy.
  5. Nasal obstruction.
POSTOPERATIVE DIAGNOSIS: Same as Preoperative.
PROCEDURES PERFORMED
  1. Bilateral endoscopic total ethmoidectomy.
  2. Bilateral endoscopic maxillary antrostomy with removal of polyps from maxillary sinus.
  3. Bilateral endoscopic sphenoidotomy.
  4. Septoplasty.
  5. Bilateral inferior turbinate overfracture.
ANESTHESIA: Endotracheal.

INDICATIONS: A 43-year-old male with history of nasal trauma that resulted in a septal deviation. He also has a history of bilateral sinonasal polyposis and has undergone prior polypectomy and sinus surgery. The patient now has recurrent disease. This was confirmed on examination and the CT scan. He also has bilateral inferior turbinate hypertrophy. The patient also has a history of severe snoring. He is to undergo correction of his nasal obstruction and sinusitis to see if that will help. If not, further evaluation of his snoring will be done.

PROCEDURE: After consent was obtained, the patient was taken to the operating room and placed on the operating table in supine position. After an adequate level of general endotracheal anesthesia was obtained, the patient was positioned for nasal and sinus surgery. The patient's nose was packed with cotton pledgets soaked with 4% cocaine. After several minutes, 1% Xylocaine with 1:100,000 epinephrine was infiltrated into the nasal portion of the polyps as well as the septum bilaterally and the inferior turbinates. Nasal hairs were trimmed. Attention was first focused on the right side. Using the 5-degree sinuscope and the microdebrider, the nasal portions of the polyps were removed. Polyps were noted both medial and lateral to the middle turbinate. There was also some scarring from the middle turbinate to the lateral nasal

PRACTICE EXERCISE 18.5   ETHMOIDECTOMY, SPHENOIDOTOMY, AND SEPTOPLASTY—cont'd

wall. This scar tissue was also removed with a microdebrider. Subsequently, polyps in the middle meatus and anterior posterior ethmoid areas were removed with microdebrider.

The maxillary sinus ostia area was cleared of polyps, and then the ostium was widened in a posterior-to-inferior direction. Polyps within the sinus near the ostia were also removed. The area was then packed with cotton pledgets soaked with 1:50,000 units of epinephrine. Attention was then focused on the left side, where a similar procedure was performed. Again, polyps were noted to be both medial and lateral to the middle turbinate remnant. Polyps were obstructing the maxillary sinus drainage area and were also cleared. The left side was packed with a pledget soaked with epinephrine solution. Attention was refocused on the right side, where further polyps were removed from the sphenoid/ethmoid area. Remnant of the superior turbinate was also cleared of polyps. The sphenoid sinus ostium was cleared of polyps. The area was then packed with cotton pledget soaked with epinephrine solution. Similar procedure was then performed on the left side. Attention was then focused on the nasal septum. Utilizing a right hemitransfixion incision, mucoperichondrium and mucoperiosteal flaps were elevated. The cartilaginous septum was noted to be severely attenuated and deviated with several fractured areas. Deviated portions were removed. This does not leave much support for the nasal tip area. If this is a problem in the future, this will need to be reconstructed. The deviated portion of the bony septum and spurs off the maxillary crest were then removed.

Attention was then focused on the inferior turbinates, which were outfractured. The hemitransfixion incision was then closed with an interrupted 4–0 chromic suture. A quilting suture of 4–0 plain gut was then performed. The pledgets in the sinus area were then removed. There was some oozing from the ethmoid as well as the sphenoid sinus areas. As such, these areas were coated with FloSeal and then packed lightly with strips of Surgicel soaked with local solutions. Bacitracin ointment was then applied. Silastic splints were then placed on both sides of the nasal septum and secured with nylon suture. The nose was then packed bilaterally. Packs consisted of a Merocel sponge with a gloved finger coated with Bacitracin ointment. It was inflated with location solution. Nasal dressing was applied.

The patient tolerated the procedure well, and there was no break in technique. The patient was extubated and taken to the postanesthetic care unit in good condition. Fluids administered included 2000 cc RL. Blood loss was less than 150 cc. Preoperative medications included 12 mg Decadron and 1 gram Ancef IV.

CPT Code(s): _____

_____

ICD-10-CM Code(s): _____

Abstracting Questions

1. Maxillary Sinus
   a. Were polyps/tissue removed? _____

   _____

   b. What additional work was done to this sinus? _____

   _____

2. Sphenoid Sinus
   a. Were polyps/tissue removed? _____

   _____

3. Ethmoid Sinus
   a. Were polyps/tissue removed? _____

   _____

   b. Was this anterior, posterior, or both? _____

   _____

4. Inferior Turbinates
   a. Was there specific work done on this area? _____

   _____

5. What modifiers were appended extensively to the majority of CPT codes that reported the services provided in this case? _____

   _____

6. What does the diagnosis "pansinusitis" indicate? _____

   _____

Surgery Section (10021-69990)

Largest CPT Section

Section Format

Divided by subspecialty, e.g., Integumentary, Cardiovascular

Notes and Guidelines

Throughout section
  Information varied and extensive
  "Must" reading
  Subsection notes apply to entire subsection
  Subheading notes apply to entire subheading
  Category notes apply to entire category
  Parenthetical information (Fig. 19.1)

Unlisted Procedure Codes

Used only when more specific code not found in Category I or Category III

Written report accompanies submission
Each unlisted code service paid on case-by-case basis

Separate Procedures

"(Separate procedure)" follows code description

Usually minor surgical procedure
Incidental to more major procedure:
  • Breast biopsy before radical mastectomy would not be reported unless results of biopsy resulted in mastectomy, modifier-59 appended to biopsy code
  • Appendectomy performed incidentally when other abdominal surgery is performed
Separate procedures reported when
  • Only procedure performed
  • With another procedure
    • On different site
    • Unrelated to major procedure

Major Guideline of Surgical Packages

Usually include
• Preoperative (before, preop)
• E/M service subsequent to decision for surgery but prior to surgery date

• Intraoperative (during, intraop)
• Postoperative (after—also known as global period, postop)
  • Post-anesthesia recovery (PAR)
  • Follow-up office visits
• Local/topical anesthesia and digital block
  To report these bundled services separately is "unbundling"
  Remember to use modifiers during global period for unrelated E/M, return to OR, etc.

Supplies

Supplies that are beyond those typically included in the procedure are reported separately
  Example: Report surgical tray with
• 99070 CPT, Medicine section
• A4550 HCPCS

Special Report

Submitting an unlisted service or one that is unusual, variable, or new may require a special report, as listed in Guidelines

Demonstrates medical necessity/appropriateness of service
Contains pertinent information describing service in terms of
  • Nature
  • Extent
  • Need for procedure
  • Time
  • Effort
  • Equipment necessary
  May also include complexity of symptoms, final diagnosis, physical findings, procedures, concurrent problems, and follow-up care

General Subsection (10021, 10022)

Fine needle aspirations with or without (w/wo) imaging guidance
  Pathology 88172, 88173, and 88177 are for evaluation of fine needle aspirate

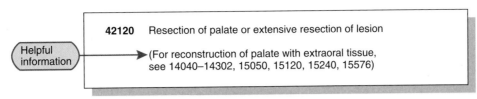

Helpful information

| 42120 | Resection of palate or extensive resection of lesion |

(For reconstruction of palate with extraoral tissue, see 14040–14302, 15050, 15120, 15240, 15576)

• **Figure 19.1** Parenthetical information in the CPT manual.

Integumentary System Subsection (10040-19499)

Often used in all specialties of medicine

Not just surgeons or dermatologists; wide range of physicians
Subheadings of Integumentary Subsection
- Skin, Subcutaneous, and Accessory Structures
- Nails
- Pilonidal Cyst
- Introduction
- Repair (Closure)
- Destruction
- Breast

Skin, Subcutaneous and Accessory Structures (10030-11646)

Introduction and Removal (10030-10036)

Report percutaneous image-guided fluid drainage of a catheter collection from soft tissue
- Example: Abscess, seroma, cyst, hematoma, or lymphocele
  Reported once for each individual collection drained
  Report codes 10035, 10036 for placement of soft tissue markers

Incision and Drainage (10040-10180)

I&D of abscess, carbuncle, boil, cyst, infection, hematoma, pilonidal cyst
- Lancing (cutting of skin)
- Aspiration (removal by puncturing lesion with a needle and withdrawing fluid)
  Gauze or tube may be inserted for continued drainage

Excision—Debridement (11000-11047)

Dead tissue cut away and washed away with sterile saline

11000, 11001 Eczematous or infected skin
11004-11006 Debridement of infected area based on location and depth of necrotizing tissue (subcutaneous tissue, muscle, and fascia)
+11008 Removal of prosthetic material or mesh from abdominal wall
11010-11012 Foreign material with open fracture or dislocation
- Skin, subcutaneous tissue, muscle fascia, muscle, and bone
  11042-11044 Subcutaneous tissue, muscle, bone

- Debridement partial thickness based on 20 square centimeters or less
11045-11047 Based on each additional 20 square centimeters

Paring or Cutting (11055-11057)

Removal by scraping or peeling (e.g., removal of corn or callus)
  Codes indicate number: 1, 2-4, 4+

Biopsy (11100, 11101)

Skin, subcutaneous tissue, or mucous membrane biopsy

Not all of lesion removed
- All lesion removed = excision
Do not use modifier -51
Codes indicate number: 1 or each additional
Tissue removed during excision, shaving, etc., and submitted to pathology is NOT reported separately as a biopsy
- Rather, it is included in the code for the excision

Skin Tag Removal (11200, 11201)

Benign lesions

Removed with scissors, blade, chemicals, electrosurgery, etc.
Do not use -51
- Codes indicate number: Up to and including 15 lesions and each additional 10 lesions or part thereof

Shaving of Lesions (11300-11313)

Removed by transverse incision or sliced horizontally

Based on
- Size (e.g., 1.1-2.0 cm)
- Location (e.g., arm, hand, nose)
Does not require suture closure
- Report most extensive lesion first with no modifier, then least extensive lesions with modifier -51

Benign/Malignant Lesions (11400-11646)

Codes divided: Benign or malignant

Physician assesses lesion as benign or malignant
Codes include local anesthesia and simple closure
Report each excised lesion separately
Lesion size
- Taken from physician's notes
- Includes greatest diameter plus narrowest margins of two sides (Fig. 19.2)

• **Figure 19.2** Calculating the size of a lesion.

Example: A benign lesion measuring 0.5 cm at widest point is removed with 0.5-cm margin at narrowest point (each side, 0.5 + 0.5 = 1.0 cm). Reported as 1.5-cm lesion excision (11402)
- Do not take size from pathology report—storage solution shrinks tissue
- Margins (healthy tissue) are also taken for comparison with unhealthy tissue
- Re-excisions following initial excision of malignant lesion coded as excision of malignant lesion

All excised tissue pathologically examined
Codes 11400-11646 report excision of lesion
Destroyed lesions have no pathology samples
Example: Laser or chemical
Lesion closure
- Simple or subcutaneous closure included in removal
- Reported separately
  - Layered or intermediate, 12031-12057 (Repair—Intermediate)
  - Complex, 13100-13153 (Repair—Complex)

Nails (11719-11765)

Includes toes and fingers

Types of services
- Trimming, debridement, removal, biopsy, repair

Pilonidal Cyst (11770-11772)

Codes divided by
- Simple
- Extensive
- Complicated

Introduction (11900-11983)

Types of services
- Lesion injections (therapeutic or diagnostic), tattooing, tissue expansion, contraceptive insertion/removal,

hormone implantation services, and insertion/removal of non-biodegradable drug delivery implant

Repair (Closure) (12001-13160)
Repair Factors in Wound Repair

As types of wounds vary, types of wound repair also vary
    Length, complexity (simple, intermediate, complex), and site must be documented
- Length measured in centimeters
- Measured prior to closure

Types of Wound Repair

Simple. Superficial, epidermis, dermis, or subcutaneous tissue
- One-layer closure
- Dermabond closure
- Medicare report Dermabond closure with G0168
Intermediate. Layered closure of deeper layers of subcutaneous tissue and superficial fascia with skin closure
- Single-layer closure can be coded as intermediate if extensive debridement required
Complex. Greater than layered; may include multiple layers of tissue and fascia or extensive debridement
Example: Scar revision, complicated debridement, extensive undermining, stents, extensive retention sutures

Included in Wound Repair Codes

Simple ligation of vessels in an open wound
Simple exploration of nerves, blood vessels, and exposed tendons
Normal debridement
- Additional codes for debridement can be used when
  - Gross contamination requires prolonged cleaning
  - Appreciable amounts of devitalized/contaminated tissue are removed to expose healthy tissue
  - Debridement is provided without immediate primary closure

Grouping of Wound Repair

Add together lengths by
- **Complexity** of Wound
  - Simple, intermediate, complex
- **Location** of Wound
  - e.g., face, ears, eyelids, nose, lips
    1 inch = 2.54 cm
      Example: **Same complexity, same codes description location:** Intermediate repairs of 2.9-cm laceration of leg and 1.1-cm laceration of buttocks. 2.9 + 1.1 = 4.0 cm (12032)
      Example: **Different complexity:** Intermediate repair of 2.9-cm laceration of leg and simple repair of 1.1-cm laceration of buttocks. 2.9-cm intermediate repair (12032) and 1.1-cm simple repair (12001)
      Example: **Same complexity, different code description locations:** Intermediate repair of 2.9-cm laceration of leg and intermediate repair

of 1.1-cm laceration of nose. 2.9-cm intermediate repair of leg (12032) and 1.1-cm intermediate repair of nose (12051)

Do Not Group Wound Repairs That Are

Different complexities

Example: Simple repair and complex repair
Different locations as stated in the code description
Example: Simple repairs of scalp (12001) and nose (12011)

Adjacent Tissue Transfer, Flaps, and Grafts (14000-15778)

Information Needed to Code Graft

Type of graft—adjacent, free flap, etc.

Donor site (from)
Recipient site (to)
Any repair to donor site
Size of graft

Adjacent Tissue Transfer/Rearrangement (14000-14350)

Includes lesion excision and/or repair (e.g., Z-plasty, W-plasty, V-plasty, Y-plasty, rotation flap, advancement flap)

Codes based on size and location of graft
Primary defect results from excision of lesion
Secondary defect results from formation of flap
To select code, add the size of the primary and secondary defects together

Skin Replacement Surgery (15002-15431)

15002-15005 Site preparation based on size and site
15040-15261 Autografts/Tissue Cultured Autografts
* 15050-15431 Autograft codes by type and size
* 15271-15278 Skin substitute grafts
  Split-thickness: Epidermis and some dermis (Fig. 19.3)
  Full-thickness: Epidermis and all dermis

Allografts (15300-15431)
Bilaminate skin substitute
* Artificial skin, such as silicone-covered biodegradable collagen matrix
  Allograft: Donor graft
  Xenograft: Nonhuman donor
  Code is based on recipient site, not donor site

Flaps (15570-15776)
Some skin left attached to blood supply
* Keeps flap viable
  Donor site may be far from recipient site
  Flaps may be in stages
  Codes divided by location and size
  Formation of flap (15570-15576)

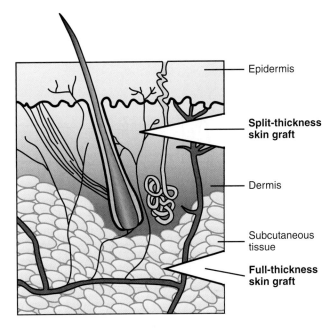

• **Figure 19.3** Split-thickness and full-thickness skin grafts.

* Based on recipient location: Trunk, scalp, nose, etc.
  Transfer of flap (15650): Previously placed flap released from donor site
* Also known as walking or walk up of flap
* 15777 is an add-on code to report soft tissue reinforcement with biological implants

Muscle, Myocutaneous, or Fasciocutaneous Flaps (15733-15738)
* Based on recipient location; head and neck, trunk, upper or lower extremity
* Repairs made with
  * Muscle
  * Muscle and skin
  * Fascia and skin
* Flaps rotated from donor to recipient site
* Includes closure donor site unless skin graft or local flaps are necessary

Other Procedures (15780-15879)

Many cosmetic procedures including:
* Dermabrasion
* Chemical peel
* Blepharoplasty
* Rhytidectomy
* Excessive skin excision

Pressure (Decubitus) Ulcers (15920-15999)

Excision and various closures
* Primary, skin flap, muscle, etc.
  Many codes "with ostectomy"
* Bone removal
  Locations
* Coccygeal (end of spine)

• **Figure 19.4** The Rule of Nines is used to calculate burn area on an adult.

Relative percentage of body surface areas (% BSA) affected by growth

	0 yr	1 yr	5 yr	10 yr	15 yr
a – 1/2 of head	9 1/2	8 1/2	6 1/2	5 1/2	4 1/2
b – 1/2 of 1 thigh	2 3/4	3 1/4	4	4 1/4	4 1/2
c – 1/2 of lower leg	2 1/2	2 1/2	2 3/4	3	3 1/4

• **Figure 19.5** Lund-Browder chart for estimating the extent of burns on children.

- Sacral (between hips)
- Ischial (lower hip)
- Trochanteric (outer hip)
  Site preparation only: 15936, 15937, 15946, 15956, or 15958
- Defect repair of donor site reported separately

Burns Local Treatment (16000-16036)

Codes for small, medium, and large
  Must calculate percentage of body burned using Rule of Nines for adults (Fig. 19.4)
- <5% small
- 5% to 10% medium
- >10% large
  Lund-Browder for children (Fig. 19.5)
- Proportions of children differ from adults
- Heads are larger
  Often require multiple debridements and redressing
  Based on
- Initial treatment of 1st-degree burn (16000)
- Size
  Report percent of burn and depth

Destruction (17000-17286)

Ablation (destruction) of tissue
- Laser, electrosurgery, cryosurgery, chemosurgery, etc.
- Benign/premalignant or malignant tissue
- Malignant tissue is based on location and size of lesion
- Benign/premalignant is based on the number of lesions removed/destroyed or size (sq cm)

Mohs Micrographic Surgery (17311-17315)

Surgeon acts as pathologist and surgeon
  Removes one layer of lesion at a time
  Continues until no malignant cells remain
  Based on stages and number of specimens per stage indicated in medical record

Other Procedures (17340-17999)

Treatment of acne
- Cryotherapy
- Chemical exfoliation
- Electrolysis
- Unlisted procedures

Breast Procedures (19000-19499)

Divided based on procedure
- Incision
- Excision
- Introduction
- Mastectomy Procedures
- Repair and/or Reconstruction
  Use excision of lesion codes if entire lesion is removed during incisional biopsy
  Use additional code for placement of radiological marker
  Mastectomies based on extent of procedure
- Wide excision
- Removal of neoplasm, capsule, and surrounding margins
- Radical
- Wide excision and anatomical structure surrounding neoplasm
  Example: Muscle or fascia

- Conservative partial mastectomy in which lesion is removed with adequate margins (19301)
- Axillary dissection and partial mastectomy, 19302
- Radical and modified radical (19305, 19306, and 19307) based on extent
  Confirm whether pectoral muscles, axillary, or internal lymph nodes were removed
  19307 most common and includes breast and axillary lymph node removal
  Code removal of lymph nodes separately unless included in code description
  Bilateral procedures, use -50

Biopsy/Removal of Lesion

Incisional biopsy: Incision made into lesion and small portion of lesion removed

Excisional biopsy: Entire lesion removed
Open incisional biopsy most complex (19101)

Percutaneous needle core biopsy without imaging guidance (19100)
- Same procedure with imaging guidance based on guidance method:
  - 19081, 19082, stereotactic
  - 19083, 19084, ultrasound
  - 19085, 19086, magnetic resonance
Complete, simple removal of a mass is reported with 19120

Lesion may be preoperatively marked with localization devices (clip, metallic pellet, wire, needle, radioactive seed) based on guidance method:
- 19281, 19282, mammographic
- 19283, 19284, stereotactic
- 19285, 19286, ultrasound
- 19287, 19288, magnetic resonance

PRACTICE EXERCISE 19.1 EXCISION, CHEEK LESION

OPERATIVE REPORT
LOCATION: Outpatient, Hospital
PATIENT: Mary Carbono
ATTENDING PHYSICIAN: Gary Sanchez, MD
SURGEON: Gary Sanchez, MD
PREOPERATIVE DIAGNOSIS: Right cheek lesion, unspecified behavior.
POSTOPERATIVE DIAGNOSIS: Right cheek lesion, unspecified behavior.
PROCEDURE PERFORMED: Excision of lesion, right cheek.
ANESTHESIA: General anesthetic by inhalational mask technique.
PROCEDURE: Following informed consent from the patient's mother, the patient was taken to the operating room and placed supine on the operating room table. The appropriate monitoring devices were placed on the patient, and general anesthesia was induced. It was maintained by inhalation mask technique. The right cheek was prepped and draped in a sterile fashion. The lesion, which was about 1.6 cm, somewhat raised, and erythematous, was injected at its base with 0.5 cc of 1% Xylocaine with 1:100,000 epinephrine. A #15-blade scalpel was used to perform a shave excision. No suture was placed. A sterile bandage was applied. The patient tolerated the procedure well. She was allowed to recover from general anesthesia and was transferred to the recovery room in good condition.
Pathology Report Later Indicated: Benign lesion of cheek.

CPT Code(s): _____

_____

ICD-10-CM Code(s): _____

_____

Abstracting Questions

1. What method was used to excise the lesion? _____

_____

2. Does the pathologic status of the report affect CPT code assignment? _____

_____

3. Does the size and location of the lesion affect CPT code assignment? _____

_____

4. Does the pathologic status of the lesion affect the diagnosis code? _____

_____

PRACTICE EXERCISE 19.2 RIGHT BREAST WIDE EXCISION

OPERATIVE REPORT
LOCATION: Outpatient, Hospital
PATIENT: Jane Doe
ATTENDING PHYSICIAN: Gary Sanchez, MD
SURGEON: Gary Sanchez, MD
PREOPERATIVE DIAGNOSIS: Mass, right breast.
POSTOPERATIVE DIAGNOSIS: Mass, right breast.
OPERATIVE PROCEDURE: Right breast mass excision.
PROCEDURE: With the patient under general anesthesia, the breast and chest were prepped and draped in a sterile manner. An elliptical incision was made about the palpated mass, including the area around the nipple. This was excised all the way down to the fascia of the breast and then submitted for frozen section. Frozen section revealed a carcinoma of the breast with what appeared to be a good margin all the way around it. We then maintained hemostasis with electrocautery and proceeded to close the breast tissue using 2-0 and 3-0 chromic. The skin was closed using 4-0 Vicryl in a subcuticular manner. Steri-Strips were applied. The patient tolerated the procedure well and was discharged from the operating room in stable condition.
Pathology Report Later Indicated: Primary, malignant neoplasm of the right breast nipple.

Continued

PRACTICE EXERCISE 19.2 RIGHT BREAST WIDE EXCISION—cont'd

CPT Code(s): _____

ICD-10-CM Code(s): _____

Abstracting Questions

1. Does the pathologic status of the lesion affect CPT code assignment? _____

2. Does the size of the lesion affect CPT code assignment?

3. Does the pathologic status of the lesion affect the diagnosis code? _____

4. Does the location of the lesion affect the diagnosis code? _____

5. Does the gender of the patient affect either code? _____

PRACTICE EXERCISE 19.3 THENAR FLAP COVERAGE

OPERATIVE REPORT

Assign an external cause code to indicate how this injury occurred in addition to the diagnosis and service codes.

LOCATION: Outpatient, Hospital
PATIENT: Leslie May
ATTENDING PHYSICIAN: Gary Sanchez, MD
SURGEON: Gary Sanchez, MD
PREOPERATIVE DIAGNOSIS: Oblique volar amputation tip, right middle finger, while working on machinery.
POSTOPERATIVE DIAGNOSIS: Oblique volar amputation tip, right middle finger, while working on machinery.
PROCEDURE: Thenar flap coverage, tip, right middle finger.
ANESTHESIA: General.
PROCEDURE: The patient was brought to the operating room, and general anesthesia was induced. Right upper extremity was prepped with Betadine and draped in a sterile fashion. The limb was exsanguinated with a tourniquet inflated to 250 mm Hg for 45 minutes. Using 4× magnification loupes, we debrided the fingertip. It was a volar oblique amputation. However, there was loss of distal phalanx down to about half of the sterile nail matrix. We trimmed the nail plate back to the level of the bone, we debrided the wound, and it was quite clean. We then fabricated a thenar flap using a piece of paper glove as a template. We traced this out on the thenar eminence. We then incised this and elevated the flap with fatty tissue. The radialward digital nerve to the index finger was exposed, and we covered this over with muscle with 4–0 Vicryl suture. We next harvested a split-thickness skin graft from the ulnar aspect of the hand using the Davol dermatome. We then placed this graft in place and sutured it over the defect in the palm with 5–0 Vicryl suture. Tegaderm was then placed over the donor site on the ulnar aspect of the hand.

We then placed the finger down in the palm and then attached the flap with interrupted 5–0 nylon sutures. This covered the defect on the finger nicely. We next applied Xeroform over all wounds and applied wet cotton balls over the graft site to hold it in place, then placed as compression a hand bandage with fluffs, Kerlix, Kling, and plaster splints immobilizing the hand in an intrinsic plus position. The tourniquet was released, and good circulation returned to the hand.

The patient tolerated the procedure well. She went to the recovery room in excellent condition. She will be dismissed as an outpatient today with plans for follow-up back in the office in appropriately 2 weeks.

CPT Code(s): _____

ICD-10-CM Code(s): _____

Abstracting Questions

1. Was this an adjacent tissue transfer flap? _____

2. Was the CPT code selection based on the recipient or donor site? _____

3. Can the split-thickness skin graft for repair of the donor site be reported separately? _____

4. What HCPCS modifier would be appropriate to append to the CPT code reported for the formation of the pedicle flap? _____

5. Does the way in which the amputation occurred affect the diagnosis code selection? _____

6. If the type of machinery used during the procedure were specified, what other type of diagnosis code would you have reported? _____

PRACTICE EXERCISE 19.4 LACERATION REPAIR

OPERATIVE REPORT

Assign an external cause code to indicate how the injury occurred.

LOCATION: Outpatient, Hospital
PATIENT: Rod Seim
ATTENDING PHYSICIAN: Gary Sanchez, MD
SURGEON: Gary Sanchez, MD
PREOPERATIVE DIAGNOSIS: Multiple simple lacerations, right middle finger due to arrow.

POSTOPERATIVE DIAGNOSIS: Multiple simple lacerations, right middle finger due to arrow.
PROCEDURE PERFORMED: Simple closure of lacerations to right middle finger.
ANESTHESIA: Ring block.
PROCEDURE: Ring block anesthesia was achieved with 1% Xylocaine without epinephrine. Once the ring block was successful, the patient was taken to the scrub sink and the finger gently scrubbed and thoroughly irrigated with water. Once the finger was cleansed, repair was performed. The

PRACTICE EXERCISE 19.4 LACERATION REPAIR—cont'd

patient had a small nick (1 cm) in the lateral band. This was tacked together with one 4–0 nylon suture. There was noted to be no dirt on the tendon after irrigating the finger. To minimize the risk for infection, it was elected to just loosely close this. The 5-cm, J-shaped wound was then closed with four 4–0 nylon sutures just to approximate the skin. Some fat at the edge of the volar wound was debrided with scissors, and some abrasion of the epidermis was also debrided with scissors. The volar wound was then closed with two 4–0 nylon sutures. Dressing and a TubeGauz dressing were then applied. The patient tolerated this well.

CPT Code(s): _____

_____

ICD-10-CM Code(s): _____

_____

Abstracting Questions

1. What type of repair was performed (simple, intermediate, complex)? _____

_____

2. Does the location on the body of the repair affect the choice of the CPT code assignment? _____

_____

3. Does the size of the repair affect the choice of CPT code?

_____

4. The 7th character on the ICD-10-CM code indicates this was a/an _____ encounter.

5. Does the repair to the nick in the tendon affect the diagnosis coding? _____

_____

PRACTICE EXERCISE 19.5 MINIMAL DEBRIDEMENT

OPERATIVE REPORT

The patient is returned to the operating room during the postoperative period of a previous procedure.
LOCATION: Inpatient, Hospital
PATIENT: Pam Tieg
ATTENDING PHYSICIAN: Leslie Alanda, MD
SURGEON: Gary Sanchez, MD
PREOPERATIVE DIAGNOSES
1. Massive abdominal wound with multiple sites of fat necrosis and retroperitoneal tissue necrosis, predominantly fat.
2. Draining sinus, anterior abdominal wall.
POSTOPERATIVE DIAGNOSES
1. Massive abdominal wound with multiple sites of fat necrosis and retroperitoneal tissue necrosis, predominantly fat.
2. Draining sinus, anterior abdominal wall.
SURGICAL FINDINGS: There are about 10 sites of fat necrosis scattered throughout the anterior abdominal wall, but the posterior aspect of the wound (i.e., in the retroperitoneal space that is obliterated by the overhang of bowel) appeared to be clean as far as we could tell, and certainly there was no odor.
SURGICAL PROCEDURE
1. Minimal debridement of anterior abdominal wall wound.
2. Collection of specimen for amylase.
ANESTHESIA: General endotracheal.

PROCEDURE: The patient's abdomen was prepped with Betadine scrub and solution and draped in the routine sterile fashion. Multiple sites of fat necrosis were debrided, and one area of protrusion of the mesh was debrided. There was some clear fluid leaking from a sinus in the anterior abdominal wall, and we collected 2 cc of fluid from this and submitted it for amylase. The wound was then repacked with Kerlix-soaked dressings using 0.5% metronidazole, and fine mesh gauze was applied to the anterior abdominal wound. The patient seemed to tolerate the procedure well and left the area in good condition. We additionally did spray Hemaseel into a pocket in the retroperitoneal area where there was some bleeding that did not respond to cautery, and it was thought that this was more the nature of generalized oozing, and therefore the Hemaseel and packing were used for control.

CPT Code(s): _____

_____

ICD-10-CM Code(s): _____

_____

Abstracting Questions

1. Was the retroperitoneum re-explored? _____

_____

2. Does the return to the operating room require a modifier appended to the surgical procedure code? _____

_____

Musculoskeletal System Subsection (20005-29999)

Subsection divided: Anatomic site, then service (e.g., excision)

Used extensively by orthopedic surgeons
• Many codes commonly used by variety of physicians
Extensive notes
Most common

• Fracture and dislocation treatments
• "General" subheading
• Arthroscopic procedures
• Casting and strapping
Eponyms are "things" named after "people"

Example: Barr procedure is a tendon transfer of the lower leg (27690-27692), and Mitchell and Chevron or concentric type procedure is a distal metatarsal osteotomy (bunion correction) (28296)

- Procedures are often referred to with eponyms
- Check the index of the CPT manual for directions to eponym codes

Fracture Treatment

Type of treatment depends on type and severity of fracture

Diagnosis codes must support the procedure codes and document the medical necessity
Open: Surgically opened to view or remotely opened to place nail across fracture site
- Open reduction with internal fixation is ORIF

Closed: Not surgically opened
Percutaneous: Insertion of devices through skin or a remote site
- Percutaneous fracture treatment neither open nor closed

Treatment terms should not be confused with **types** of fractures:
- Open fracture: Fractured bone penetrates skin
- Closed fracture: Fractured bone does not penetrate skin

Traction

- Application of force to align bone
- Force applied by internal device (e.g., wire, pin) inserted into bone (skeletal fixation)
- Application of force by means of adhesion to skin (skin traction)

Manipulation

Use of force to return bone back to normal alignment by manual manipulation (reduction) or temporary traction
    Codes often divided based on whether manipulation was or was not used

Dislocation

Bone displaced from normal joint position
    Treatment: Return bone to normal joint location

Subheading "General"

Begins "Incision" (20005)

Depth: Difference between Integumentary and Musculo-skeletal incision codes
Musculoskeletal used when underlying bone or muscle is involved or procedure is deep subcutaneous

Wound Exploration (20100-20103)

Traumatic penetrating wounds

Divided by wound location
Includes
- Enlargement
- Debridement

- Foreign body(ies) removal
- Ligation
- Repair of tissue and muscle

Use additional code for repair of major structures or blood vessels
Not used for integumentary repairs
- Unless the repair requires extension, enlargement, or exploration

Repair of major structure is reported instead when exploration leads to repair

Excision (20150-20251)

Biopsies for bone and muscle

Divided by
- Type of biopsy (bone/muscle)
- Depth
- Some by method

Can be percutaneous needle or excisional
Does not include tumor excision, which is coded separately
Biopsy with excision: Code only excision

Introduction or Removal (20500-20697)

Codes for
- Injections
- Aspirations
- Insertions
- Applications
- Removals
- Adjustments

Therapeutic sinus tract injection procedures
- Not nasal sinus
- Abscess or cyst with passage (sinus tract) to skin
- Antibiotic injected with use of radiographic guidance

Removal of foreign bodies lodged in muscle or tendon sheath
Integumentary removal codes for removal from skin
Injection into
- Tendon sheath
- Tendon origin
- Ligament
- Ganglion cyst
- Trigger points

Placement of needles or catheters into muscle and/or soft tissue
- For interstitial radioelement application

Arthrocentesis: Injection "and/or" aspiration of a joint
- Both aspiration and injection reported with one code (20600-20611)
- Codes based on joint size: Small, intermediate, major and with or without guidance
- Do not unbundle and report aspiration/injection with two codes

External Fixation

Device that holds bone in place

- Application, adjustment, removal under anesthesia
  Code fracture treatment and external fixation device (EFD)
- Unless treatment and fixation both included in fracture care code description
- Adjustment to (20693) and removal of (20694 [under anesthesia]) EFD are coded separately

Replantation (20802-20838)

Used to report reattachment of amputated limb
  Code by body area

Grafts (or Implants) (20900-20938)

Autogenous Grafts

Used to report harvesting through separate incision of
- Bone
- Cartilage
- Tendon
- Fascia lata
- Tissue
  Fascia lata grafts: From upper lateral thigh where fascia is thickest
  Some codes include obtaining grafting material (not coded separately)
  Some grafts are add-on codes for spine surgery only (20930-20938)

Other Procedures (20950-20999)

Monitoring interstitial fluid pressure (interstitial for compartment syndrome, etc.)
- Pressure increases due to increased accumulation of fluids, causing blood supply to be compromised
  Bone grafts identified by donor site
  Free osseocutaneous flaps: Bone grafts
- Taken along with skin and tissue overlying bone
  Electrical stimulation
- Used to speed bone healing
- Placement of stimulators externally or internally
- Ultrasound also used externally

Soft Tissue Tumors

Codes identify excision of soft tissue and subfascial (intramuscular) tumors
- Subcutaneous soft tissue tumors: Below skin but above deep fascia
- Fascial or subfascial soft tissue tumors: Within or below deep fascia (not bone)
- Soft tissue tumors: May involve resection from one or more layer (i.e., subcutaneous, subfascial)
  Example: 21011-21016 to report subcutaneous, subfascial, and soft tissue tumors

Arthrodesis

Fixation of joint (arthro = joint, desis = fusion)

- Bony structures of joint fused together to form one solid bone
- Fixation with pins, wires, rods, etc. to hold the joint immobile
  Often performed with other procedure such as fracture repair
- Arthrodesis of the spine is also called spinal fusion

Subsequent Subheadings

After General subheading, divided by anatomic location
- Anatomic subheadings divided by type procedure
  Example: Subheading "Head" divided by procedure
- Incision
- Excision
- Manipulation
- Head Prosthesis
- Introduction or Removal
- Repair, Revision, and/or Reconstruction
- Fracture and/or Dislocation
- Other Procedures

Spine and Spinal Instrumentation

Insertion of spinal instrumentation reported in addition to arthrodesis (fusion)

Many add-on codes reported in addition to definitive procedure
Spine (Vertebral Column), 22100-22899, divided by repair location (Fig. 19.6)
- Cervical (C1-C7)
  C1 = Atlas
  C2 = Axis
- Thoracic (T1-T12)
- Lumbar (L1-L5)
- Sacral (S1-S5)
- Coccyx (tailbone)
  Vertebral segment: Single complete vertebral bone with articular processes and laminae
  Vertebral interspace: Non-bony compartment between two vertebral bodies which contains the disc
  Single level = two vertebrae and the disc that separates them
  Percutaneous vertebroplasty
- Use of polymethylmethacrylate injected into the vertebral space
  - Polymethylmethacrylate is a type of bone cement/glue similar to texture of silicone
  - Adheres bone fragments together
  - Fills vertebral body defects

Types of Spinal Instrumentation
Segmental: Devices at each end of repair area + at least one other attachment
Nonsegmental: Devices at each end of defect only
Approach: Pay special attention to the approach used to perform the surgery
- Several different approaches to spine: Most common are anterior (front) and posterior (back)

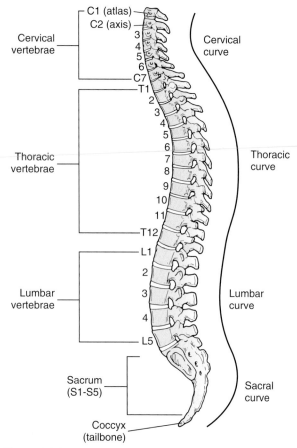

C1 (atlas)
C2 (axis)
Cervical vertebrae
3
4
5
6
C7
Cervical curve

T1
2
3
4
5
6
7
8
9
10
11
T12
Thoracic vertebrae
Thoracic curve

L1
2
3
4
L5
Lumbar vertebrae
Lumbar curve

Sacrum (S1-S5)
Sacral curve

Coccyx (tailbone)

• **Figure 19.6** The spinal cord is part of the central nervous system (CNS) and extends from the brain to the lower back.

- Most spinal instrumentation codes divided based on approach

Casts and Strapping (29000-29799)

Replacement procedure or initial placement to stabilize without additional restorative treatment

Example: Application of wrist splint or cast for wrist sprain
Initial fracture treatment includes placement and removal of first cast
- Subsequent cast applications coded separately
- Payers have strict individual reimbursement policies for subsequent casting
Application not coded when part of surgical procedure
Example: Application of wrist splint or cast for wrist sprain
Initial fracture treatment includes placement and removal of first cast
Elastic bandage application is not billed separately
Removal bundled into surgical procedure
Supplies reported separately

Endoscopy/Arthroscopy (29800-29999)

Surgical arthroscopy always includes diagnostic arthroscopy

Codes divided by joint
- Subdivided by procedure
Be aware of subterms and bundled procedures within code descriptions
Note: Parenthetical information following codes indicates codes to use if procedure was an open procedure

---

PRACTICE EXERCISE 19.6   STEROID INJECTION

LOCATION: Outpatient, Clinic
PATIENT: Kim Ortega
PRIMARY CARE PHYSICIAN: Frank Gaul, MD
SURGEON: Mohomad Almaz, MD
PROCEDURE PERFORMED: Steroid injection.
INDICATIONS: Left shoulder subacromial bursitis.
PROCEDURE: This procedure was done in the procedure area in the hospital.
   After obtaining consent, area of the left shoulder was prepped in the usual fashion with Betadine; 6 cc of 1% lidocaine with 1 cc of Kenalog was injected without guidance in the left subacromial bursa without difficulty. The patient tolerated the procedure well without immediate complications. There was moderate relief of pain afterward.
   The patient was advised to call me if she experiences any signs of infection, such as fever, chills, erythema, or swelling. She will call me in 3 days and tell me how she is doing.

CPT Code(s): _____

ICD-10-CM Code(s): _____
_____

Abstracting Questions

1. What is the medical term for inserting a needle into a joint?
_____
_____

2. Would the joint into which the needle is inserted affect CPT code assignment? _____
_____

PRACTICE EXERCISE 19.7   ARTHROPLASTY AND SPUR EXCISION

LOCATION: Outpatient, Hospital
PATIENT: Merry Hoffert
PRIMARY CARE PHYSICIAN: Frank Gaul, MD
SURGEON: Mohomad Almaz, MD
PREOPERATIVE DIAGNOSIS: Arthritis, secondary impingement, right ankle.

POSTOPERATIVE DIAGNOSES
1. Osteoarthritic change, grade 3/4 tibia, medial shoulder of the talus, right ankle.
2. Osteophytic spurring with secondary impingement, both hard and soft tissue anterior talotibial articulation, right ankle.

PRACTICE EXERCISE 19.7 ARTHROPLASTY AND SPUR EXCISION—cont'd

3. Impinging soft tissue entity, anterolateral aspect of the ankle.

PROCEDURES PERFORMED
1. Abrasion arthroplasty, right ankle.
2. Excision of osteoarthritic spurs of the anterior articular margin, distal tibia.

PROCEDURE: After a satisfactory level of general anesthesia and the patient in a supine position, the extremity was prepped and draped in a routine sterile manner. At this time we proceeded with the establishment of routine arthroscopic portals. We entered from an anteromedial direction with camera, anterolateral direction with camera, and anterolateral direction with in-cutting device. At this setting there was a proud prominence of secondary scar tissue formation. We proceeded with its resection at this time. There were also areas of secondary eburnation change diffusely of grade 2/3 about the lateral aspect of the talus and focally grade 3/4 changes about the medial shoulder of the talus and the tibia as they articulate. There was also the demonstration with dorsiflexion of secondary abutment of soft tissue and proud tibial spurring. At this setting, with use of mechanical in-cutting device, we reamed back the abutment of the diarticular tibia and also at this time proceeded with abrasion chondroplasty and arthroplasty procedures where appropriate of the distal articular tibial plafond and the talus proper.

Medial and lateral recesses were evaluated at this time and were otherwise unremarkable. The posterior confines of the ankle other than the areas of graded arthritic change as noted above were otherwise unremarkable. With completion of this element of the procedure we simply proceeded with closure of portal sites. Both preprocedure and postprocedure arthroscopic photos were obtained for documentation purposes. The patient tolerated the procedure well and was transported to the recovery room in a stable manner.

CPT Code(s): _____

_____

ICD-10-CM Code(s): _____

_____

Abstracting Questions

1. What approach was used for this procedure? _____

_____

2. Was the procedure limited or extensive? _____

_____

PRACTICE EXERCISE 19.8 FASCIAL SLING ARTHROPLASTY

LOCATION: Outpatient, Hospital
PATIENT: Becky Wellington
PRIMARY CARE PHYSICIAN: Ronald Green, MD
SURGEON: Mohomad Almaz, MD
PREOPERATIVE DIAGNOSIS: Degenerative arthritis carpometacarpal joint, left thumb.
POSTOPERATIVE DIAGNOSIS: Same as Preoperative.
PROCEDURES PERFORMED: Fascial sling arthroplasty, left thumb.
ANESTHESIA: General.

PROCEDURE: The patient was brought to the operating room and a general anesthetic was induced. The left upper extremity was prepped with Betadine and draped in a sterile fashion. The limb was exsanguinated and tourniquet inflated to 250 mm Hg for 40 minutes. With 4× magnification loupes, we made a Chevron incision at the base of the thumb metacarpal. Dissection was carried down to the CMC joints, preserving subcutaneous nerves and vessels. We made a longitudinal arthrotomy incision and exposed the trapezium. We then morselized the trapezium and slowly removed the pieces with the rongeur. We carefully removed the entire trapezium, preserving the underlying FCR tendon. There was eburnated bone at the base of the first metacarpal. We then placed a drill hole through the base of the first metacarpal from its dorsal surface to its volar ulnar base. We opened this up to accept the tendon transfer. We next harvested the flexor carpi radialis tendon through two incisions, a short 1-cm incision over the tendon at the distal wrist flexor crease and an incision parallel to this 10 cm up the forearm at the myotendinous junction, where the FCR was transected at the floor of the thumb. Both volar forearm wounds were then closed with 5–0 nylon suture.

We next transferred the FCR tendon through the hole at the base of the first metacarpal, which effectively slung the first metacarpal up to the second metacarpal. We then pinned this to the second metacarpal with a 0.045-inch Kirchner wire bent and cut off outside the skin. We next sutured the tendon to the hole in the first metacarpal with 4–0 Vicryl sutures and packed bone graft into the hole to secure this. We then placed a 4–0 Vicryl suture in the floor of the wound, placed two Bunnell needles over the limbs of this, and then threaded the tendon onto this in an accordion fashion. We tied this Vicryl, pulled the tendon down into the defect, where the trapezium was excised, and filled this nicely. We then proceeded with capsular closure, imbrication of the capsule, and closed this with 4–0 Vicryl sutures. The appearance was excellent. We irrigated the wound with sterile saline and closed the skin with interrupted 5–0 nylon sutures. Next, we applied Xeroform, and a thumb spica compression hand bandage was then applied with plaster splints immobilizing the thumb. The tourniquet was released, and good circulation returned to the hand.

The patient tolerated the procedure well and went to the recovery room in excellent condition. She will be dismissed as an outpatient today with plans for follow-up back in the office in approximately 2 weeks.

DISCHARGE MEDICATION: Lorcet, 30 tablets.
Pathology Report: No specimen was sent.

CPT Code(s): _____

_____

ICD-10-CM Code(s): _____

_____

Abstracting Questions

1. On what area of the body was the arthroplasty performed?

_____

2. Was the tendon transfer bundled into the arthroplasty?

_____

3. Are modifiers reported with these procedures? _____

_____

PRACTICE EXERCISE 19.9   EXCISION BONE TUMOR

LOCATION: Outpatient, Hospital
PATIENT: Tyron Banks
PRIMARY CARE PHYSICIAN: Leslie Alanda, MD
SURGEON: Mohomad Almaz, MD
PREOPERATIVE DIAGNOSIS: Bone tumor, distal lateral right femur.
POSTOPERATIVE DIAGNOSIS: Same as Preoperative.
PROCEDURES PERFORMED: Excision bone tumor, distal right femur.
ANESTHESIA: General.
PROCEDURE: The patient was brought to the operating room and a general anesthetic was induced. Right lower extremity was prepped with Betadine and draped in a sterile fashion. The limb was exsanguinated, and tourniquet was inflated to 300 mm Hg for 25 minutes. Ioban drape was applied. A standard 4-inch longitudinal anterolateral incision was made beginning at the lateral patellar region and extending proximally. Dissection was carried down through the lateral parapatellar region and lateral parapatellar arthrotomy was performed. We entered down to the lateral femur where the tumor was palpable. This appeared to represent a chondroma on the lateral femur. We elevated the soft tissue and periosteum off of this and then used osteotomes to sharply excise this and gradually take this down to its base. It appeared to be bleeding normal bone, and at that point we did put bone wax on the bone. We then closed the periosteum with a running 0 Vicryl suture, then closed the fascia and joint with a running 0 Vicryl suture, and then closed the skin with a

subcuticular 2–0 Vicryl suture and a running 4–0 Monocryl suture. Steri-Strips were applied with gauze dressing, Kling, ABD, Kerlix, and a Coban. The tourniquet was released, and good circulation returned to the leg.

The patient tolerated the procedure well. He will be dismissed as an outpatient today with plans for follow-up in the office in approximately 2 weeks.

DISCHARGE MEDICATIONS: Tylenol #3, 30 tablets.
Pathology Report Later Indicated: Benign neoplasm.

CPT Code(s): _____

_____

ICD-10-CM Code(s): _____

_____

Abstracting Questions

1. From what body part was the bone tumor excised? _____
_____

2. Was a graft required to repair the defect? _____
_____

3. Was any fixation required? _____
_____

4. What report is required to correctly assign a diagnosis to the excision? _____
_____

PRACTICE EXERCISE 19.10   EXCISION OF MASS, BURSA

LOCATION: Outpatient, Hospital
PATIENT: Brittany Lionel
PRIMARY CARE PHYSICIAN: Ronald Green, MD
SURGEON: Mohomad Almaz, MD
PREOPERATIVE DIAGNOSIS: Mass, left prepatellar bursa.
POSTOPERATIVE DIAGNOSIS: Same as Preoperative.
PROCEDURES PERFORMED: Excision of mass, left prepatellar bursa.
ANESTHESIA: Local infiltration with 1% Xylocaine, supplemented with IV sedation.
PROCEDURE: The patient was placed in the supine position on the operating room table. She pointed out the mass on the anterior aspect of her left knee, which was a very small mass, perhaps 2 or 3 mm in diameter. This bothers her when she kneels on her left knee, and she wanted it removed. We therefore marked it with a marking pen since it was not a large mass but was still nevertheless fairly easily palpable.

We then prepped her left knee with Betadine and draped it in a sterile fashion. She was given IV sedation. We then infiltrated the area around the mass with 1% Xylocaine. Once adequate anesthesia had been achieved, we exsanguinated the left leg with Esmarch bandage and inflated a tourniquet to 225 mm Hg. The total tourniquet time was about 6 minutes.

We created an incision in a longitudinal fashion directly over this mass and carried it down through the subcutaneous tissue. We very quickly found this mass, which was perhaps half the size of a pea (0.5 cm). It was fairly firm, and we sent it

to pathology. It appears to be part of the left prepatellar bursa. We then excised some of the adjacent bursal tissue. We found this was located directly over the left patella and the patella was very visible underneath this mass. We then probed the area, looking for any other masses. We then thoroughly irrigated the area and closed the subcutaneous tissue with 2–0 Vicryl and the skin with 3–0 nylon suture. Pressure was applied to this area, and the tourniquet was released after 6 minutes of tourniquet time. We then applied a 4 × 4 dressing and an Ace wrap over this. She was then awakened and taken from the operating room in good condition, breathing spontaneously. The final sponge and needle counts were correct. She tolerated this procedure very well.

Pathology Report Later Indicated: Benign mass of left prepatellar bursa.

CPT Code(s): _____

_____

ICD-10-CM Code(s): _____

_____

Abstracting Questions

1. What was the body location of the tumor? _____
_____

2. What was the size of the mass? _____
_____

Respiratory System Subsection (30000-32999)

Anatomic site arrangement, such as:
- Nose
- Larynx
  Further subdivided by procedure, such as:
- Incision
- Excision

Endoscopy

Endoscopy in all subheadings except Nose
  Each preceded by "Notes"

Endoscopy Rule One

Code full extent of endoscopic procedure performed
  Example: Procedure begins at mouth and ends at bronchial tube
- Bronchial tube = full extent

Endoscopy Rule Two

Code correct approach
  Example: For removal:
- Interior lung lesion via endoscope inserted through mouth
- Exterior lung lesion via endoscope inserted through skin into chest
  Incorrect approach = incorrect code = incorrect or no reimbursement

Endoscopy Rule Three

Diagnostic endoscopy always included in surgical endoscopy
  Examples:
- Diagnostic bronchial endoscopy begins
- Identified foreign body
- Removed foreign body (surgical endoscopy)
- Only surgical endoscopy reported

Multiple Procedures

Frequent in respiratory coding
- **Watch for bundled services**
  Sequence primary procedure first, no modifier
  Sequence secondary procedures next, with -51
  Bilateral procedures often performed, use -50
  Format for reporting chosen by payer
  Example: Nasal lavage
- 31000 × 2
- 31000 and 31000-50
- 31000-50
- 31000-RT and 31000-LT

Nose (30000-30999)

Used extensively by otorhinolaryngologists (ear, nose, and throat [ENT] specialists)

Also used by wide variety of physicians in other specialties
Approach to nose
- External approach, use Integumentary System
- Internal approach, use Respiratory System

Incision (30000-30020)

Bundled into Incision codes are drain or gauze insertion and removal
  Supplies reported separately

Excision (30100-30160)

Contains intranasal biopsy codes

Polyp excision, coded by complexity
- Excision includes any method of destruction, even laser
- Use -50 (bilateral) for both sides
Turbinate excision and resection
- Three turbinates: Superior, middle, inferior
- Excision of inferior turbinate, 30130
- Excision of superior or middle turbinate, 30999
- Submucous resection of inferior turbinate, 30140
- Submucous resection of superior or middle turbinate, 30999

Introduction (30200-30220)

Common procedures
  Example: Injections to shrink nasal tissue or displacement therapy (saline flushes) to remove mucus
- Displacement therapy performed through nose

Removal of Foreign Body (30300-30320)

Distinguished by the site of removal, whether at office or hospital (requires general anesthesia)

Repair (30400-30630)

Many plastic procedures
- Rhinoplasty (reshaping nose internal and/or external)
- Septoplasty (rearrangement or repair of nasal septum)

Destruction (30801-30802)

Use of ablation (removing by cutting)

Used for removal of excess nasal mucosa or to reduce turbinate inflammation
Based on intramural or superficial extent of destruction
- **Intramural:** Deeper mucosa
- **Superficial:** Outer layer of mucosa

Other Procedures (30901-30999)

Control of nasal hemorrhage
- Packing
- Ligation
- Cauterization
- The packing may be anterior or posterior

Accessory Sinuses (31000-31299)

Subheadings include:

Incision (31000-31090)
Excision (31200-31230)
Endoscopy (31231-31297)
Other Procedures (31299)
Codes for lavage (washing) of sinuses
- Cannula (hollow tube) placed into sinus
- Sterile saline solution flushed through

Procedures may involve multiple codes when multiple locations are accessed

Example: 31020, Sinusotomy, maxillary, can be coded with 31050 sinusotomy, sphenoid, and 31070 sinusotomy, frontal

Use -50 (bilateral) for both sides

Maxillary sinusotomy may use an external and intranasal approach to creating passage between sinus and nose
- Used to clear blocked or infected sinus
- Intranasal sinusotomy, 31020
- External sinusotomy, radical (such as Caldwell-Luc)

Access through mouth
Incision above eyetooth
Sinus is cleaned
New opening created or existing opening enlarged

Repair of fractures occurring during procedure may be coded separately if not included in code description

Larynx (31300-31599)

Excision (31300-31420)

Laryngotomy: Open surgical procedure to expose larynx
- For removal procedure (e.g., tumor)
  May be confused with Trachea/Bronchi codes for tracheostomy used to establish airflow

Introduction (31500-31502)

Used to establish, maintain, and protect air flow
  Endotracheal intubation, establishment of airway
  Based on planned (ventilation support) or emergency procedure

Endoscopy (31505-31579)

Uses terms *indirect* and *direct*
- **Indirect:** Tongue depressor with mirror used to view larynx
- **Direct:** Endoscopy passed into larynx; physician directly views vocal cords

Repair (31580-31592)

Several plastic procedures and fracture repairs
  Laryngoplasty procedures based on purpose
  Fracture code is open reduction code

Trachea and Bronchi (31600-31899)

Incision (31600-31614)

Most codes: Tracheostomy divided by
- Planned (ventilation support), based on age
- Emergency
  Divided by type
- Transtracheal or cricothyroid (location of incision)

Endoscopy (31615-31661)

Bronchoscope may be inserted into nose or mouth
  Rigid endoscopy performed under general anesthesia
  Flexible endoscopy usually performed under local or moderate (conscious) sedation

Bronchial Thermoplasty (31660, 31661)

- Treatment for severe asthma in which radiofrequency is utilized to produce heat in the airways that results in reduction of the airway smooth muscles

Introduction (31717-31730)

Catheterization
  Instillation
  Aspiration
  Tracheal tube placement

Excision, Repair (31750-31830)

Repairs of trachea and bronchi

Lungs and Pleura (32035-32999)

Incision (32035-32225)

Thoracotomy
Surgical opening of chest to expose to view.

Used for
- Biopsy
- Cyst
- Foreign body removal
- Cardiac massage, etc.

Excision/Removal (32310-32540)

Biopsy codes in both Excision and Incision categories
- Excisional biopsy with percutaneous needle
- Incisional biopsy with chest open
  Also services of pleurectomy, pneumocentesis, and lung removal
- **Segmentectomy:** 1 segment
- **Lobectomy:** 1 lobe
- **Bilobectomy:** 2 lobes
- **Total Pneumonectomy:** 1 lung

Thoracentesis
Needle inserted into pleural space for aspiration (withdrawal) of fluid and/or air (32554, 32555)

Introduction and Removal (32550-32557)

- Insertion of indwelling tunneled pleural catheter (removal 32552)
- Tube thoracostomy
- Placement of interstitial device(s) for radiation therapy guidance
- Thoracentesis and percutaneous pleural drainage

Destruction (32560-32562)

- Chemical pleurodesis
- Fibrinolysis, initial day, subsequent day

Cardiovascular System Subsection

CV coding may require codes from
- **Radiology:** Diagnostic studies
- **Medicine:** Nonsurgical and percutaneous
- **Surgery:** Open and percutaneous
  Both Medicine and Surgery sections contain invasive procedures

Cardiology Coding Terminology

Invasive: Enters body
- Incision
  Example: Opening chest for removal (e.g., tumor on heart)
- Percutaneous
  - Placement of catheter into artery or vein through the skin by means of wire threaded through needle and catheter slid over wire
  Example: PTCA (percutaneous transluminal coronary angioplasty) procedure
  Percutaneous—wire threaded through needle placed through skin into vessel and catheter placed over wire
- Cut down—small nick made into vessel under direct vision and catheter inserted
  Example: Catheter inserted into femoral or brachial artery
  Common catheters are:
- Broviac
- Hickman
- HydroCath
- Arrow multi-lumen
- Groshong
- Dual-lumen
- Triple-lumen
  Noninvasive: Procedures that do not break skin
  Example: Electrocardiogram
  Electrophysiology (EP): Study of electrical system of heart
  Example: Study of irregular heartbeat (arrhythmia)
- EP studies are in Medicine section, 93600-93662
- Electrophysiologic Operative Procedures are in Surgery section, 33250-33266

Nuclear Cardiology: Diagnostic and treatment specialty; uses radioactive substances to diagnose cardiac conditions
Example: Myocardial perfusion and cardiac blood pooling imaging studies

Cardiovascular in Surgery Section (33010-37799)

Codes for Procedures

Heart/Pericardium (33010-33999)
- Pacemakers, valve disorders
  Arteries/Veins (34001-37799)

Heart/Pericardium (33010-33999)

Both percutaneous and open surgical
- Cardiologists often use percutaneous intervention; cardiovascular or thoracic surgeons often use open surgical procedures
  Extensive notes throughout
  Frequent changes with medical advances
  Examples of categories of Heart/Pericardium subheading
- Pericardium
- Cardiac Tumor
- Pacemaker or Implantable Defibrillator
  Examples of services
- Pericardiocentesis: Percutaneous withdrawal of fluid from pericardial space (pericarditis) (33010-33011)
- Cardiac Tumor: Open surgical procedure for removal of tumor on heart (33130)

Pacemaker or Implantable Defibrillator (33202-33273)

Devices that assist heart in electrical function
- Differentiate between temporary and permanent devices
- Differentiate between one-chamber and dual-chamber devices
  Divided by where pacer placed, approach, and type of service
  Patient record indicates revision or replacement
- Pacemaker pulse generator is also called a battery
- Pacemaker leads are also called electrodes
  Usual follow-up 90 days (global period)

Placed
Atrium (single chamber)
- Pulse generator and one or more electrodes in atrium (single-chamber pacemaker)
  Ventricle (single chamber)
- Pulse generator and one or more electrodes in ventricle (single-chamber pacemaker)
  Both (dual chamber)
- Pulse generator and one electrode in right ventricle and one electrode in right atrium

Biventricular, right ventricle, right atrium, and coronary sinus
- Pulse generator and one electrode in right ventricle, one electrode(s) may be placed in right atrium, and one electrode in the coronary sinus over the left ventricle

Approach
Epicardial: Open procedure to place electrodes on heart
Transvenous: Through vein to place in heart (endoscopic)

Type of Service
Initial placement or replacement of all or part of device
    Number of leads placed is important in code selection

Electrophysiologic Operative Procedures (33250-33266)
Surgeon repairs defect causing abnormal rhythm

Chest opened to full view
- Cardiopulmonary (CP) bypass usually used

Endoscopy procedure
- Without cardiopulmonary bypass

Codes based on reason for procedure and if CP bypass used

Patient-Activated Event Recorder (33282-33284)
Also known as cardiac event recorder or loop recorder
    Internal surgical implantation required
    Divided based on whether device is being implanted or removed

Cardiac Valves (33361-33478)
Divided by valve
- Aortic, mitral, tricuspid, pulmonary
    Subdivided by whether replacement, repair, resection, and use of bypass machine
    33361-33369 report transcatheter aortic valve replacement and implant

Coronary Artery Bypass Graft (CABG)
CABG performed for bypassing coronary arteries severely obstructed as in atherosclerosis or arteriosclerosis

Determine what was used in repair
- Vein (33510-33516)
- Artery (33533-33536)
- Both artery and vein (33517-33523 and 33533-33536)

Based on number of bypass grafts performed and if combined venous and arterial grafts are used
Example: Three venous grafts

Venous Grafting Only for Coronary Artery Bypass (33510-33516)
Based on number of grafts being replaced

Combined Arterial-Venous Grafting (33517-33530)
Divided based on number of grafts and whether initial procedure or reoperation

Procuring saphenous vein included, unless performed endoscopically
These codes are never used alone
- Arterial-Venous codes (33517-33523) report only **venous** graft portion of procedure
- Always used with Arterial Grafting codes (33533-33536)

Example: 3 vein grafts and 2 arterial grafts = 33519 and 33534

Open procurement of saphenous vein is included in procedure (not coded separately)
Code harvesting of saphenous vein graft separately when endoscopic video-assisted procurement is performed (33508)
Code harvesting separately for upper extremity or femoral vein

Arterial Grafting for Coronary Artery Bypass (33533-33548)
Divided based on number of grafts

Obtaining artery for grafting included in codes, except
- Procuring upper-extremity artery (e.g., radial artery), coded separately (35600)

Several codes (33542-33548) for myocardial resection, repair of ventricular septal defect (VSD), and ventricular restoration

Endovascular Repair of Descending Thoracic Aorta (33880-33891)
Placement of an endovascular aortic prosthesis for repair of descending thoracic aorta
- Less invasive than traditional approach of chest or abdominal incision
    Synthetic aortic prosthesis placed via catheter
- Report fluoroscopic guidance separately 75956-75959
    Fluoroscopic guidance codes includes diagnostic imaging prior to placement and intraprocedurally
    Stent-graft (endoprosthesis) is deployed to reinforce weakened area

Extracorporeal Membrane Oxygenation and Extracorporeal Life Support Services (33946-33989)
Cardiac and/or respiratory support to the heart and/or lungs
- Provide cardiac and respiratory support for patients whose heart and lungs are diseased or damaged beyond function

Arteries and Veins Subheading (34001-37799)
Only for noncoronary vessels
- Divided based on whether artery or vein involved
    Example: Different codes for embolectomy, depending on artery or vein
    Catheters placed into vessels for monitoring, removal, repair
    Nonselective or selective catheter placement

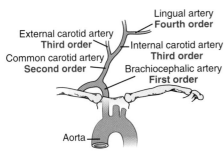

• **Figure 19.7** Brachiocephalic vascular family with first-, second-, third-, and fourth-order vessels.

- Nonselective: Direct placement without further manipulation
- Selective: Place and then manipulate into further order(s) Catheter Placement Example
- Nonselective: 36000 Introduction of needle into vein
- Selective: 36012 Placement of catheter into second-order venous system

Vascular Families Are Like a Tree

First-order (main) branch (tree trunk)
Second-order branch (tree limb)
Third-order branch (tree branch)
Brachiocephalic vascular family (Fig. 19.7)
- Report farthest extent of catheter placement in a vascular family; labor intensity is increased with the extent of catheter placement

Embolectomy and Thrombectomy (34001-34490)

Embolus: Dislodged thrombus
Thrombus: Mass of material in vessel located in place of formation
- May be removed by dissection or balloon

Balloon: Threaded into vessel, inflated under mass, pulled out with mass
- Codes are divided by site of incision and whether artery or vein

Venous Reconstruction (34501-34530)

Types of Repairs
- Valve of the femoral vein
- Vena cava
- Saphenopopliteal vein anastomosis

Aneurysm

Aneurysm: Weakened arterial wall causing a bulge or ballooning
Repair by removal, bypass, or coil placement
Endovascular repair (34701-34848) from inside vessel
Direct (35001-35152) from outside vessel

Endovascular Repair of Abdominal Aortic Aneurysm (34701-34706)

Reported separately; introduction of guideline and catheters

Other procedures performed at same time coded separately

Endovascular Repair of Iliac Aneurysm (34707-34708)

Extensive notes preceding codes—"must" reading
Includes introduction, positioning, and deployment of graft, stent and balloon angioplasty
Reported separately: Introduction of guidewire and catheters

Repair Arteriovenous Fistula (35180-35190)

Abnormal passage from artery or vein

Divided based on fistula type
- Congenital
- Acquired/traumatic
- By site
Repair methods
- Autogenous graft—fistula created artery to vein
- Non-auto fistula—biocompatible tube connecting artery to vein

Angioplasty

Divided as open or percutaneous and by vessel
- **Transluminal:** By way of vessel
- **Transluminal Angioplasty:** Catheter passed into vessel and a balloon is inflated to crush/flatten fatty deposits in vessel
  - Placement of eluting or non-eluting stents coded in addition to catheter placement
- Reported with codes 36902, 36905, 36907, and 37246-37249

Noncoronary Bypass Grafts (35500-35671)

Divided by
- Vein
- In-Situ Vein (veins repaired in their original place)
- Other Than Vein
Code by type of graft and vessels being used to bypass
Example: 35506 Bypass graft, with vein; carotid-subclavian
- Graft attached to carotid and to subclavian, bypassing defect of subclavian
Procurement of saphenous vein graft is included and not reported separately
Harvesting of upper-extremity vein (35500) or femoropopliteal vein (35572) is reported separately

Vascular Injection Procedures (36000-36598)

Divided into
- Intravenous
- Intra-arterial—Intra-aortic
- Venous
- Central venous access procedures
  Used for many procedures, including
- Local anesthesia
- Introduction of needle

- Injection of contrast material
- Preinjection and postinjection care related to injection procedure
  Example: Injection of opaque substance for venography (radiography of vein)

Central Venous Access (CVA) Procedures

Long-term use for medication/chemotherapy administration and short term use for monitoring

Approach
- Central: jugular, subclavian, or femoral vein
- Peripheral: basilic or cephalic vein

Categories
1. Insertion
2. Repair
3. Replacement, partial or complete
4. Removal
5. Other central venous access procedure
6. Guidance for vascular access

Insertion (36555-36571)

Insertion of newly established venous access
- Tunneled under skin (e.g., Hickman, Broviac, Groshong)
- Nontunneled (e.g., Hohn catheter, triple lumen, PICC)
- Central (e.g., subclavian, internal jugular, femoral, inferior vena cava)
- Peripheral (basilic or cephalic vein)
  Codes divided by tunneled/non-tunneled, with/without port, central/peripheral, and age

Repair (36575-36576)

Repair of malfunction without replacement with or without subcutaneous port or pump
  Repair of central venous access device
  No differentiation between age of patient or central/peripheral insertion

Replacement (Partial or Complete) (36578-36585)

Partial (36578) is replacement of catheter only
  Complete (36580-36585) is replacement through same venous access site
  Differentiated by tunneled/non-tunneled, central/peripheral, and with or without subcutaneous port or pump

Removal (36589, 36590)

To be used for tunneled catheter
  Removal of non-tunneled catheter is not reported separately

Other Central Venous Access Procedures (36591-36598)

Collection of blood specimen
  Declotting of catheter or access device by thrombolytic agent
  Mechanical removal of obstructive material from around catheter or within lumen

Guidance for Vascular Access

77001, Fluoroscopic guidance for central venous access device placement, replacement, or removal
- Reported in addition to primary procedure

76937, Ultrasound guidance for vascular access
- Reported in addition to primary procedure

Transcatheter Procedures (37184-37218)

Arterial Mechanical Thrombectomy (37184-37186)

- Removal of thrombus by means of mechanical device
  From artery or arterial bypass graft

Venous Mechanical Thrombectomy (37187-37188)

- Removal of a thrombus by means of a mechanical device
  From vein

Arterial and venous mechanical thrombectomy may be performed as primary procedure or add-on
- Includes
  Introduction of device into thrombus
  Thrombus removal
  Injection of thrombolytic drug(s), if used
  Fluoroscopic and contrast guidance
  Follow-up angiography
- Report separately
  Diagnostic angiography
  Catheter placement(s)
  Diagnostic studies
  Pharmacologic thrombolytic infusion before or after (37211-37214, 75898)
  Other interventions

Other Procedures (37195-37218)

- Used to report a variety of transcatheter procedures
  Example: Transcatheter biopsy, therapy, infusion for thrombolysis or antispasmotic treatment of a vessel, retrieval of foreign object, occlusion or embolization, and intravascular stents

Endovascular Revascularization (Open or Percutaneous, Transcatheter) (37220-37235)

Lower extremity codes

Cardiovascular in Medicine Section (92920-93799)

Services can be
- Invasive or noninvasive
- Diagnostic or therapeutic
  Subheadings
- Therapeutic Services and Procedures
- Cardiovascular Monitoring Services
- Implantable and Wearable Cardiac Device Evaluations
- Cardiography
- Echocardiography
- Cardiac Catheterization

- Intracardiac Electrophysiologic Procedures/Studies
- Peripheral Arterial Disease Rehabilitation
- Noninvasive Physiologic Studies and Procedures
- Other Procedures

Therapeutic Services and Procedures (92920-92998)

Types of services
- Cardioversion
- Infusions
- Thrombolysis
- Catheter placement
  Codes divided by
- Method (e.g., balloon, blade)
- Location (e.g., aortic or mitral valve)
- Number (e.g., single or multiple vessels)

Intracoronary Brachytherapy (92974)

Uses radioactive substances to destroy re-stenosis of coronary vessel
  Patients have had stent placed in coronary vessel
  Stent "re-stenosis" (re-formation of plaque)
  Add-on code
  Cardiologist: Places guidewire and catheter
  Radiation oncologist: Places radioactive elements

Cardiography (93000-93050)

Types of services
- Stress tests
- Holter monitor
- Electrocardiogram
  Separate codes for components of study, such as
- 93000 global
- 93005 tracing only
- 93010 interpretation and report only
  Codes report professional and/or technical components, so do not append -26 or -TC

Cardiovascular Monitoring Services (93224-93278)

Diagnostic procedures in-person or by means of remote technology to assess cardiovascular rhythm via ECG
- Holter monitors, 93224-93227
- Mobile telemetry, 93228, 93229
- Event monitors, 93268-93272
  - Patient depresses a button on portable monitor when feeling a sensation (event), such as a flutter or dizziness
    Codes divided based on type of monitoring and time

Implantable and Wearable Cardiac Device Evaluations (93279-93299)

Diagnostic medical procedures for cardiac rhythm devices
- Devices are internal or external
- In-person or remote assessments
  Codes divided by

- Type of Service
  Implantation
  Interrogation
  Programming
- Devices such as:
  Implantable defibrillator
  Implantable loop recorder
- Number of leads or chambers
- Monitoring period must exceed 10 days
  Implantation procedures (93279-93291)
- Reported once per procedure
  Interrogation device evaluation of implantable defibrillator (ICD) or pacemaker (93293-93296)
  - ICDs may act as defibrillator or pacemaker
  - Report interrogation or monitoring once per 90-day period
  Interrogation device evaluation implantable cardiovascular monitor system (93297-93299)
- Report interrogation or monitoring once per 30-day period

Echocardiography (93303-93355)

Noninvasive Diagnostic Procedure

Ultrasound detects presence of cardiac or vascular disease

Codes divided by
- Approach
- Extent of study (e.g., limited, complete)
- Service provided (e.g., probe only, interpretation and report)

Cardiac Catheterization (93451-93572)

Used to identify valve disorders, abnormal blood flow

Many bundled services in catheterization codes
Examples:
- Introduction
- Positioning/Repositioning of catheter
- Pressure readings inside heart or vessels
- Blood samples
- Rest/Exercise studies
- Final evaluation and report
- Many codes are -51 exempt
- Many codes include moderate (conscious) sedation

Three Components of Coding Cardiac Catheterization

1. Placement of catheter
2. Injection
3. Imaging supervision, interpretation, and report
   Most codes have all three components in the code
   - Example: 93456 includes catheterization, injection, imaging
   Some codes require multiple codes
   - Example: 93531 reports catheterization for congenital cardiac anomalies, injection code (93563/93564) must be added

Intracardiac Electrophysiologic Procedures/ Studies (93600-93662)

Services to diagnose and treat conditions of electrical system of heart
- Arrhythmic induction
- Mapping
- Ablation

EP System of Heart

Electrical conduction system
> Electrical recording codes divided based on location of recording device
> ***Example:*** Bundle of His or right ventricle
> Pacing: Temporary pacing to stabilize beating of heart
> ***Example:*** Intraventricular or intra-arterial pacing

Peripheral Arterial Disease (PAD) Rehabilitation (93668)

Rehabilitation sessions: 45-60 minutes
> Use of motorized treadmill/track/bicycle to build patient's CV function
> Supervised by exercise physiologist or nurse
> If E/M is provided by physician, service is reported separately

Noninvasive Physiologic Studies and Procedures (93701-93790)

Category contains codes for services such as
- **Plethysmography:** Recordings of changes in size of body part when blood passes through it
- **Electronic Analysis:** Checks electronic function of devices, such as pacemakers
- **Ambulatory Blood Pressure Monitoring:** Outpatient basis over 24-hour period
- **Thermograms:** Visual recordings of body temperature

Other Procedures (93797-93799)

Codes 93797 and 93798 report professional outpatient cardiac rehabilitation services, per session
- With or without ECG monitoring

Cardiovascular in Radiology Section (75557-75774)

Radiology section, Heart (75557-75574) and Aorta/Arteries (75600-75774) subsections

Prior to 1992, Radiology section contained codes for entire CV procedures
Major revision to CV radiology codes 1992
Divided complete procedures into two components: technical and professional
Example: Angiography
- Technical component angiography—remains in Radiology section
- Professional component injection—moved to Surgery section

Complete angiography requires radiology code and surgery code
Reflects common practice of cardiologist's performing injection and radiologist's performing angiography

Contrast Material

Often radiologic procedures use contrast material to improve image

Many codes have contrast material bundled into service
- "with contrast" or "with or without contrast"

Only injected contrast qualifies as "with contrast"
Contrast not included in description but used in procedure:
> Code contrast material and injection separately
- Specify site where service is received to differentiate between global (total), technical, and professional components of the procedure

Non-hospital-based (not employed by hospital) physician usually performs procedure in hospital outpatient department: Use -26 to report only professional component

---

EXAMPLE

Component Coding

Two physicians (cardiologist and radiologist from same facility) perform angiography of third-order brachiocephalic artery with contrast
- Cardiologist places catheter (36217), Surgery section
- Radiologist performs angiography (75710), Radiology section
- Supply of contrast material (99070), Medicine section

Hemic and Lymphatic System Subsection (38100-38999)

Divisions

- Spleen
- General
- Lymph Nodes and Lymphatic Channels

Spleen Subheading (38100-38200)

Spleen easily ruptured, causing massive and potentially lethal hemorrhage

Excision:
- Splenectomy: Total or partial/open or laparoscopic

Often done as part of more major procedure
- Bundled into major procedure
- Repair
- Laparoscopy

General (38204-38243)

Bone Marrow

Codes divided based on
- Preservation
- Preparation
- Purification
- Aspiration
- Biopsy
- Harvesting
- Transplantation

Hematopoietic Progenitor Cell (HPC)

- Obtained from bone marrow, peripheral blood apheresis, umbilical cord blood

Types of Cells

Allogenic: Same species (38240)
Autologous: Patient's own (38241)

Lymph Nodes and Lymphatic Channels Subheading (38300-38999)

Two types of lymphadenectomies:

1. **Limited:** Pelvic and para-aortic lymph nodes only for neoplasm staging
2. **Radical:** Aortic and/or splenic lymph nodes and surrounding tissue for neoplasm staging
   Often bundled into more major procedure (e.g., prostatectomy)
   Do not unbundle and report lymphadenectomy separately

Mediastinum and Diaphragm Subsection (39000-39499)

Incision codes for foreign body removal, biopsy, or drainage
  Excision codes for removal of cyst or tumor

Diaphragm (39501-39599)

Only two categories: Repair and Other Procedures
  Includes hernia and laceration repairs

PRACTICE EXERCISE 19.11   ANGIOGRAM

Assign the codes for the catheterizations only.

RADIOLOGY REPORT
LOCATION: Inpatient, Hospital
PATIENT: Joy Gigel
ORDERING PHYSICIAN: John Hodgson, MD
ATTENDING/ADMIT PHYSICIAN: Frank Gaul, MD
RADIOLOGIST: Morton Monson, MD
PERSONAL PHYSICIAN: Frank Gaul, MD
EXAMINATION: Carotid/cerebral angiogram.
CLINICAL SYMPTOMS: Intracranial bleed.
  CAROTID/CEREBRAL ANGIOGRAM: The patient is a 54-year-old female who was found to have an intracranial bleed. Carotid/cerebral angiogram was requested by Dr. Hodgson, neurosurgery.
APPROACH: Right common femoral artery.
VESSELS INJECTED
  1. Proximal thoracic aorta.
  2. Right common carotid artery.
  3. Right internal carotid artery.
  4. Left common carotid artery.
  5. Left vertebral artery.
  FOLLOW-UP: Dr. Hodgson.
  Prior to the start of the study, the procedure was explained to the patient's husband by Dr. Hodgson, including risks, complications, and alternatives. The patient's husband understood and consented to the exam. This study was performed on an emergency basis.
  The patient was prepped and draped in the usual sterile fashion. Utilizing single wall technique following administration of local anesthesia (1% lidocaine), a #5 French flush catheter was introduced into the right common femoral artery through a vascular sheath, and the tip was advanced into the proximal thoracic aorta. Contrast was injected, and sequential digital subtraction angiography films were obtained.

  The flush catheter was then exchanged for a #4 French Osborne catheter for select evaluation of both common carotid arteries, as well as the right internal carotid artery and the left vertebral artery. Again, contrast was injected, and multiple views of the carotid bifurcations and cerebral vessels were obtained.
  On arch injection, there is no significant stenosis at the origin of the great vessels. There is an antegrade flow in both vertebral arteries. Please note that the right vertebral artery is somewhat smaller when compared to the left.
  On evaluation of the carotid bifurcations, there is no evidence of narrowing or irregularity.
  On evaluation of cerebral vessels, there is no evidence of aneurysm, extravasation, or arteriovenous malformation. Please note that there is marked medial and superior displacement of the vessels in the right middle cerebral artery distribution. There is also midline shift of all the cerebral structures of the left as well as midline shift to the left of the anterior cerebral arteries. These findings are consistent with the patient's intraparenchymal bleed predominantly in the right temporal lobe seen on CT study from an outside institution.
  The patient tolerated the procedure well. The puncture site was closed with sutures utilizing the Perclose device. There was no evidence of bleeding, hematoma, or change in peripheral pulses at the termination of the study.
  IMPRESSION: Carotid/cerebral angiogram with multiple findings as described above.
  Dr. Hodgson was present during this examination.

CPT Code(s): _____

_____

ICD-10-CM Code(s): _____

_____

Continued

PRACTICE EXERCISE 19.11 ANGIOGRAM—cont'd

Abstracting Questions

1. What CPT Appendix could you reference to understand how to code the procedure performed in the report? _____

_____

2. What vessels were evaluated? _____

_____

3. Are right and left HCPCS modifiers appended to the catheter insertion codes? _____

_____

4. Are both the right common carotid and right internal carotid reported? _____

_____

5. Is the left common carotid reported? _____

_____

6. Is the left vertebral artery reported? _____

7. Why does the proximal thoracic aorta not get reported?

_____

PRACTICE EXERCISE 19.12 DIALYSIS CATHETER REPLACEMENT

LOCATION: Outpatient, Hospital
PATIENT: Sally Perez
ATTENDING PHYSICIAN: George Orbitz, MD
SURGEON: George Orbitz, MD
PREOPERATIVE DIAGNOSIS: ESRD.
POSTOPERATIVE DIAGNOSIS: ESRD.
PROCEDURE PERFORMED: Dialysis catheter replacement.
ANESTHESIA: Local.
   DESCRIPTION OF PROCEDURE: After obtaining consent, the 46-year-old patient was put in the Trendelenburg position. The area of the right IJ vein where the catheter was placed was prepped in the usual fashion. A guidewire was advanced without difficulty. The old dialysis catheter was taken out. Tip was sent for culture. A new 11.5 French 13.5-cm temporary dialysis catheter was advanced through the right IJ vein over the guidewire using the Seldinger technique without difficulty. Both ports had good blood return. Both ports were flushed with saline and heparin. The catheter was secured to the skin. The patient tolerated the procedure well without immediate complications.

CPT Code(s): _____

_____

ICD-10-CM Code(s): _____

_____

Abstracting Questions

1. Was the catheter placement venous or arterial? _____

_____

2. Was this an open or percutaneous insertion? _____

_____

3. Was the catheter a central or peripheral insertion? _____

_____

4. Was this reported as an insertion or a replacement? _____

_____

5. What was the principal reason for the encounter? _____

_____

PRACTICE EXERCISE 19.13 CATHETER PLACEMENT

Report the services, diagnosis(es), and any sedation provided to this patient by the interventional radiologist.
LOCATION: Outpatient, Hospital
PATIENT: John Cane
PRIMARY CARE PHYSICIAN: Rapheal White, MD
INTERVENTIONAL RADIOLOGIST: Edward Riddle, MD
EXAMINATION: Right IVJ Port-a-Cath placement.
CLINICAL SYMPTOMS: Primary lung cancer. Access required for chemotherapy.
   PORT-A-CATH PLACEMENT: Informed consent was obtained from this 26-year-old patient. The right neck and infraclavicular region were prepped and draped in the usual sterile fashion. Skin and subcutaneous tissues were infiltrated with 1% lidocaine with epinephrine. Under ultrasound guidance, access was obtained into the right jugular vein, and over a 0.035 J-tip guidewire the needle was exchanged for a 10 French peel-away sheath. A subcutaneous pocket was created in the right infraclavicular region using blunt dissection. A #9.6 French Bard single-lumen Port-a-Cath was placed into the pocket and a subcutaneous tunnel created from the pocket to the right IJV puncture site. The #9.6 French catheter was advanced through the tunnel and placed through the peel-away sheath. The sheath was removed. Under fluoroscopic

observation the distal tip of the catheter was positioned in the right atrium. The pocket was closed using subcutaneous interrupted sutures with 4–0 Vicryl and a subcuticular stitch with 4–0 Vicryl. The right neck incision site was closed using vertical mattress suture technique with 3–0 Ethilon.

   Patient received conscious sedation for 45 minutes. The patient's pulse oximeter and vital signs were monitored throughout the exam. There were no complications. The patient tolerated the procedure well and left the radiology department in stable condition.

   A single digital spot radiograph obtained demonstrates the single-lumen port placed via a right IJV approach with the distal tip of the catheter in the right atrium.

CPT Code(s): _____

_____

ICD-10-CM Code(s): _____

_____

Abstracting Questions

1. Was the catheter inserted by the radiologist? _____

_____

PRACTICE EXERCISE 19.13 CATHETER PLACEMENT—cont'd

2. Was the catheter inserted into the venous or arterial system? _____

3. Was the catheter inserted centrally or peripherally? _____

4. Was the catheter tunneled? _____

5. Was a subcutaneous port/pump inserted? _____

6. Does the age of the patient affect code assignment? _____

7. What were the two types of guidance used? _____

8. The catheter inserted was used for access for what purpose? _____

PRACTICE EXERCISE 19.14 AORTOGRAM

LOCATION: Outpatient, Hospital
PATIENT: Theodore Lambert
PRIMARY CARE PHYSICIAN: Ronald Green, MD
INTERVENTIONAL RADIOLOGIST: Edward Riddle, MD
EXAMINATION: Arch aortogram with bilateral carotid and cerebral arteriograms.
CLINICAL SYMPTOMS: Previous stroke; carotid artery stenosis.

AORTOGRAPHIC TECHNIQUE: Informed consent was obtained. The right groin was prepped and draped in the usual sterile fashion. Skin and subcutaneous tissues were infiltrated with 1% lidocaine. Access was obtained of the right common femoral artery, and over a 0.035 Bentson guidewire the needle was exchanged for a 5 French sheath. Over the guidewire a #5 French Pigtail catheter was threaded to the aortic arch and angiography was performed in the LAO projection during mechanical injection of contrast through the catheter. The catheter was exchanged for a #5 French H1H catheter. The right vertebral artery was selectively catheterized using the H1H and a 0.035 angled Glidewire. Posterior fossa arteriogram was performed during hand injection of contrast through the catheter. This was performed in AP and lateral projections.

The right common carotid artery was selectively catheterized using the Glidewire and H1H catheter. Right carotid arteriogram was performed in three projections during mechanical injection of contrast through the catheter. AP and lateral cerebral arteriography on the right was performed during mechanical injection of contrast through the catheter.

The left common carotid artery was selectively catheterized using the Glidewire and H1H. Left carotid arteriogram was performed during hand injection of contrast through the catheter. Cerebral arteriogram was performed on the left during hand injection of contrast through the catheter.

Catheter and sheath were removed. Hemostasis was obtained using a 6 French AngioSeal device. The patient received conscious sedation. His pulse oximeter and vital signs were monitored throughout the exam. There were no complications. He tolerated the procedure well and left the radiology department in stable condition.

ARCH AORTOGRAM: The arch is unremarkable. Origins of the great vessels are normal in caliber with no stenosis seen. Subclavian arteries are patent. Bilateral vertebral arteries are patent. Left common carotid artery is small in caliber and indicates that the left internal carotid artery is completely occluded.

POSTERIOR FOSSA ARTERIOGRAM: Visualized distal right vertebral artery is patent. Basilar artery is unremarkable, as are the bilateral posterior cerebral arteries. No aneurysm is seen. No anterior cerebral arterial circulation is noted on this posterior fossa injection.

RIGHT CAROTID ARTERIOGRAM: Calcified atheromatous disease of the carotid bulb and proximal internal carotid artery is noted. There is approximately 30-40% diameter narrowing of the carotid bulb, with no significant stenosis seen involving the proximal internal carotid artery. There is a 90-95% diameter narrowing of the proximal external carotid artery.

LEFT CAROTID ARTERIOGRAM: The common carotid artery is small in caliber, with the distal common carotid artery demonstrating a high-grade stenosis with a "string sign." The internal carotid artery is completely occluded.

RIGHT CEREBRAL ARTERIOGRAM: The distal internal carotid artery and the intracranial internal carotid artery are widely patent. The right anterior and middle cerebral artery and their distribution are unremarkable, with no stenosis seen. No hypervascular or hypovascular mass is present. No aneurysm is seen. The left anterior and middle cerebral arterial supply is provided via a patent anterior communicating artery. No abnormalities are seen on the left anterior or middle cerebral arterial supply.

LEFT CEREBRAL ARTERIOGRAM: As discussed above, the left cerebral anterior circulation is provided from the right cerebral anterior circulation. There is no intracranial supply on the left seen via external carotid branches. No reconstitution of the left internal carotid artery is seen.

IMPRESSION

1. Negative arch aortogram with a small-caliber left common carotid artery.
2. Negative posterior fossa arteriogram.
3. 30-40% diameter narrowing of the carotid bulb on the right, with no significant stenosis of the right internal carotid artery seen.
4. Complete occlusion of the left internal carotid artery.
5. The left anterior and middle cerebral arteries receive their supply via patent anterior communicating artery from the right anterior arterial circulation.

CPT Code(s): _____

ICD-10-CM Code(s): _____

_____

Abstracting Questions

1. What does LAO stand for? _____

_____

2. In the Left Carotid Arteriogram section of the report, the radiologist refers to a "string sign." What is a string sign?

_____

PRACTICE EXERCISE 19.15 EXTREMITY ANGIOGRAM

LOCATION: Outpatient, Hospital
PATIENT: George Ball
PRIMARY CARE PHYSICIAN: Ronald Green, MD
SURGEON: Gary Sanchez, MD
INTERVENTIONAL RADIOLOGIST: Edward Riddle, MD
EXAMINATION: Right lower extremity angiogram and thrombolysis.
CLINICAL SYMPTOMS: Cold right foot.

RIGHT LOWER EXTREMITY ANGIOGRAM AND THROMBOLYSIS: This 62-year-old male presented a month ago with ischemic changes below the knee of the right lower extremity. Some years earlier, the patient had a femoral-popliteal Gore-Tex graft placed. At the time of the angiogram a month ago, there was clot of virtually all the arteries commencing in the distal external iliac artery. We saw very few collateralizations extending into the right lower extremity. Subsequent lytic procedure cleared the Gore-Tex graft and the popliteal artery, but there was then very hard material in the distal popliteal artery that was resistant to the tPA lysis. Subsequently, the patient was taken to the operating room by Dr. Sanchez, where he placed a vein graft from the proximal third of the Gore-Tex graft and inserted it into the posterior tibial artery. The patient then did very well. He now presents acutely with ischemic changes of the right foot.

The patient is on heparin and had been taking Plavix and aspirin as an outpatient. The present procedure was performed via the left femoral artery with single-wall micropuncture entry and placement of a #5 French sheath. A #5 French Omni Flush catheter was then positioned into the right external iliac artery for examination of the right lower extremity.

There is a patency of the right external iliac artery to the junction with the common femoral artery. The common femoral artery is virtually occluded. One or two proximal branches are arising from the artery. The superficial femoral artery and the Gore-Tex graft are occluded. There was also no visualization of the saphenous vein graft. Some collaterals from the deep femoral artery can be visualized at the level of the knee. Although these are scant, they are certainly more than we appreciated when the patient initially arrived here last month.

Utilizing a long Glidewire, I obtained access into the Gore-Tex graft. While traversing the Gore-Text graft, I kept the curve of the wire pointed anteromedially, hoping that we might enter the vein graft. I was able to extend the Glidewire all the way to the knee. Subsequently, a Mewissen catheter with 15 cm of holes was placed proximally with the most proximal hole in the beginning of the clot in the common femoral artery. Coaxially, a Katzen wire with 12 cm of holes was positioned into the graft. tPA was then commenced through both catheters. The patient was medicated with intravenous Versed and fentanyl. He will return to the angiographic suite in the morning.

IMPRESSION: Complete occlusion of the patient's superficial femoral artery, Gore-Tex femoral-popliteal graft, and saphenous graft that extends from the Gore-Tex graft to the posterior tibial artery. Coaxial system has been appropriately placed and tPA lysis started.

CPT Code(s): _____

_____

ICD-10-CM Code(s): _____

_____

Abstracting Question

1. The furthest extent of this selective catheterization was to the _____ artery and to this order? _____

_____

_____

Digestive System Subsection (40490-49999)

Divided by anatomic site from mouth to anus + organs that aid digestive process

Example: Liver and gallbladder
Many bundled procedures

Endoscopy

Diagnostic procedure always bundled into surgical endoscopic
Code to furthest extent of procedure

Endoscopy Terminology

Notes define specific terminology
Code descriptions are specific regarding
- Technique and depth of scope
Esophagoscopy: Esophagus only
Esophagogastroscopy: Esophagus and past diaphragm
Esophagogastroduodenoscopy: Esophagus and beyond pyloric channel

- Proctosigmoidoscopy: Rectum and sigmoid colon (6-25 cm)
- Sigmoidoscopy: Entire rectum, sigmoid colon, and may include part of descending colon (26-60 cm)
- Colonoscopy: Entire colon, rectum to cecum, and may include terminal ileum (greater than 60 cm)

Laparoscopy and Endoscopy

Some subheadings have both laparoscopy (outside) and endoscopy (inside) procedures
Example: Subheading Esophagus
- Endoscopy views inside
- Laparoscopy—scope inserted through umbilicus; views from outside

Hemorrhoidectomy and Fistulectomy Codes (46200-46320)

Divided by
- Location
  - Internal
  - External

- Complexity
  - Simple: No repair procedure involved
  - Complex: Includes repair procedure and fissurectomy
- Anatomy
  - Subcutaneous: No muscle involvement
  - Submuscular: Sphincter muscle
- Complex fistulectomy involves excision/incision of multiple fistulas

Hernia Codes (49491-49659)

Divided by
- Type of hernia
  Example: Inguinal, femoral
- Initial or subsequent repair
- Age of patient determines code choice
- Clinical presentation
  - **Strangulated:** Blood supply cut off
  - **Incarcerated:** Cannot be returned to cavity (not reducible)
    Additional code is used for implantation of mesh or prosthesis for incisional or ventral hernias only
- Open or laparoscopic surgical approaches

PRACTICE EXERCISE 19.16 OROGASTRIC TUBE PLACEMENT

OPERATIVE REPORT
The intraoperative KUB was provided by the radiologist, and you are only reporting the services of Dr. Friendly.
LOCATION: Outpatient, Hospital
PATIENT: Otto Garth
ATTENDING/ADMIT PHYSICIAN: Alma Naraquist, MD
SURGEON: Larry P. Friendly, MD
INDICATION: Feeding, patient with gastroparesis.
PROCEDURE: The patient was placed in the sitting position and then tilted to the right with a wedge. CORFLO was placed at the level of 19 cm without any complications. KUB was then done demonstrating the tip of the CORFLO in the third portion of the duodenum. After confirmation of postpyloric position of the CORFLO, the patient was started on UltraCal at 10 cc/hour.

CPT Code(s): _____

_____

ICD-10-CM Code(s): _____

_____

Abstracting Questions

1. What does KUB stand for? _____

_____

2. What type of tube is a CORFLO? _____

_____

PRACTICE EXERCISE 19.17 GASTROJEJUNOSTOMY PLACEMENT

Because this is an interventional radiologist performing the procedure, report both the procedure and the radiology services.
RADIOLOGY REPORT
LOCATION: Outpatient, Hospital
PATIENT: Betty Frye
ORDERING PHYSICIAN: Ronald Green, MD
ATTENDING/ADMIT PHYSICIAN: Ronald Green, MD
INTERVENTIONAL RADIOLOGIST: Monica Hamilton, MD
EXAMINATION: Gastrojejunostomy placement.
CLINICAL SYMPTOMS: Malnutrition needing nutritional support.
INDICATION: The patient is a 69-year-old female requiring tube feeding. Placement of a #14 French Shetty gastrojejunostomy catheter was requested by Dr. Green for nutritional support.

Prior to the start of the study, the procedure was explained to the patient, including the risks, complications, and alternatives. The patient understood and consented to the procedure.
PERCUTANEOUS GASTROJEJUNOSTOMY PLACEMENT: The patient was prepped and draped in the usual sterile fashion. Using ultrasound guidance, we localized the edge of the liver. Through a previously placed nasogastric tube, the stomach was distended with air.

Using fluoroscopic guidance following administration of local anesthesia (1% lidocaine), we performed gastropexy utilizing four Medi-Tech T-tacks at the mid- to distal aspect of the stomach.

Using multiple wires and catheters, an extra-stiff guidewire was ultimately placed with the tip in the proximal jejunum. Following multiple dilatations, a #14 French Shetty gastrojejunostomy catheter was placed with the tip in the proximal jejunum. A small amount of contrast was administered, which revealed adequate placement. There is no evidence of extravasation or other significant abnormalities.

The patient tolerated the procedure well. There was no evidence of bleeding at the termination of the study.
IMPRESSION: Placement of a #14 French Shetty gastrojejunostomy catheter with the tip in the proximal jejunum, as described above.

CPT Code(s): _____

_____

ICD-10-CM Code(s): _____

_____

Abstracting Questions

1. What was the approach for insertion of the gastrostomy tube? _____

_____

2. Was the ultrasonic guidance separately reported? _____

3. Was the radiology service to check placement separately reported? _____

_____

PRACTICE EXERCISE 19.18 CYSTOTOMY

OPERATIVE REPORT

Dr. Martinez operated on this patient yesterday. The patient presents to the emergency department with an acute abdomen. You are to report only Dr. Martinez's services.

LOCATION: Inpatient, Hospital
PATIENT: Patti Bryan
ATTENDING PHYSICIAN: Gary Sanchez, MD
SURGEONS: Paula Smithson, MD, and Andy Martinez, MD
PREOPERATIVE DIAGNOSES
1. Acute abdomen.
2. Hematuria with suspected bladder injury.

POSTOPERATIVE DIAGNOSES
1. Iatrogenic cystotomy with urine extravasation into the peritoneal cavity.
2. Peritonitis.
3. Extensive intestinal adhesions.

PROCEDURES PERFORMED
1. Exploratory laparotomy.
2. Closure of cystotomy.
3. Extensive intestinal adhesiolysis.

SURGICAL INDICATIONS: This patient is a 32-year-old female who had undergone a Hasson laparoscopy that I performed yesterday. She presented to the emergency department last night with abdominal pain and findings of an acute abdomen. She also had a leukopenia. She was not running a fever. She was noted on insertion of the catheter into the bladder to have some grossly bloody urine.

OPERATIVE FINDINGS: There was less than 1-cm laceration in the dome of the bladder that was extravasating through the bladder. There was a large amount of urine in the peritoneal cavity and some slightly foul-smelling purulent fluid as well. This looked relatively murky and was just not plain urine. There were multiple intestinal adhesions, mostly involving the small bowel. No perforation of the bowel could be detected. The appendix was normal.

OPERATIVE DESCRIPTION: After induction of general anesthesia with patient in the supine position, the abdomen was prepped and draped. The abdomen was opened through a midline hypogastric incision excising her old scar on the way

in. The above findings were noted initially, and Dr. Smithson was able to isolate the small bladder dome laceration. This was smaller than one would expect if a 5-mm laparoscopic trocar had gone through the bladder. I believe that the edge of the bladder probably was nicked. Dr. Smithson will dictate her note concerning the cystotomy repair. We then ran the bowel in its entirety from the ligament of Treitz on down to the ileocecal junction. There were multiple interloop adhesions, which were lysed by Dr. Smithson. She will dictate her note separately. Some omental adhesions were also lysed. After copious irrigation of the abdominal cavity, we then irrigated with heparinized lactated Ringer's and left some of the Ringer's in the abdomen. The peritoneum was closed with a running 2–0 Vicryl. The fascia was closed with interrupted figure-of-eight 0 Vicryl, and the skin closed with staples. Blood loss estimation was 100 cc. The patient received 3000 cc of lactated Ringer's during the case.

Specimens to pathology were cultures of the peritoneal fluid. A Foley catheter was changed at the end of the case. The patient was returned to the recovery room in stable condition.

CPT Code(s): _____

_____

ICD-10-CM Code(s): _____

_____

Abstracting Questions

1. What procedures were performed during this operative session? _____

_____

2. Which procedure did Dr. Martinez perform? _____

_____

3. Were any modifiers required for the two surgeons involved in the same session, and if so, which modifier? _____

_____

PRACTICE EXERCISE 19.19 SMALL-BOWEL ANASTOMOSIS

OPERATIVE REPORT
LOCATION: Inpatient, Hospital
PATIENT: Dona Kelly
ATTENDING PHYSICIAN: Ronald Green, MD
SURGEON: Daniel G. Olanka, MD
PREOPERATIVE DIAGNOSIS: Multiple intestinal fistulas.
POSTOPERATIVE DIAGNOSIS: Multiple intestinal fistulas.

PROCEDURE PERFORMED: Excision of abdominal wall and small bowel with primary anastomosis of small bowel.

PRELIMINARY NOTE: This patient is well known to us. She has had multiple abdominal procedures to try to repair a very large abdominal wall hernia. She is outside the postoperative period of the hernia repair. She basically has no abdominal cavity left, and all her intestine resides outside the abdomen. There is such a drag on her abdominal wall that she has developed fistulas at the base of where the bowel rests against the mesh, and these have become unmanageable in the home setting. On this basis, we take this very high-risk patient to the operating room, with appropriate counseling for the family about the dire consequences.

OPERATIVE NOTE: With the patient under general anesthesia, the abdomen was prepped and draped in a sterile manner. A long incision was made above the area of the

fistulas, and we began to work our way down onto the mesh. Unfortunately, we entered the bowel at multiple points and had multiple enterotomies into the small bowel *(small intestine)* and colon *(large intestine)*. Finally we got everything freed up and were able to resect some of the abdominal wall that had adherent small bowel to it *(this indicates that part of the small intestine was removed)*. We were able to repair all of the enterostomies and a right colotomy using two layers of suture, an inner layer of Vicryl, and an outer layer of silk. We then copiously irrigated the abdominal field and used some large retention-type sutures to bring the wound together for partial closure. It is our hopes that the bowel that remains is viable *(this indicates that part of the bowel was removed)*. This procedure took substantially greater time than typically would be required. *(This statement indicates -22 may be assigned.)* We measured it at approximately 200 cm of length of her small bowel, and we are hopeful that this will be enough for her to nourish adequately.

CPT Code(s): _____

_____

ICD-10-CM Code(s): _____

_____

PRACTICE EXERCISE 19.19 SMALL-BOWEL ANASTOMOSIS—cont'd

Abstracting Questions

1. Was a portion of the large or small intestine removed?_____
_____

2. What statement indicates that modifier -22 would be appended to the CPT code? _____
_____

PRACTICE EXERCISE 19.20 PYLOROPLASTY

OPERATIVE REPORT

Report only Dr. White's surgical services. Note in this case that the surgeon began the procedure as a percutaneous liver biopsy, but because the patient could not hold his breath long enough for the biopsy to be obtained, Dr. White decided to discontinue the percutaneous biopsy and take the patient directly to the operating room for an open procedure. Two surgeons (co-surgeons) are performing this case. Dr. Sanchez, in his operative report, states that the patient was turned to a lateral position, prepped, and draped and the chest was opened to expose the esophagus. The distal esophagus was mobilized under direct vision and divided above the diseased segment. The distal esophagus and the attached proximal stomach were removed. The remaining stomach was pulled into the chest and connected to the stump of the proximal esophagus. Drains were placed and a chest tube inserted and the incision was closed.

LOCATION: Inpatient, Hospital
PATIENT: Ted Boyd
ATTENDING PHYSICIAN: Larry Friendly, MD
PRIMARY CARE PHYSICIAN: Ronald Green, MD
SURGEONS: Loren White, MD, and Gary Sanchez, MD
PREOPERATIVE DIAGNOSIS: Barrett's esophagus with severe dysplasia, possible carcinoma.
POSTOPERATIVE DIAGNOSIS: Barrett's esophagus with severe dysplasia, possible carcinoma, hemangioma liver.
PROCEDURES PERFORMED
1. Exploratory laparotomy.
2. Biopsy of liver lesion.
3. Immobilization of stomach with pyloroplasty.
4. Placement of feeding tube.

PRELIMINARY NOTE: This patient is a 63-year-old man who has been referred by Dr. Green for a bleeding esophageal lesion. This was seen and scoped, and the patient was markedly anemic. Biopsies showed it to be severe dysplasia with possible cancer present. He has had a rather extensive workup including complete cardiac workup. CT of the abdomen showed some lesions within the liver, which we tried to have biopsied percutaneously, but the patient could not hold his breath well enough and the lesions were too close to the diaphragm, so we do not have a tissue diagnosis on these. After all this workup we are taking the patient to the operating room for exploration. Assuming that he does not have disease metastatic to the liver, we will proceed with an esophagogastrectomy in the Ivor-Lewis technique. The abdominal portion of the procedure, which I am dictating, will be done by myself, and then Dr. Sanchez will do the chest portion of the procedure.

OPERATIVE NOTE: With the patient under general anesthesia, the abdomen was prepped and draped in a sterile manner. Midline incision was made from the xiphoid to below the pubis. Sharp dissection was carried down into the peritoneal cavity, and hemostasis was maintained with electrocautery. We began by exploring the abdominal cavity. The liver was carefully palpated. The area that had been identified on CT was at the very apex of the right lobe of the liver, we could feel this area; it did not have a thickened feel to it but was more consistent with an area of hemangioma. There

was a small secondary lesion on the undersurface of the right lobe. A **wedge biopsy** of this was taken and it did return a diagnosis of hemangioma. The rest of the liver appeared normal, and I thought that we did not need to proceed with anything further. We thus began with mobilization of the stomach, taking down the greater curvature vessels, preserving the gastroepiploica. We carried our dissection all the way up into the hiatal hernia, preserving the blood supply to the spleen and not injuring it. We were then able to detach the left gastric artery such that the stomach was tethered on its other vasculature but appeared completely viable. All these vessels were taken down with clamps and ligatures of 2–0 silk. We then circumferentially went around the esophagus and carried our dissection all the way back toward the pylorus. We then had the entire stomach freed up from pylorus all the way up to the diaphragm. *(The esophagus has been mobilized where it passes through the diaphragm and the stomach has been totally freed up so that when the chest is opened Dr. Sanchez will perform the remaining part of the surgery.)* The stomach appeared viable with reasonable circulation. A Heineke-Mikulicz **pyloroplasty** was then performed opening the pylorus in one direction and closing it in another using interrupted 3–0 silk sutures to complete the pyloroplasty. With this accomplished, we then picked up the **jejunum** approximated 40 or 50 cm beyond the ligament of Treitz and placed a red rubber **feeding tube** using a Witzel technique; this was a number 18-2. This was attached to the skin and brought out through a separate stab incision. The abdominal cavity was then checked for hemostasis and everything appeared to be intact. We then closed the incision using running 0–loop nylon. We closed the skin with staples. A sterile dressing was applied. With all this completed, the patient remained in the operating room and will be positioned by Dr. Sanchez for the thoracic portion of the procedure.

Pathology Report Later Indicated: Hemangioma.

CPT Code(s): _____
_____

ICD-10-CM Code(s): _____
_____

Abstracting Questions

1. Can the discontinued percutaneous liver biopsy be reported? _____
_____

2. If reporting the percutaneous liver biopsy, what modifier(s) is/are required? _____
_____

3. Was the wedge biopsy reported? _____

4. Dr. White performed an immobilization and what other procedure? _____
_____

5. Was the Barrett's and hemangioma reported separately?
_____

Urinary System Subsection (50010-53899)

Anatomic division
- Kidney
- Ureter
- Bladder
- Urethra
  Further divided by procedure such as:
- Incision
- Excision
- Introduction
- Repair
- Laparoscopy
- Endoscopy

Kidney Subheading (50010-50593)

Endoscopy codes are for procedure performed through previously established stoma or incision

Caution: Codes may be unilateral or bilateral

Introduction Category (50382-50435)

Codes divided by renal pelvis catheter procedures or other introduction procedures
  Renal pelvis catheters further divided; internally dwelling or externally accessible
  Catheters for drainage and injections and for radiography
  Aspirations
  Insertion of guidewires
  Tube changes
  Usually reported with radiology component

Ureter Subheading (50600-50980)

Caution: Codes may be unilateral or bilateral
  Divided by type of procedure
- Incision
- Excision
- Introduction
- Repair
- Laparoscopy
- Endoscopy

Bladder Subheading (51020-52700)

Includes codes for
- Incision
- Removal
- Excision
- Introduction
- Urodynamics
- Repair
- Laparoscopy
- Endoscopy

- Cystoscopy
- Urethroscopy
- Cystourethroscopy
- Transurethral surgery
  Vesical Neck and Prostate
  Many bundled codes
  Example: Urethral dilation is included with insertion of cystoscope
  Read all descriptions carefully

Urodynamics (51725-51798)

Procedures relate to motion and flow of urine
  Used to diagnose urine flow obstructions
  Bundled: All instruments, equipment, fluids, gases, probes, catheters, technician's fees, medications, gloves, trays, tubing, and other sterile supplies

Vesical Neck and Prostate (52400-52700)

Contains codes for transurethral resection of the prostate (TURP)

Example: 52601 reports a complete transurethral electrosurgical resection of the prostate and includes vasectomy, meatotomy, cystourethroscopy, urethral calibration and/or dilation, internal urethrotomy, and control of any postoperative bleeding
Other approaches are reported with 55801-55845
Example: 55801 reports a removal of the prostate gland (prostatectomy) through an incision in the perineum and includes vasectomy, meatotomy, urethral calibration and/or dilation, internal urethrotomy, and control of any postoperative bleeding

Male Genital System Subsection (54000-55899)

Penis
Testis
Epididymis
Tunica Vaginalis
Scrotum
Vas Deferens
Spermatic Cord
Seminal Vesicles
Prostate

Biopsy Codes

Located in anatomical subheading to which the codes refer

Example: Biopsy codes in subheadings
- Epididymis (Excision)
Example: 54800, needle biopsy of epididymis
- Testis (Excision)
Example: 54500, needle biopsy of testis

Penis (54000-54450)

Incision codes (54000-54015) differ from Integumentary System codes
- Penis incision codes assigned for deeper structures

Destruction (54050-54065)

Codes divided by
- Extent: Simple or extensive
- Method of destruction, e.g., chemical, cryosurgery
  Extensive destruction can be by any method

Excision (54100-54164)

Commonly used codes for biopsy and circumcision

Introduction (54200-54250)

Many procedures for corpora cavernosa (spongy bodies of penis)
- Injection procedures for Peyronie disease (toughening of corpora cavernosa)
- Treatments for erectile dysfunction (ED)

Repair (54300-54440)

Many plastic repairs
  Some repairs are staged (more than one procedure)
- Stage indicated in code description

Reproductive System Procedures (55920)

Code 55920 reports the placement of catheters/needles into pelvic organs/genitalia
  For subsequent interstitial radioelement application

Intersex Surgery Subsection (55970-55980)

Only 2 codes within subsection
1. Male to female
2. Female to male
   Complicated procedures completed over extended period of time
   Performed by multiple physicians with extensive specialized training

Female Genital System Subsection (56405-58999)

Anatomic division: From vulva to ovaries
- Many bundled services

Vulva, Perineum, and Introitus (56405-56821)

Skene's gland reported with Urinary System, Incision or Excision codes
- Group of small mucous glands, lower end of urethra
- Paraurethral duct

Incision (56405-56442)

I&D of abscess of vulva, perineal area, or Bartholin's gland

Marsupialization (56440)

Cyst incised
  Drained
    Edges sutured to sides to keep cyst open, creating a pouchlike repair

Destruction (56501, 56515)

Lesions destroyed by variety of methods
- Destruction = Eradication (not to be confused with excision; excision is removal)
  Divided by simple or extensive destruction
- Complexity based on physician's judgment
- Stated in medical record
  Destruction has no pathology report

Excision (56605-56740)

Biopsy includes
- Local anesthetic
- Biopsy
- Simple closure
  Code based on number of lesions biopsied

Vulvectomy

Surgical removal of portion of vulva (56620-56640)

Based on extent and size of area removed
Extent
- Simple: Skin and superficial subcutaneous tissues
- Radical: Skin and deep subcutaneous tissues
Size
- Partial: <80% vulvar area
- Complete: >80% vulvar area
Extent and size indicated in operative report

Repair (56800-56810)

Includes plastic repair

Read notes following category
- If repair procedure for wound of genitalia, use Integumentary System code

Endoscopy (56820-56821)

By means of a colposcope with or without biopsy(ies)

Vagina (57000-57426)

Codes divided based on service, e.g., incision, excision

Introduction (57150-57180)

Includes vaginal irrigation, insertion of devices, diaphragm, cervical caps
  Report device inserted separately

- 99070 or HCPCS National Level II codes, such as A4261 (cervical cap)

Repair (57200-57335)

For nonobstetric repairs
- Obstetric repairs, report Maternity Care and Delivery codes

Manipulation (57400-57415)

Dilation: Speculum inserted into vagina, which is enlarged by dilator

Endoscopy/Laparoscopy (57420-57426)

Colposcopy codes based on purpose
- e.g., biopsy, diagnostic
  Includes code for laparoscopic approach for repair of paravaginal defect

Cervix Uteri (57452-57800)

Cervix uteri, narrow lower end of uterus
  Services include endoscopy, excision, repair, manipulation

Excision (57500-57558)

Conization codes
  Conization: Removal of cone of tissue from cervix
  LEEP (loop electrocautery excision procedure) technology may be used for conizations or loop electrode biopsies

Corpus Uteri (58100-58579)

Many complex procedures
- Often very similar wording in code descriptions
- Requires careful reading and specific documentation in the medical record

Excision (58100-58294)

Dilation and curettage (D&C, 58120) of nonobstetric uterus
- After dilation, curette used to scrape uterus
- Coded according to circumstances: Obstetrical or nonobstetrical
  Do not report postpartum hemorrhage service with 58120
- Report 59160—Maternity and Delivery code
  Many hysterectomy codes
- Based on approach (vaginal, abdominal), extent (uterus, fallopian tubes, etc.), and weight of uterus
  Often secondary procedures performed with hysterectomy
  Do not report secondary, related minor procedures separately

Introduction (58300-58356)

Common procedures
- e.g., insertion of an IUD
  Report supply of device separately
  Specialized services

- e.g., artificial insemination procedures
  Used to report physician component of service
  Component coding
- Necessary with catheter procedures for hysterosonography
- Notes following codes indicate radiology guidance component codes

Laparoscopy/Hysteroscopy (58541-58579)

Laparoscopic approach for:
- Removal of myomas
- Radical hysterectomy
- Supracervical and laparoscopic vaginal hysterectomies
  Codes divided by tissue removed and weight of uterus
- Hysteroscopy codes divided on procedure performed (e.g., lysis of uterine adhesions, endometrial ablation)

Oviduct/Ovary (58600-58770)

Oviduct. Fallopian tube
  Incision category contains tubal ligations
- When during same hospitalization (but not at same session as delivery), is reported separately

Laparoscopy (58660-58679)

Through abdominal wall
  Codes in the laparoscopy and hysteroscopy section are divided by procedure performed (e.g., lysis of adhesions, removal adnexal structures)
  Caution: If only diagnostic laparoscopy
- Do not report Female Genital System codes
- Report 49320, Digestive System
  Many codes can be reported separately with appropriate modifiers
  Example: 58660 Laparoscopy, surgical, with lysis of adhesions, can be reported with any of the indented codes that follow 58660 (58661-58673)

Ovary (58800-58960)

Two categories only: Incision and Excision

Incision: Primarily for drainage of cysts and abscesses
- Divided by surgical approach
Excision: Biopsy, wedge resection, and oophorectomy

In Vitro Fertilization (58970-58976)

Specialized codes used by physicians trained in fertilization procedures
- Codes divided by type of procedure and method used

Maternity Care and Delivery Subsection (59000-59899)

Divided by service, such as:
- Antepartum and Fetal Invasive Services

Amniocentesis
Fetal non-stress test
Fetal monitoring during labor
- Type of delivery
Vaginal delivery
C-section
Delivery after previous C-section
- Abortion

Gestation

Fetal gestation: Approximately 266 days (40 weeks)
EDD: Estimated Date of Delivery
- 280 days from last menstrual period (LMP)

Trimesters

First, LMP to less than 14 weeks 0 days
  Second, 14 weeks 0 days to less than 28 weeks 0 days
  Third, 28 weeks 0 days until deliver

Global Package and Delivery

Uncomplicated maternity care includes
- Antepartum care = Before delivery
- Delivery
- Postpartum care = After delivery

Antepartum Care Includes

Initial and subsequent H&P (history and physical)

Blood pressures
Weight
Routine chemical urinalysis
Fetal heart tones
Monthly visits to 28 weeks
Twice-a-month visits, weeks 29 to 36
Weekly visits from week 37 to delivery
Listed in notes preceding 59000
- Services not related to antepartum care are reported separately

Example: Pregnant female with complaint of suspicious mole on left shoulder
- Visits OB/GYN physician, who provides antepartum care
- Service regarding mole, not antepartum care, requires good documentation in the maternity record and a specific diagnosis relative to the treatment provided

Delivery Includes

Admission to hospital with admitting H&P

Management of uncomplicated labor
Vaginal or cesarean section delivery
- Complications coded separately
- Listed in notes preceding 59000

Postpartum Care Includes

Normal follow-up care for 6 weeks after delivery
- Hospital visits, office visits
- Listed in notes preceding 59000

Antepartum and Fetal Invasive Services (59000-59076)

Amniocentesis: Insertion of needle into pregnant uterus, withdrawal of fluid (59000, 59001)
- Ultrasound guidance with 59000 (76946)
- Ultrasound guidance included with 59001
- Component coding often part of services in subheading

Fetal services: Include stress tests, blood sampling, monitoring, and therapeutic procedures

Excision (59100-59160)

Postpartum curettage: Removes remaining pieces of placenta or clotted blood (59160)
Nonobstetric curettage: 58120 (Corpus Uteri, Excision)

Introduction (59200)

Insertion of cervical dilator: Used to prepare and soften the cervix for an abortive procedure or delivery (for abortive procedure, see 59855)
  Cervical ripening agents may be introduced to prepare cervix
- Separate procedure and not reported when part of more major procedure

Repair (59300-59350)

Only for repairs during pregnancy
  Repairs done as a result of delivery or during pregnancy
  Episiotomy or vaginal repair by other than attending physician
  Suture closure (cerclage) of cervix or repair of uterus (hysterorrhaphy)

Routine Global Obstetric Care

Includes antepartum care, delivery, and postpartum care
  59400, Vaginal delivery
  59510, Cesarean delivery
  59610, Vaginal delivery after previous cesarean delivery (VBAC)
  59618, Cesarean delivery following attempted vaginal delivery after previous cesarean delivery

Note: Take care when assigning diagnosis codes for normal versus complicated delivery. ICD-10-CM states specific guidelines for a normal delivery.

Episiotomies and Use of Forceps

Included in delivery
Not reported separately

Physician Provides Only Portion of Global Routine Care, Delivery

59409, Vaginal delivery only
59514, Cesarean delivery only
59612, Vaginal delivery only, after previous cesarean delivery
59620, Cesarean delivery only, following attempted vaginal delivery after previous cesarean delivery

Delivery of Twins

Payers differ on reporting format

- -22 (Unusual Procedural Services)
- -51 (Multiple Procedures)

Abortion Services (59812-59857)

Spontaneous: Happens naturally (for a complete spontaneous abortion, report with a code from the E/M section [99201-99233])
Incomplete: Requires medical intervention
Induced: Intentional termination of pregnancy
Missed: Fetus dies naturally but does not abort during first 22 weeks of gestation
Septic: Abortion with infection
Medical intervention
- Dilation and curettage or evacuation (suction removal)
- Intra-amniotic injections (saline or urea)
- Vaginal suppositories (prostaglandin)

PRACTICE EXERCISE 19.21   RENAL TUMOR EXCISION

LOCATION: Inpatient, Hospital
PATIENT: Brian Eberhoft
ATTENDING PHYSICIAN: Leslie Alanda, MD
SURGEON: Ira Avila, MD
PREOPERATIVE DIAGNOSIS: Right renal tumor.
POSTOPERATIVE DIAGNOSIS: Complex right renal cyst (acquired).
PROCEDURE PERFORMED: Right renal exploration; de-roofing of right renal cyst.
ANESTHESIA: General.

CLINICAL NOTE: Mr. Eberhoft is a 78-year-old gentleman found to have an enlarging right complex renal mass. This does not enhance but has irregular boundaries and has increased in size over the past year. It is located on the medial posterior part of the right kidney adjacent to the renal hilum. Options were discussed with the patient, and he elected to proceed with exploration and possible partial nephrectomy or radical nephrectomy depending on findings.

PROCEDURE: The patient was given a general endotracheal anesthetic as well as an epidural for intraoperative and postoperative analgesia. An incision was made over the tip of the 10th rib and the tip of the 10th rib excised. A small hole in the pleura was created, which was closed at the end of the case.

The patient has very poor fascial structures and very poor superficial muscle development. The peritoneal space was entered and the kidney identified. The Omni retractor was used for exposure. The ascending color was reflected off of Gerota's fascia. The duodenum had made a large turn over top of the renal hilum, and the duodenum was kocherized carefully. The renal vein and renal artery were identified, isolated, and surrounded with vessel loops.

The kidney was mobilized. The adrenal was quite superficial within Gerota's fascia, and the fascia was accidentally torn during the mobilization of the kidney. This was controlled with hemoclips. There was a large perinephric fat pad that was mobilized with the kidney initially, and then Gerota's fascia opened posteriorly. The area in question was identified. The patient had some reaction around the area, but this was not significant. There was a lot of fat adherent to the kidney that was dissected off the posterior region around the renal hilum to identify the mass. The mass

appeared to be cystic in origin. A total of 3 cc of cyst fluid was aspirated from this and sent for cytology.

The cyst room was then opened. There was only a very small part of the cyst visible at the renal surface. Inspection of the cyst wall showed it to be smooth without masses. A small vessel was seen coursing inferiorly. This was cauterized. The renal pelvis was identified and Jelco catheter placed, and 5 cc of methylene blue–stained saline was injected through this to ensure that there was no communication with the cyst cavity and the renal pelvis. There was none.

The entire cyst wall was then cauterized. It was packed with Surgicel. Surgicel was also placed over the adrenal gland to help ensure hemostasis. Hemostasis was ensured. Vessel loops were removed. The kidney was then returned to renal fossa. A 10-mm Jackson-Pratt drain was left through a left lower quadrant stab wound and was placed adjacent to the de-roofed renal cyst.

The peritoneum was inspected, and there was no other abnormality identified on laparotomy.

The abdominal wall was then closed with three layers of 1 Vicryl. The skin was closed with surgical clips. A dressing was applied. Abdominal binder was applied. Prior to beginning closure of the abdominal wall, the rent in the pleura was closed with 3–0 Vicryl. Air was removed using a red rubber catheter in the usual fashion.

Sponge and needle counter were reported correct. The patient had a Foley catheter placed intraoperatively, and he had good urine output throughout the case. Estimated blood loss was 300 cc. He was transferred to the recovery room in good condition.

CPT Code(s): _____

_____

ICD-10-CM Code(s): _____

_____

Abstracting Questions

1. Was this procedure reported as an excision, even though the cyst was drained and the cyst wall retained? _____

_____

PRACTICE EXERCISE 19.21   RENAL TUMOR EXCISION—cont'd

2. Was de-roofing of renal cyst the same as an excision?

_____

3. Did the accidental tear of the fascia require a separate, reportable repair? _____

_____

4. Was a modifier reported? _____

_____

5. Was the diagnosis for an acquired or congenital renal cyst?

_____

PRACTICE EXERCISE 19.22   RENAL MASS

LOCATION: Inpatient, Hospital
PATIENT: Myra Grossman
ATTENDING PHYSICIAN: Ronald Green, MD
SURGEON: Ira Avila, MD
PREOPERATIVE DIAGNOSIS: Right renal mass.
POSTOPERATIVE DIAGNOSIS: Right renal cyst (acquired).
PROCEDURE PERFORMED: Laparoscopic exploration of kidneys, de-roofing, and biopsy of right renal mass.
ANESTHESIA: General.
  SURGICAL INDICATIONS: This is a 20-year-old female who has a complex right renal cyst. She has been evaluated and worked up by Dr. Green. Options have been discussed, and she has elected to proceed with the exploration.
  PROCEDURE: The patient was prepped and draped in the right flank position. A Foley catheter was placed. An incision was made. A retroperitoneal laparoscopic approach was used to approach the kidney, the cyst isolated, vessels identified and surrounded with vessel loops. The cyst was then aspirated and contents sent for cytology. The roof was ablated

free and the base biopsied. There was some bleeding from the bases, which was controlled with 3–0 Chromic suture ligature. 3–0 Chromic sutures were used to close the cyst defect. A 10-mm flat Jackson-Pratt drain was left through a separate stab wound and sutured to the skin. The wound was closed with Vicryl and skin with clips. The patient tolerated the procedure well and was transferred to the recovery room in good condition. Estimated blood loss was 100 cc.
  Pathology Report Later Indicated: Both pathology and cytology reports demonstrating benign cyst.

CPT Code(s): _____

ICD-10-CM Code(s): _____

_____

Abstracting Question

1. What surgical approach was used for this procedure?

_____

PRACTICE EXERCISE 19.23   ABDOMINAL HYSTERECTOMY

OPERATIVE REPORT
LOCATION: Inpatient, Hospital
PATIENT: Maggie Brock
ATTENDING PHYSICIAN: Andy Martinez, MD
SURGEON: Andy Martinez, MD
PREOPERATIVE DIAGNOSES
  1. Chronic menorrhagia.
  2. Uterine fibroids.
POSTOPERATIVE DIAGNOSES
  1. Chronic menorrhagia.
  2. Uterine fibroids.
  PROCEDURE PERFORMED: Total abdominal hysterectomy and bilateral salpingo-oophorectomy.
  ANESTHESIA: General endotracheal.
  SURGICAL INDICATION: This patient is a 48-year-old multiparous female who had had problems with chronic menorrhagia, unsuccessfully treated with hormone manipulation. She had known fibroids as well. Endometrial biopsy preoperatively was benign.
  OPERATIVE FINDINGS: The uterus was about 10- to 12-week size with multiple leiomyomas. There was a functional-appearing cyst on the left ovary that contained some clear fluid. The right ovary was normal. The appendix was retrocecal but otherwise unremarkable.
  OPERATIVE DESCRIPTION: After induction of general anesthesia, the patient was in the supine position. The abdomen and vagina were prepped, and Foley catheter placed; the patient was then draped. The abdomen was

opened through a midline hypogastric incision, excising the old skin scar on the way in. Bowel was then packed out of the pelvis and a self-retaining Balfour retractor was placed. The uterus was elevated with clamps at the cornual areas. The left round ligament was clamped, divided, suture ligated with 0 Vicryl. All sutures were 0 Vicryl unless otherwise indicated. The peritoneal lateral to the left infundibulopelvic ligament was opened with Metzenbaum scissors, isolated in the left ovarian vasculature. This pedicle was isolated, clamped, divided, and doubly ligated. An identical procedure was carried out in the structures on the right side. The anterior and posterior leaves of the broad ligament were taken down with Metzenbaum scissors. There was some abnormal scarring and retraction of the bladder flap on the left side due to her prior cesarean sections. We then skeletonized the uterine artery pedicles on either side. The uterine artery pedicles were clamped with curved Rogers clamps, cut, and suture ligated. The cardinal ligaments and paracervical tissue were taken with two bites of straight Heaney-Ballantine clamps and suture ligated. The vaginal angle was then clamped with curved Rogers clamps, cut and held. The anterior vagina was opened with scalpel; then the upper vagina was incised circumferentially with right-angled scissors. The uterus was then removed and handed off. The vaginal angles were sutured with 0 Vicryl, and the vaginal cuff was closed with a series of interrupted figure-of-eight 0 Vicryl sutures. There was a small bleeding area on one of the cardinal ligament pedicles on the left side. This was isolated with an Allis clamp and secured with a

Continued

PRACTICE EXERCISE 19.23 ABDOMINAL HYSTERECTOMYC—cont'd

suture ligature. Sponges were then removed. Sponge and needle counts were correct. The abdominal fascia was closed with interrupted 0 Ethibond sutures and the skin with staples. Blood loss estimation by anesthesia was 250 cc. Specimen to pathology: Uterus, tubes, and ovaries. Final sponge and needle counts were correct.

CPT Code(s): _____

_____

ICD-10-CM Code(s): _____

_____

Abstracting Questions

1. What factors affect CPT code assignment for the abdominal hysterectomy? _____

_____

2. What factors affect the diagnosis code selection for the uterine leiomyoma? _____

3. What is another name for leiomyoma? _____

_____

PRACTICE EXERCISE 19.24 CESAREAN SECTION

OPERATIVE REPORT

The physician who performs the cesarean section will also provide the postpartum care in this case.

LOCATION: Inpatient, Hospital
PATIENT: Joan Tisdale
ATTENDING PHYSICIAN: Andy Martinez, MD
SURGEON: Andy Martinez, MD
PREOPERATIVE DIAGNOSES
1. Intrauterine pregnancy at 31 weeks and 6 days.
2. Abruptio placentae.

POSTOPERATIVE DIAGNOSES
1. Intrauterine pregnancy at 31 weeks and 6 days.
2. Abruptio placentae.

PROCEDURE PERFORMED: Primary low transverse cervical cesarean section.

ANESTHESIA: General endotracheal.

SURGICAL INDICATIONS: The patient is a 31-year-old woman, gravida 4, para 3, at 31 weeks 6 days by menstrual dates, who was transferred on an emergency basis because of uterine bleeding. She had an apparent abruption on ultrasound, and the vagina was filled with blood clot. For these reasons, she was taken to surgery for an emergency cesarean section.

OPERATIVE FINDINGS: The infant is female, born at 2007 hours, weighing 2125 grams (4 lb 10 ounces), with Apgar scores of 8 at 1 minute and 9 at 5 minutes. There was a lot of blood in the uterine cavity and some adherent clot to the placenta, estimated to be less than 10% abruption. The tubes and ovaries were normal.

PROCEDURE: The abdomen was prepped and draped. A Foley catheter was in. The patient was then given a general endotracheal anesthetic, and the abdomen was opened through a Pfannenstiel incision. Bladder flap was opened transversely with scissors, and bladder was dissected downward bluntly with a hand. A small incision was made in the myometrium of the lower uterine segment, and then entry into the uterus was accomplished bluntly with a Kelly clamp. Low transverse incision was made with bandage scissors. The infant was delivered without undue difficulty. The infant's mouth

and nose were suctioned with a bulb syringe, the cord was clamped and cut, and the infant was handed to Dr. Ortez and the ICN staff. A segment of the cord was taken for cord blood gases, and the placenta was then delivered manually. Inspection of the uterine incision revealed there was a brisk bleeder near the left corner of the incision, and this was oversewn initially and the first layer was a running locked 0 Vicryl. The second layer was a running horizontal Lembert 0 Vicryl. The pelvis was irrigated with saline. The uterine incision was inspected, and there was a small amount of oozing from the incision, which was controlled with a single figure-of-eight 0 Vicryl suture. When hemostasis was adequate and lap sponges were correct, attention was directed toward closure. The peritoneum was loosely approximated in the midline with a couple of mattress sutures of 2–0 Vicryl. A medium Hemovac drain was placed subfascially to exit below the right side of the incision. The fascia was closed with running 0 Vicryl using two strands, one from either side to the middle and tied independently. The skin was closed with staples and the drain sutured to the skin with silk. Estimated blood loss was 1200-1500 cc.

Specimen to pathology was placenta. Final sponge and needle counts were correct.

CPT Code(s): _____

_____

ICD-10-CM Code(s): _____

_____

Abstracting Questions

1. What factor in this case determines the appropriate C-section code? _____

_____

2. In addition to the placental abruption, what other two diagnoses must be reported? _____

and _____

PRACTICE EXERCISE 19.25 LABIAL EXCISION

OPERATIVE REPORT
LOCATION: Inpatient, Hospital
PATIENT: Mary Brown
ATTENDING PHYSICIAN: Andy Martinez, MD
SURGEON: Andy Martinez, MD
PREOPERATIVE DIAGNOSIS: Vulvar intraepithelial neoplasia III of the right labia.
POSTOPERATIVE DIAGNOSIS: Vulvar intraepithelial neoplasia III of the right labia.
PROCEDURE PERFORMED: Radical excision, right labia.
PREAMBLE: The patient is a 47-year-old woman who presented with a right labial lesion. This was biopsied and reported as being VIN-III; invasion cannot be ruled out. The decision was therefore made to proceed with radical excision of the right vulva.
PROCEDURE: The patient was taken to the operating room and general anesthetic was administered. The patient was then prepped and draped in the usual manner in lithotomy position, and the bladder was emptied with a straight catheter. The vulva was then inspected. On the right labia majora at approximately the 11 o'clock position, there was a multifocal lesion present. A marking pen was then used to mark out an elliptical incision leaving a 1-cm border on all sides. The skin ellipse was then excised using the knife. Bleeders were cauterized with electrocautery. A running locked suture of 2–0

Vicryl was then placed in the deeper tissues. The skin was finally reapproximated with 4–0 Vicryl in an interrupted fashion. Good hemostasis was thereby achieved. The patient tolerated this procedure well. There were no complications. Estimated blood loss was 75 cc.

Pathology Report Later Indicated: Neoplasia III, carcinoma in situ.

CPT Code(s): _____

_____

ICD-10-CM Code(s): _____

Abstracting Questions

1. In what area of the female genital anatomy is the labia located? _____

_____

2. CPT code assignment was affected by the extent (partial/complete) and what other factor? _____

_____

3. Define "in situ." _____

_____

Endocrine System Subsection (60000-60699)

Nine glands in endocrine system; only four included in subsection
1. Thyroid
2. Parathyroid
3. Thymus
4. Adrenal

Pituitary and Pineal

See Nervous System subsection

Pancreas

Digestive System

Ovaries and Testes

Respective genital systems

Divided into two subheadings
- Thyroid Gland
- Parathyroid, Thymus, Adrenal Glands, Pancreas, and Carotid Body

Carotid Body

Refers to area adjacent to the bifurcation of the carotid artery
    Can be site of tumors

Thyroid Gland, Excision Category (60100-60281)

- **Lobectomy:** Partial or subtotal (something less than total)

- **Thyroidectomy:** Total (all)
  Thyroid, 1 gland with 2 lobes

Nervous System Subsection (61000-64999)

Divided anatomically
- Skull, Meninges, and Brain
- Spine and Spinal Cord
- Extracranial Nerves, Peripheral Nerves, and Autonomic Nervous System

Skull, Meninges, and Brain (61000-62258)
Category Examples:

Injection, Drainage, or Aspiration
    Twist Drills, Burr Hole(s), or Trephine

Conditions That Require Openings Into Brain to

Relieve pressure
    Insert monitoring devices
    Place tubing
    Inject contrast material

Craniectomy or Craniotomy (61304-61576)

Craniectomy involves removal of portion of skull, at operative site, performed emergently to prevent herniation of brain into the brainstem

Craniotomy—bone flap is replaced after surgery
Codes divided by site and condition for which procedure is performed

Surgery of Skull Base (61580-61619)

Skull base: Area at base of cranium
- Lesion removal from this area very complex

Surgery of Skull Base Terminology

Approach procedure used to gain exposure of lesion
Definitive procedure is what is done to lesion
Repair/reconstruction procedure reported separately only if extensive repair
Approach procedure and definitive procedure coded separately
Example: Removal of an intradural lesion using middle cranial fossa approach
- 61590 approach procedure, middle cranial fossa and
- 61608 definitive procedure of intradural resection of lesion

Cerebrospinal Fluid (CSF) Shunt Category (62180-62258)

Performed to drain fluid

Codes describe, e.g.:
- Placement of devices
- Reprogramming
- Replacement
- Removal of shunting devices

Spine and Spinal Cord (62263-63746)

Codes divided by condition and approach
Often used are
- Unilateral or bilateral procedures (-50)
- Multiple procedures (-51)
- Radiologic supervision and fluoroscopic guidance coded separately

Includes codes for
- Myelography injections 62302-62305
  - Spinal or steroid anesthetic injections 62320-62326
  - Intrathecal or epidural catheter placement/implantation 62350-62355

Extracranial Nerves, Peripheral Nerves, and Autonomic Nervous System (64400-64999), Introduction/Injection of Anesthetic Agent (Nerve Block), Diagnostic or Therapeutic Category (64400-64530)

Includes codes for
- Nerve blocks 64486-64489, 64505-64530
  - Bundled when used as anesthesia for procedure
- Paravertebral facet joint injections 64490-64495, diagnostic or therapeutic
- Epidural injections 64479-64484
  - Used to provide pain relief
  - As compared with an epidural catheter placement used for anesthetic purposes

Eye and Ocular Adnexa Subsection (65091-68899)

Terminology extremely important
- Code descriptions often vary only slightly
  Understanding of eye anatomy is necessary for proper coding in this subsection
  Codes divided anatomically, e.g.,
- Eyeball
- Anterior segment
- Posterior segment
- Ocular adnexa
- Conjunctiva
  Some codes specifically for previous surgery
  Example: Insertion of ocular implant, secondary (65130)
  Much bundling
  Example: Subheading Posterior Segment, Prophylaxis category notes indicate:
- "The following descriptors (67141, 67145) are intended to include all sessions in a defined treatment period."

Cataracts

Method used depends on type of cataract and surgeon preference
  Nuclear cataract: Most common, center of lens (nucleus), due to aging process
  Cortical cataract: Forms in cortex of lens and extends outward; frequent in diabetics
  Subcapsular cataract: Forms at back of lens, increased rate in diabetics, those who take steroid medications, certain genetic factors, and eye trauma

Removal and Lens Replacement (66830-66986)

- Extracapsular cataract extraction (ECCE)
  Patient retains posterior outer shell of the lens
  Soft cortex and rest of shell is removed in multiple pieces
  Posterior shell helps prevent vitreous prolapse
- Intracapsular cataract extraction (ICCE) is total removal
  Removes lens and capsule in one piece
- Phacoemulsification
  Small incision into eye and introduction of probe
  High-frequency waves fragment cataract (extracapsular); then suctioned out
  Lens placed through same small incision

Eyelids (67700-67999)

Blepharotomy (67700)
- Incision into eyelid for drainage of abscess
  Blepharoplasty
- Repair of eyelid
- Codes in Integumentary System (15820-15823), report removal of excess skin
- Codes in Eye and Ocular Adnexa (67916, 67917, 67923, 67924), report muscle repairs and slings
  Selection of code depends on technique used to repair eyelid
- Blepharoplasty codes with specific techniques, 67901-67908

Auditory System Subsection (69000-69979)

Codes divided by
- External Ear (69000-69399)
- Middle Ear (69420-69799)
- Inner Ear (69801-69949)
- Temporal Bone, Middle Fossa Approach (69950-69979)
  Understanding of ear anatomy is necessary for proper coding in this subsection
  External, middle, and inner ear further divided by procedure, such as
- Incision
- Excision
- Removal
- Repair
  Myringotomy and tympanostomy
- Eustachian tube connects middle ear to back of throat for drainage
- Fluid collects in middle ear when tube does not function properly
- Prevents air from entering middle ear and pressure builds
- Surgical intervention
  Myringotomy (incision into tympanic membrane)
  Tympanostomy (placement of PE [pressure equalization] tube)

Operating Microscope Subsection (+69990)

Employed with procedures using microsurgical techniques

Code in addition to primary procedure performed
Do not report separately when primary procedure description includes microsurgical techniques
Example: 15758 Free fascial flap with microvascular anastomosis
Note that following 15758 is the statement:
- "(Do not report code 69990 in addition to code 15758)" indicating to the coder not to report the use of the operating microscope separately
Do not report 69990 when magnifying loupes are used

PRACTICE EXERCISE 19.26   INTRACEREBRAL HEMATOMA

OPERATIVE REPORT
LOCATION: Inpatient, Hospital
PATIENT: Suzy Kunklemann
ATTENDING PHYSICIAN: Gary Sanchez, MD
SURGEON: Gary Sanchez, MD
PREOPERATIVE DIAGNOSIS: Intracerebral hematoma (nontraumatic), right temporal lobe.
POSTOPERATIVE DIAGNOSIS: Intracerebral hematoma (nontraumatic), right temporal lobe.
PROCEDURE PERFORMED: Osteoplastic craniotomy, right temporal area; evacuation of intracerebral hematoma.
ANESTHESIA: General.
  PROCEDURE: Under general anesthesia, the patient's head was placed in the Mayfield pins. The right frontal temporoparietal area was prepped and draped in the usual manner. A linear incision was made extending from the midline of the temporal fossa up to the midportion of the scalp. The skin was incised. The temporalis muscle was separated and divided off the bone. I did a craniotomy here the size of a half-dollar and made a burr hole. I utilized the craniotome to elevate the bone flap, and this was a free bone flap. This was then removed. We placed the Weitlaners into the wound and then incised the dura in a cruciate fashion over the temporal lobe. I then entered the middle temple gyrus and irrigated much of the clot from the temporal and posterior parietal areas, and evacuated the clot from the area. This took copious irrigation. We used cotton balls for hemostasis. I did this

numerous times until all the bleeders were coagulated. I then lined the cystic cavity with Gelfoam and coagulated the edges of the raw brain. I closed the dura with 4–0 Vicryl. This was closed in a watertight fashion. I used 2–0 Vicryl to elevate the dura to the bone flap with Wurzburg plates, two of them, utilizing plates and screws. I then closed the scalp in one layer using 0 Vicryl on the temporalis muscle and fascia, and the skin was approximated with 2–0 nylon interrupted mattress sutures. Dressing was applied, and the patient was on the ventilator and discharged to the surgical intensive care unit.

CPT Code(s): _____

_____

ICD-10-CM Code(s): _____

Abstracting Questions

1. Was the procedure performed a surgical craniotomy?

_____

2. Does the area of the skull being opened affect the code?

_____

3. What was the purpose of the procedure? _____

_____

4. Does the purpose of the procedure affect the CPT code?

_____

PRACTICE EXERCISE 19.27   PARIETAL BURR HOLES

OPERATIVE REPORT
LOCATION: Inpatient, Hospital
PATIENT: Reed Scaleni
ATTENDING PHYSICIAN: Gary Sanchez, MD
SURGEON: Gary Sanchez, MD
PREOPERATIVE DIAGNOSIS: Subacute subdural hematoma (nontraumatic), right side.

POSTOPERATIVE DIAGNOSIS: Subacute subdural hematoma (nontraumatic), right side.
PROCEDURE PERFORMED: Burr hole times two, right frontal and right posterior parietal.
ANESTHESIA: General.
  PROCEDURE: Under general anesthesia, the patient's head was prepped and draped in the usual manner. The

Continued

PRACTICE EXERCISE 19.27   PARIETAL BURR HOLES—cont'd

incision was made. Straight line linear incisions over the frontal and posterior parietal areas were made on the right side. Retractors were placed. Burr holes remained. The dura was visualized. The bony edges were waxed with beeswax. The dura was incised, both the frontal and the parietal holes. Serosanguineous fluid and clouded blood exuded. I cleaned it out until the supernatant was clear. The brain was found to be pulsating beneath. We then placed two medium-size Penrose drains and closed the galea with 2–0 Vicryl. The skin was approximated with surgical staples, and the Penrose drains were anchored with sutures. A dressing was applied. The patient was discharged to the PAR.

CPT Code(s): _____

_____

ICD-10-CM Code(s): _____

_____

Abstracting Questions

1. What determines the code assignment for burr holes of the skull? _____

_____

2. Does the location of the hematoma being drained/aspirated make a difference in the CPT code assignment? _____

_____

3. Was this CPT code reported twice for the two burr holes?

_____

4. Was a modifier reported to indicate which side of the skull was drilled? _____

_____

PRACTICE EXERCISE 19.28   CARPAL TUNNEL

OPERATIVE REPORT
LOCATION: Outpatient, Hospital
PATIENT: Judy Burns
ATTENDING PHYSICIAN: Gary Sanchez, MD
SURGEON: Gary Sanchez, MD
PREOPERATIVE DIAGNOSIS: Left carpal tunnel syndrome.
POSTOPERATIVE DIAGNOSIS: Left carpal tunnel syndrome.
PROCEDURE PERFORMED: Carpal tunnel released, left wrist.
ANESTHESIA: Regional.
   PROCEDURE: After a satisfactory level of regional anesthesia, the extremity was addressed once it had been sterilely prepped and draped. Throughout the procedure the patient needed some focal augmentation for sharp pain characteristics at the level of the skin most distally about the skin wound. Sharp dissection was conducted down to the palmaris fascia. We identified the deep transverse ligament. In a blunt manner, we undermined this, and with use of a Freer interposing between deep transverse carpal ligament and the medial nerve, sharply dissected over the Freer, releasing the

impinging structures about the carpal canal. The probe palpation, the tendinous structures, and the floor of the carpal canal were otherwise unremarkable. She has at this time an exiting thenar motor branch, which was not obscured. There is an hourglass deformity of the median nerve as noted. At completion of this the wound was irrigated, followed by closure of the dermal planes and application of a splint. The patient tolerated the procedure well and was transported to the recovery room in a stable manner.

CPT Code(s): _____

_____

ICD-10-CM Code(s): _____

_____

Abstracting Question

1. Release of the carpal tunnel has what effect on the median nerve? _____

_____

PRACTICE EXERCISE 19.29   REPAIR OF PSEUDOMENINGOCELE

OPERATIVE REPORT
   This patient is returned to the operating room during the postoperative period for a decompression laminectomy performed by the same physician who now performs the pseudomeningocele repair.
LOCATION: Inpatient, Hospital
PATIENT: Debbie Smith
ATTENDING PHYSICIAN: Gary Sanchez, MD
SURGEON: Gary Sanchez, MD
PREOPERATIVE DIAGNOSIS: Pseudomeningocele.
POSTOPERATIVE DIAGNOSIS: Pseudomeningocele.
PROCEDURE PERFORMED: Repair of pseudomeningocele at the L4-5 level just to the left of the midline.
   PROCEDURE: The patient was taken to the operating room and underwent placement of a spinal drain by the anesthesiologist. She then underwent induction of a general endotracheal anesthesia. She was flipped to the prone position

and was thoroughly prepped and draped. The previous incision was reopened and was extended approximately 1 inch both superiorly and inferiorly. A large amount of spinal fluid came forth. There was a well-epithelialized membrane underneath the subcutaneous tissue extending deep to the muscle. This was excised as much as possible. I first dissected the paraspinal muscles laterally on each side along the L2 vertebra. I identified epithelial lining consistent with a pseudomeningocele. I saw a small leak and thought that I saw spinal fluid coming from the small defect. I gave a Valsalva maneuver, but it was not crystal clear whether this was spinal fluid or merely epidural blood. Anyway, I packed this off with Surgicel, placed a small fat graft, and secured it with a 4–0 Nurolon. I then used the FloSeal and Duragen to seal off the defect. I began reapproximating the muscle when I then noticed that there was spinal fluid again coming from the inferior portion of the incision. I exposed the lamina of L5

PRACTICE EXERCISE 19.29 REPAIR OF PSEUDOMENINGOCELE—cont'd

bilaterally and placed a retractor. I then noticed that there was a dural defect just to the left of the midline between the L4 and L5 laminae. I did a partial hemilaminectomy of L5 on the left side and was able to place three separate 4–0 Nurolon sutures through the dural defect. Care was taken to depress the nerve within the dural sac with a #4 Penfield. I then directly repaired the dura and did not see any further spinal fluid leakage with a Valsalva maneuver. I then used some FloSeal and strategically placed pieces of Surgicel to cover the defect. I then placed a small piece of Duragen on top of this as well. I irrigated with copious amounts of saline. I then closed the muscle in the deep fascia with interrupted 2–0 Vicryls, which were very closely approximated. I then used interrupted 2–0 Vicryl to close the subcutaneous tissue. The skin was closed with a running 4–0 nylon interlocking stitch. A sterile dressing was placed.

The patient tolerated the procedure well without apparent complications. The spinal drain was sutured in by me at the end of the procedure. She was taken to the recovery room in stable condition. Sponge, instrument, and needle counts were correct times two.

CPT Code(s): _____

ICD-10-CM Code(s): _____

Abstracting Questions

1. Repair of the pseudomeningocele is repair of what? _____
_____

2. What procedure was performed to clear the approach for the repair of the dura tear? _____

3. Does the pseudomeningocele make a difference in the CPT code assignment? _____

4. What modifiers are required? _____
_____

PRACTICE EXERCISE 19.30 LAMINECTOMY WITH FORAMINOTOMY

OPERATIVE REPORT
LOCATION: Inpatient, Hospital
PATIENT: Karen Origami
ATTENDING PHYSICIAN: Gary Sanchez, MD
SURGEON: Gary Sanchez, MD
PREOPERATIVE DIAGNOSIS: Severe spinal stenosis from L3 through L5.
POSTOPERATIVE DIAGNOSIS: Severe spinal stenosis from L3 through L5 without neurogenic claudications.
PROCEDURES PERFORMED
1. Bilateral L3 laminectomy with foraminotomy.
2. Bilateral L4 laminectomy with foraminotomy.
3. Bilateral L5 laminectomy with foraminotomy.
   INDICATION: This patient is a 79-year-old female who presented with severe neurogenic claudication, left greater than right. Workup included an MRI scan, which showed severe spinal stenosis from L3 through L5. After discussion of the options, she elected to undergo surgery. She was informed that this was an elective surgery and was not life or limb threatening. The risks of the procedure were thoroughly discussed, and the patient consented to proceed.
   PROCEDURE: The patient was taken to the operating room and underwent induction after general endotracheal anesthesia in the supine position. She was then flipped to the prone position on the operating room table and the knees were flexed. The lower lumbar spine was thoroughly prepped and draped, and a vertical midline skin incision was made from the L3 to the S1 spinous processes. The skin was infiltrated with local anesthetic prior to making the incision. Using the monopolar cautery, I identified the spinous processes of L2 through S1 bilaterally. Then using the periosteal elevator, I retracted the paraspinal muscles laterally bilaterally. Deep retractors were placed. At this point, I used the handheld rongeur and removed the spinous processes of L4 and L3. An intraoperative x-ray was done to verify the location. At this, the L5 spinous process was then removed. I then alternated between the rongeurs and the high-speed burr, and drilled down the medial facets and the lamina of L5, L4, and L3. I then began using the Kerrison and removed the inferior lamina of L5 and proceeded from a caudal to cephalad direction. I alternated between the high-speed drill and the Kerrison

rongeurs and eventually removed the lamina and the medial facets bilaterally of L3 through L5. There was noted to be very severe compression of the thecal sac at the L4-5 level as there was a grade 1 spondylolisthesis at that level. There was also noted to be severe spinal stenosis at the L3-4 level. After an adequate decompression, I made sure that the decompression extended laterally out to the exiting nerve roots on each side bilaterally. The nerve roots were particularly tight at the L4-5 level, where the spondylolisthesis was located. At no time was there a dural tear or spinal fluid leak. I irrigated with copious amounts of saline. Bleeding bone edges were waxed. The gutters were lined with Surgicel, and a piece of Gelfoam was placed over the exposed dura. I irrigated again. I closed the wound in layers with interrupted 0 and 2–0 Vicryl. Skin was closed with a running 3–0 Vicryl subcuticular stitch. Benzoin and one-half-inch Steri-Strips and a sterile dressing were placed.

The patient tolerated the procedure well without apparent complication. She will go to the recovery room after the surgery. Sponge, instrument, and needle counts were correct.

CPT Code(s): _____

ICD-10-CM Code(s): _____
_____

Abstracting Questions

1. In addition to the laminectomy with foraminotomy, what other procedure was performed? _____
_____

2. Which vertebrae were addressed? _____

3. How many codes are necessary to report all three vertebrae? _____

4. What modifiers are required? _____
_____

20
Radiology Section (70010-79999)

Radiology: Branch of medicine that uses radiant energy to diagnose and treat patients

Specialist in radiology: Radiologist (doctor of medicine)

Radiology Subsections

1. Diagnostic Radiology
2. Diagnostic Ultrasound
3. Radiologic Guidance
4. Breast, Mammography
5. Bone/Joint Studies
6. Radiation Oncology
7. Nuclear Medicine

Procedures

Fluoroscopy views inside of body, projects onto television screen

Live images by which physician can view function, structure, and defects or anomalies within an organ

Example: 71047, 76000 chest x-ray with fluoroscopy

Magnetic Resonance Imaging (MRI)

Example: 72148 MRI of spinal canal

Tomography or Computed Axial Tomography (CAT or CT Scan)

Example: 70450 tomographic scan of head or brain

Planes of Body (Fig. 20.1)

Position and Projection

Position = method of positioning patients for examination

Projection path = pathway traveled by x-ray beam

Component Coding

Three component terms
1. Professional
2. Technical
3. Global

Professional Component

Physician portion of service, includes
- Supervision of technician
- Interpretation of results, including written report

Technical Component

- Technologist's services
- Equipment, film, and supplies

Global Procedure

Both professional and technical portions of radiology service

Component Modifiers

If only professional component of radiology service provided: add modifier -26

If only technical component provided: add modifier -TC
- -TC HCPCS modifier used with CPT and HCPCS codes

If both professional and technical components of radiology service are provided by physician who owns equipment and facility, pays technician and supplies (global), no modifier is needed

Example: Chest x-ray
- Professional component: 71048-26 (supervision and final report)
- Technical component: 71048-TC (technician, supplies, equipment)
- Global procedure: 71048 (both professional and technical)

Third-party payers usually reimburse
- 40% professional component
- 60% technical component
- 100% global procedure

Contrast Material

Statement "with contrast" indicates injection service included in code

Oral or rectal contrast does not qualify for "with contrast"

Notes indicate codes for components

Example: 75801, Lymphangiography, parenthetical note above code indicates: "For injection procedure for lymphatic system, use 38790"

Interventional Radiologist

Combination radiologist and surgeon

Provides total procedure for cystography with contrast

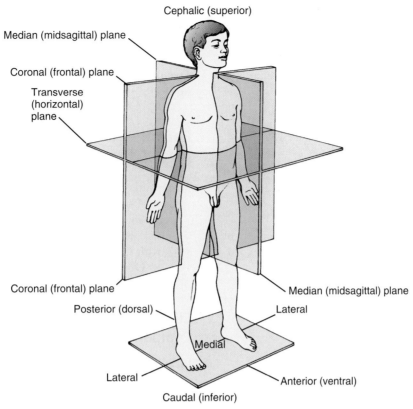

Cephalic (superior)

Median (midsagittal) plane

Coronal (frontal) plane

Transverse (horizontal) plane

Coronal (frontal) plane

Median (midsagittal) plane

Posterior (dorsal)

Lateral

Medial

Lateral

Anterior (ventral)

Caudal (inferior)

• **Figure 20.1** Planes of the body.

- Report 74430, x-ray portion
- 51600 for injection procedure
- Plus code for supply of contrast material (e.g., 99070)

Diagnostic Radiology Subsection (70010-76499)

Most standard radiographic procedures
  Codes often divided by whether contrast material used
  Codes further divided by number of views
  Example: 71048, Chest x-ray, 4 views or more
  Used to:
  - Diagnose disease
  - Monitor disease process—progression or remission
  - Therapeutic procedures (guidance)

Diagnostic Procedures Include

X-ray
  Computerized axial tomography (CAT or CT scan)
  Magnetic resonance imaging (MRI)
  Angiography
    Fluoroscopy
    3D rendering

Computed Axial Tomography (CAT or CT)

X-ray image taken in sections
  Computer reconstructs and enhances image

Magnetic Resonance Imaging (MRI)

Uses magnetic fields to produce an image displayed on computer screen
  Codes of same area (e.g., spine) divided by whether or not contrast material used

Angiography

Used to view vessel obstructions
  Dye injected into vessel
  Radiologist uses angiography to diagnose vascular conditions
  Example:
  - Malformation
  - Stroke (cerebrovascular accident, CVA)
  - Myocardial infarction (MI)

> **NOTE**
>
> **Remember**
> If fewer than total number of views specified in code provided: Report -52, Reduced Service

Diagnostic Ultrasound Subsection (76506-76999)

Uses high-frequency sound waves to image anatomic structures
  Nine subheadings of Diagnostic Ultrasound
  Primarily based on anatomy

A-Mode (A = Amplitude)

Technique used to map structure outline in one-dimensional image

M-Mode (M = Motion)

Technique used to display one-dimensional movement of structure

B-Scan (B = Brightness)

Technique used to display two-dimensional movement of tissues and organs
  Known as gray scale ultrasound

Real-Time Scan

Technique used to display both structure and motion with time of organ and tissues in a two-dimensional image

Extent of Study

Codes often divided on extent of study
  Example: Extent of scan as follows
  • **Complete:** Scans entire body or body region
  • **Limited:** Scans part of body, e.g., one organ
  • **Follow-up/repeat:** Limited study of part of body that was scanned previously

Three Locations for Ultrasound Services

76506-76999: Radiology codes for diagnostic ultrasound services
93875-93990: Medicine codes for non-invasive vascular studies
93303-93355: Medicine codes for echocardiography

Radiologic Guidance Subsection (77001-77022)

Guidance
  • Fluoroscopic
  • Computed tomography
  • Magnetic resonance
  • Other

Breast Mammography Subsection (77051-77063)

Example: Computer-aided detection and screening
  Some codes specify unilateral/bilateral

Bone/Joint Studies Subsection (77071-77086)

Example: Bone density, bone mineral density, and joint survey

Radiation Oncology Subsection (77261-77799)

Therapeutic use of radiation
  Codes both professional and technical services
  Subheadings divided based on treatment
  Initial consultation, prior to decision to treat, reported with E/M code
  • **Outpatient:** 99241-99245
  • **Inpatient:** 99251-99255

Clinical Treatment Planning—Professional Component (77261-77299)

Includes
  • Interpretation of special testing
  • Tumor localization
  • Determination of treatment volume
  • Choice of treatment method
  • Determination of number of treatment ports
  • Selection of treatment devices
  • Other necessary procedures
    Clinical Treatment Planning consists of
  • Planning
  • Simulation

Three Levels of Planning (77261-77263)

1. **Simple:** One treatment area, one port, or one set of parallel ports
2. **Intermediate:** Three or more ports, two separate treatment areas, multiple blocking
3. **Complex:** Complex blocking, custom shielding blocks, tangential ports, special wedges, 3+ treatment areas, special beams

Simulation (77280-77293)

Determining placement of treatment areas/ports for radiation treatment
  Does not include administration of radiation

Definitions of Simulation

1. **Simple:** 1 treatment area with 1 port or pair of ports
2. **Intermediate:** 3+ ports, 2 separate treatment areas, multiple blocking
3. **Complex:** Tangential ports, 3+ treatment areas, complex blocking
4. **Computer-generated 3D:** reconstruction of volume of tumor and critical structures

Medical Radiation, Physics, Dosimetry, Treatment Devices, and Special Services (77295, 77300-77370)

Decision making services of physicians
- Treatment types
- Dose calculation and placement (dosimetry)
- Development of treatment device

Stereotactic Radiation Treatment Delivery (77371-77373)

Delivers large radiation dose to specific tumor sites
- Computer(s) map location
- Radiation delivered to one or more sites

Radiation and Neutron Beam Treatment Delivery (77401-77525)

Technical component of actual delivery of radiation

Information Needed to Code Radiation Treatment Delivery

Amount of radiation delivered
    Type of radiation—electron (most common), neutron, or proton
    Number of
- Areas treated (single, two, three or more)
- Ports involved (single, three or more, tangential)
- Blocks used (none, multiple, custom)

Reporting Radiation Treatment Management (77427-77499)

Professional (physician) portion of services, including
- Review port films
- Review dosimetry, dose delivery, treatment parameters
- Treatment set-up
- Patient examination for medical E/M

Report in units of five fractions, unless last 3-4 fractions are at the end of the treatment; then you can count the last 3-4 as an additional fraction

Hyperthermia (77600-77615)

Use of heat by means of ultrasound, probes, microwave, etc.
    Treatment delivered at three levels:
- External (superficial and deep)
- Interstitial
- Intracavitary

Used in addition to radiation therapy or chemotherapy
Includes three months follow-up after procedure

Clinical Brachytherapy (77750-77799)

Placement of radioactive material into or around site of tumor
- Intracavitary (within body cavity)
- Interstitial (within tissues)

Source

Radioactive element delivers radiation dose over time
    Example: Seeds, ribbons, or capsules
- **Ribbons:** Seeds embedded on tape and inserted into tissue
- Tape is cut to desired length, thereby controlling amount of radiation

Clinical Brachytherapy Codes Divided Based on

Number of sources applied
- Simple 1-4
- Intermediate 5-10
- Complex 11+

Nuclear Medicine Subsection (78012-79999)

Placement of radioactive material into body and measurement of emissions
    Used for both diagnosis and treatment
    Codes divided primarily on organ system
- Except "Therapeutic," which is for radiopharmaceutical therapies

PRACTICE EXERCISE 20.1 CRANIAL CT

RADIOLOGY REPORT
LOCATION: Inpatient, Hospital
PATIENT: Bill Arnold
ORDERING PHYSICIAN: Timothy L. Pleasant, MD
ATTENDING/ADMIT PHYSICIAN: Timothy L. Pleasant, MD
RADIOLOGIST: Morton Monson, MD
PERSONAL PHYSICIAN: Ronald Green, MD
EXAMINATION: Cranial CT.
CLINICAL SYMPTOMS: Altered mental status.
TECHNIQUE: Axial noncontrast CT scan of the head.
   INTERPRETATION: There is diffuse mild enlargement of the sulci and ventricles. Periventricular diminished density is present bilaterally and is prominent near the trigones of the lateral ventricles. There is a 1-mm high-density area seen on image 10 in the left posterior temporal occipital region.
   In the posterior fossa the fourth ventricle is normal in position. Mildly prominent cerebellar folia are present.
   No abnormalities of the orbits, paranasal sinuses, or temporal bone can be seen.
   There is a small amount of calcification in the paraclinoid and carotid arteries.
CONCLUSIONS
   1. Mild diffuse cerebral atrophy.

   2. Periventricular changes consistent with age-related ischemic change.
   3. Tiny calcification in the left posterior temporal occipital region. Finding is nonspecific and could reflect previous granulomatous calcification, intraluminal calcification, Pantopaque, or calcification in a lesion. Recommend clinical correlation and cranial MRI if appropriate.
   4. Vascular calcifications are present.
   CPT Code(s): _____

_____

ICD-10-CM Code(s): _____

Abstracting Questions

1. What was the clinical symptom that prompted this CT?

_____

2. Sulci were referred to in the Interpretation section. What are sulci? _____

_____

PRACTICE EXERCISE 20.2 GALLBLADDER ULTRASOUND

RADIOLOGY REPORT
LOCATION: Outpatient, Hospital
PATIENT: Dan Diel
ORDERING PHYSICIAN: Daniel G. Olanka, MD
ATTENDING/ADMIT PHYSICIAN: Daniel G. Olanka, MD
RADIOLOGIST: Morton Monson, MD
PERSONAL PHYSICIAN: Ronald Green, MD
EXAMINATION: Gallbladder ultrasound.
CLINICAL SYMPTOMS: Increased bilirubin.
   GALLBLADDER ULTRASOUND: Examination was technically difficult with some limitations due to overlying leads. Large right pleural effusion identified. Gallbladder is visualized. No obvious gallstones or gallbladder wall thickening. Only short portions of the common hepatic duct and common bile duct are visualized. Common hepatic duct measures 3.6 mm, and common bile duct measures 5.2 mm. These values are within normal limits. There is limited assessment of the liver, which is grossly unremarkable.
   IMPRESSION: Gallbladder ultrasound with limitations as discussed above. Grossly unremarkable sonographic appearance of the gallbladder. No obvious dilatation of the common duct. Large right pleural effusion identified.

CPT Code(s): _____

_____

ICD-10-CM Code(s): _____

_____

Abstracting Questions

1. What subcategory within Radiology in the CPT was referenced for assignment of a code for this case? _____

_____

2. What body area was evaluated? _____

_____

3. What code range in the CPT was reviewed to select the ultrasound code? _____

4. What modifier was appended to the CPT code? _____

_____

PRACTICE EXERCISE 20.3 STRESS TEST

RADIOLOGY REPORT
LOCATION: Outpatient, Hospital
PATIENT: Harry Stein
ORDERING PHYSICIAN: James Noonar, MD
ATTENDING/ADMIT PHYSICIAN: James Noonar, MD
RADIOLOGIST: Morton Monson, MD
PERSONAL PHYSICIAN: Ronald Green, MD
   EXAMINATION: Adenosine stress test and resting Myoview, left ventricle, with estimate of left ventricular ejection fraction.

CLINICAL SYMPTOMS: Chest pain.
   ADENOSINE STRESS AND RESTING MYOVIEW EVALUATION, LEFT VENTRICLE, WITH ESTIMATE OF LEFT VENTRICULAR EJECTION FRACTION: Clinical information states chest pain. This is a patient with known coronary artery disease. The patient has had prior replacement of aortic and mitral valve 3 to 4 years ago by history. The patient has a previous Cardiolite scan from December 24 two years ago that showed "fixed posterior/inferior wall perfusion defect extending into the cardiac apex." On September 12 of

PRACTICE EXERCISE 20.3   STRESS TEST—cont'd

this year, the patient was given adenosine challenge under the supervision of Dr. Dawson, who will report on that portion of the evaluation. On September 12, the patient was injected with 27.2 mCi of technetium-99m–tagged tetrofosmin. Views of the left ventricle were then acquired with a SPECT nuclear medicine camera and reformatted into the standard projections. On September 13, the patient was returned to the nuclear medicine department for resting or redistribution scan and injected with 26.2 mCi of technetium-99m–tagged tetrofosmin. Again, views of the left ventricle were acquired with the SPECT nuclear medicine camera and reformatted into standard projections. Comparison of the stress and resting images shows no area to suggest perfusion defect. Nothing to suggest ischemia or infarct is seen. All segments of the left ventricle are perfused.

IMPRESSION

1. Adenosine challenge as the stress. That will be reported by Dr. Dawson.

2. Normal adenosine stress and resting Myoview evaluation, left ventricle. No region suggesting ischemia or infarct.
   ADDENDUM: Previously described fixed perfusion defect involving posterior/inferior wall and apex is no longer seen.
   Left ventricular ejection fraction estimated at 66%. This is normal. Normal is 50% or greater.

CPT Code(s): _____

_____

ICD-10-CM Code(s): _____

_____

Abstracting Questions

1. Does use of the SPECT camera affect code assignment? _____

2. Were the left ventricular perfusion and ejection fractions reported separately? _____

_____

PRACTICE EXERCISE 20.4   HEAD ULTRASOUND

LOCATION: Inpatient, Hospital
PATIENT: Jason Whittle
ATTENDING PHYSICIAN: Rolando Ortez, MD
CLINICAL SYMPTOMS: Premature, weight 1800 grams.

HEAD ULTRASOUND: Sonographic evaluation of the newborn brain was performed through the anterior fontanel. The study was performed in the coronal and sagittal planes. There is a hyperechoic area seen within the right subependymal region. This measures $0.6 \times 0.4 \times 0.5$ cm. I suspect this is a subependymal hemorrhage. There is also an area within the left intraparenchymal region measuring $0.9 \times 1.0 \times 1.4$ cm. This is a hyperechoic area, which may represent an intraparenchymal hemorrhage on the left parietal/occipital region. There is also question of a small septum cavum pellucidum. This is difficult to state for certain, however.

CONCLUSION

1. What appears to be a right subependymal hemorrhage, as discussed above.
2. Hyperechoic area within the left intraparenchymal region. It may also represent a focal area of hemorrhage measuring 1 cm in greatest diameter.

3. Question of small septum cavum pellucidum as a congenital variation. This is very questionable and difficult to assess for the patient's age. The ventricles themselves do not appear to be grossly dilated.

CPT Code(s): _____

_____

ICD-10-CM Code(s): _____

_____

Abstracting Questions

1. In what CPT section was the code to report this service located? _____

_____

2. In what CPT category of codes was the code to report this service located? _____

_____

PRACTICE EXERCISE 20.5   NEONATAL CYSTOURETHROGRAM

LOCATION: Inpatient, Hospital
PATIENT: Crystal Morgan
ATTENDING PHYSICIAN: Rolando Ortez, MD
RADIOLOGIST: Morton Monson, MD
CLINICAL SYMPTOMS: Congenital hydronephrosis.

VOIDING URETHROCYSTOGRAPHY: The study is technically limited due to the infant's inability to cooperate. The urinary bladder was filled to presumed capacity before spontaneous voiding. The bladder capacity is estimated at 25 cc. No immediate, delayed, or voiding reflux is demonstrated.

IMPRESSION: No definite vesicoureteral reflux demonstrated.

CPT Code(s): _____

_____

ICD-10-CM Code(s): _____

_____

Abstracting Questions

1. Was this an acquired or congenital condition? _____

_____

2. What type of evaluation was performed? _____

_____

21

Pathology and Laboratory Section (80047-89398)

- Organ or Disease-Oriented Panels
- Drug Assay
- Therapeutic Drug Assays
- Evocative/Suppression Testing
- Consultations (Clinical Pathology)
- Urinalysis
- Molecular Pathology
- Multianalyte Assays with Algorithmic Analyses
- Chemistry
- Hematology and Coagulation
- Immunology
- Transfusion Medicine
- Microbiology
- Anatomic Pathology
- Cytopathology
- Cytogenetic Studies
- Surgical Pathology
- In Vivo (Transcutaneous) Laboratory Procedures
- Other Procedures
- Reproductive Medicine Procedures

Pathology and Laboratory

Codes for laboratory test only
    Specimen collection coded separately
    Example: Venous blood draw reported with 36415
    (Surgery section)

Facility Indicators

Allow additional tests without physician written order
    Example: Urinalysis positive for bacteria, built-in indicator for culture

Pathology/Laboratory Caution

Report second or subsequent tests without -51, multiple procedures

Organ or Disease-Oriented Panels (80047-80081)

Groups of tests often ordered together

Examples:
- Basic Metabolic Panel
- General Health Panel
- Electrolyte Panel

Rules of Panels

All tests must have been conducted

Do not use -52, Reduced Service
Additional tests, over those in panel, reported separately
If all tests in panel not done
- List each test separately
- Do not use panel code

Drug Assay

Presumptive Drug Class Screening (80305-80307)

Identifies presence or absence of drug
Chromatography procedure in which single or multiple drugs identified
- Reports thin layer chromatography procedure(s)
- Screening(s) is presumptive
Code by method performed
Example:
- Chemical analyzers = 80307
- Read by instrument = 80306
Does not identify amount of drug present
- Only presence or absence

Therapeutic Drug Assays (80150-80299)

Reports the presence and amount (quantitative)
Material examined can be from any source

Drugs listed by generic names
Example: Amitriptyline, generic name for brand name Elavil

Evocative/Suppression Testing (80400-80439)

Measures stimulating (evocative) or suppressing agents

Codes report only technical component of service
Additional services reported
- Supplies and/or drugs used in testing (99070 or HCPCS code)

E/M code reported for physician monitoring of test

Consultations (Clinical Pathology) (80500, 80502)

At request of physician
Additional information about specimen
Consultant prepares written report

Levels

Limited without review of medical record
Comprehensive with review of medical record

More Consultation Codes (88321-88334)

Surgical Pathology
Used when pathologist either
- Reviews slides, material, or reports
- Provides consultation during surgery

Reported by number of specimens

Urinalysis (81000-81099)

Tests on Urine

Method of test
- e.g., tablet, reagent, or dipstick

Reason for test
- e.g., pregnancy

Constituents being tested for
- e.g., bilirubin, glucose

Equipment Used

Automated or nonautomated
With or without microscope

Molecular Pathology (81161, 81200-81479)

- 81105-81383 are Tier 1 procedures that report molecular assay
  - More common gene procedures
  - Example, breast cancer gene—81211 (BRCA1 or BRCA2)
- 81400-81408, 81479 are Tier 2 procedures to report less commonly performed analyses

Multianalyte Assays With Algorithmic Analyses (81490-81599)

Analyses that use the results of various measures and patient information to predict probabilities in a numeric form
CPT notes an Appendix O provide further detail

Chemistry (82009-84999)

Specific tests on any bodily substances
- Urine
- Blood
- Breath
- Feces
- Sputum
Most are for quantitative (amount of) screenings only
Few report qualitative (presence of) screenings
Samples from different sources reported separately, e.g., blood, feces
Samples taken different times of day reported separately

Hematology and Coagulation (85002-85999)

Laboratory procedures on blood

Example:
- Complete blood count (CBC)
- White blood cell count (WBC)
Codes divided based on method of
- Blood draw
- Test being conducted

Immunology (86000-86849)

Identifying immune system conditions caused by antibodies and antigens
Example: Hepatitis C antibody screening

Tissue Typing (86805-86849)

Compatibility test on tissue
- Match donor to recipient
- Measure/monitor cytotoxic reactions

Transfusion Medicine (86850-86999)

Blood bank codes
Tests performed on blood or blood products
Identifies
- Collection
- Processing
- Typing

Microbiology (87003-87999)

Study of Microorganisms

Identification of organism
Sensitivities of organism to antibiotics

Anatomic Pathology (88000-88099)

Postmortem examinations

- Autopsies

  Reports only physician service

  Codes divided on extent of exam and type of examination—gross versus gross and microscopic

  Example: Gross examination without central nervous system (88000)

Cytopathology (88104-88199)

Identifies cellular changes

Common laboratory procedures, e.g., Pap smear

Codes divided by

- Type of procedure
- Technique used

Cytogenetic Studies (88230-88299)

Branch of genetics concerned with cellular abnormalities and pathologic conditions

  Example: Chromosomes

Surgical Pathology (88300-88399)
Pathology Terminology

Specimen sample of tissue of suspect area

- Basis of reporting determined by number of labeled specimens

  Block: Frozen piece of specimen

  Section is a slice of frozen block

Evaluation of Specimens to Determine Disease Pathology

Tissue removed during procedures undergoes pathology evaluation

Operative report usually coded after pathology report received

Pathology reports usually coded with operative report

Unit of measure (88300-88309), specimen

- 2 separately identifiable anus tags, each examined, 88304 × 2
- 1 anus tag examined in 2 different areas of tag, 88304

Types of Pathologic Examination

Microscopic: With microscope

Gross: Without microscope

- 88300, only gross exam code
- Other codes are gross and microscopic

Six Levels of Surgical Pathology

Based on specimen examined, e.g., breast, prostate, lung, and reason for evaluation, e.g., radical procedure for suspected carcinoma

  Levels divided on complexity of examination

Example:

  88305, Colon, Biopsy

  88307, Colon, Segmental Resection, Other than for Tumor

  88309, Colon, Total Resection

Level I

- Specimen can be accurately diagnosed without microscopic examination

Level II

- Gross and microscopic examination is performed on the specimen

Levels III, IV, V, and VI

- Include gross and microscopic examination and additional ascending levels of physician work (increasing difficulty)

  Based upon method of or need for removal

  Same anatomical site can be listed in each level

  Additional service codes 88311-88399 are not included in codes 88300-88309

  Example: Special stains (88312)

PRACTICE EXERCISE 21.1 L3-4 DISC

LOCATION: Outpatient, Hospital
PATIENT: Corrine Wilson
ATTENDING PHYSICIAN: Timothy Pleasant, MD
SURGEON: Timothy Pleasant, MD
PATHOLOGIST: Grey Lonewolf, MD
CLINICAL HISTORY: Lumbar disc L3-4 herniation.
SPECIMEN RECEIVED: L3-4 disc.

GROSS DESCRIPTION: The specimen is labeled with the patient's name and "lumbar disc L3-4" and consists of fibrillary pink-tan tissue fragments. Representative section in one cassette.

MICROSCOPIC DIAGNOSIS: Fragments of fibrocartilage, consistent with herniated disc L3-4.

CPT Code(s): _____

_____

ICD-10-CM Code(s): _____

_____

Abstracting Questions

1. How would the code for this service be referenced in the CPT index? _____

_____

2. Was the examination gross, microscopic, or both? _____

_____

3. What was the level of surgical pathology? _____

_____

4. Does the pathologic status of the tissue affect the diagnosis code? _____

_____

PRACTICE EXERCISE 21.2 UTERUS, BILATERAL TUBES, AND OVARIES

LOCATION: Outpatient, Hospital
PATIENT: Tina Highdorn
ATTENDING PHYSICIAN: Ira Avila, MD
SURGEON: Ira Avila, MD
PATHOLOGIST: Grey Lonewolf, MD
CLINICAL HISTORY: Menorrhagia.
SPECIMEN RECEIVED: Uterus, bilateral tubes, and ovaries.

GROSS DESCRIPTION: The specimen is labeled with the patient's name and "uterus, bilateral tubes, and ovaries" and consists of 370 gm; this includes the complete uterus with tubes and ovaries. The uterus measures 14 cm in length × 10 cm in fundal diameter. The specimen is distorted by several bulging areas on the surface. The cervix is transverse. The endometrium is up to 0.3 cm thick and composed of pale tan color. Cut section of the myometrium reveals multiple whirling masses, up to 3 cm in diameter, consisting of white whirling tissue. The fallopian tubes have been surgically divided. The left ovary measures 5 × 4 cm and contains a central cystic structure with smooth lining. A section of the left tube and ovary is placed in cassette labeled 7. The right ovary measures 3 × 2 × 1.5 cm and is composed of wrinkled tan tissue. A section of the right tube and ovary is placed in cassette labeled 8.

MICROSCOPIC DIAGNOSIS: Sections of cervix show squamous metaplasia. Sections of endometrium show tubular glands lined by pseudostratified columnar epithelium. Small nests of endometrial glands and stroma are noted in the superficial myometrium. Sections of myometrium show masses, consisting of interdigitating bands of smooth muscle. Section of left fallopian tube is unremarkable. Section of left ovary shows a follicle cyst. Sections of right fallopian tube are unremarkable. Section of right ovary shows physiologic structures.

DIAGNOSIS
Complete uterus, tubes, and ovaries showing:
1. Squamous metaplasia, cervix.
2. Proliferating endometrium.
3. Adenomyosis, uterus.
4. Multiple intramural leiomyomata.
5. Status post surgical division of fallopian tubes.
6. Follicle cyst, left ovary.

CPT Code(s): _____

_____

ICD-10-CM Code(s): _____

_____

Abstracting Questions

1. When you reference "Metaplasia, cervix" in the Index of the ICD-10-CM, you are referred to what code? _____

_____

2. The clinical history was menorrhagia. What is menorrhagia? _____

_____

3. Why was it not correct to report menorrhagia as the diagnosis? _____

_____

PRACTICE EXERCISE 21.3 PLACENTA

LOCATION: Inpatient, Hospital
PATIENT: Cindy Kretchenhoff
ATTENDING PHYSICIAN: Ira Avila, MD
SURGEON: Ira Avila, MD
PATHOLOGIST: Grey Lonewolf, MD
CLINICAL HISTORY: 31 weeks, 6 days' gestation, possible placental abruption.
SPECIMEN RECEIVED: Placenta.

GROSS DESCRIPTION: Submitted in formalin, labeled with the patient's name, and "placenta" is 600 gm. Discoid placenta measuring 18 × 17 × 3 cm, with three centrally attached vessels and 5 cm long umbilical cord. The umbilical cord shows no knots or gross abnormalities (cassette 1). The membranes are tan and opaque and show no significant exudates, nodules, or green discoloration (cassette 2). The fetal surface of placenta shows a normal vascular pattern. The maternal surface features multiple intact cotyledons. No

Continued

PRACTICE EXERCISE 21.3 PLACENTA—cont'd

significant adherent blood clot or cotyledon compression is seen. Sectioning reveals dark red to purple spongy parenchyma without significant scarlike areas or masses. Representative sections of central and peripheral placenta are submitted in cassettes 3 and 4, respectively (two separate specimens, placenta and umbilical cord).

MICROSCOPIC DIAGNOSIS: Sections are umbilical cord showing three vessels. No significant inflammatory infiltrates are seen. Sections of membranes feature intact chorionic and amnionic membranes. Focal mild neutrophilic infiltrates are identified within chorionic membranes. Sections of placenta show multiple chorionic villi with villous architecture consistent with 32 weeks' gestational age. Villous vascularity is within normal limits. There is mild intervillous fibrin deposition. No significant large vessels lesions are seen. Minimal neutrophilic infiltrates are present within the fibrin beneath the chorionic plate.

DIAGNOSIS: Placenta, delivery; early third-trimester placenta, membranes, and umbilical cord showing mild early placentitis.

COMMENTS: While no gross pathologic changes of placental abruption are seen, acute abruption may not be accompanied by demonstrable placental changes at the time of pathologic examination.

CPT Code(s): _____

_____

ICD-10-CM Code(s): _____

_____

Abstracting Questions

1. How many specimens were examined? _____

_____

2. According to the notes in the CPT manual before 88300, the unit of services for codes 88300 through 88309 is the what? _____

3. Also in the notes of the CPT manual before 88300, a specimen is defined as tissue(s) submitted for individual and separate attention, requiring individual examination and pathologic _____

_____.

PRACTICE EXERCISE 21.4 CERVICAL DISC

LOCATION: Outpatient, Hospital
PATIENT: Sally Reagon
ATTENDING PHYSICIAN: Timothy Pleasant, MD
SURGEON: Timothy Pleasant, MD
PATHOLOGIST: Grey Lonewolf, MD
CLINICAL HISTORY: Severe cervical spinal stenosis.
SPECIMEN RECEIVED: Cervical disc.
GROSS DESCRIPTION: The specimen is labeled with the patient's name and "cervical disc" and consists of approximately 5 grams of tan fibrous fragments.
MICROSCOPIC DIAGNOSIS: Sections show disc tissue.
DIAGNOSIS: Disc tissue (cervical).

CPT Code(s): _____

_____

ICD-10-CM Code(s): _____

_____

Abstracting Question

1. What statement in the code description for 88304 identifies cervical disc pathological examination? _____

_____

PRACTICE EXERCISE 21.5 CEREBRAL HEMATOMA

LOCATION: Inpatient, Hospital
PATIENT: Daniel Smithson
ATTENDING PHYSICIAN: Timothy Pleasant, MD
SURGEON: Timothy Pleasant, MD
PATHOLOGIST: Grey Lonewolf, MD
CLINICAL HISTORY: Nontraumatic cerebral bleeding.
SPECIMEN RECEIVED: Cerebral hematoma.
GROSS DESCRIPTION: Submitted in formalin and labeled with the patient's name and "cerebral hematoma" are fragments of reddish brown blood clot measuring approximately 4.5 × 3.5 × 1.5 cm in aggregate. Representative fragments are submitted in one cassette.
MICROSCOPIC DIAGNOSIS: Sections show fragments of fresh blood clot and a single fragment of brain parenchyma featuring intact cortex and underlying white matter and mild-to-moderate edema. No neoplasm is identified.

DIAGNOSIS: Cerebral hematoma, evacuation: Recent blood clot and benign brain parenchyma.

CPT Code(s): _____

_____

ICD-10-CM Code(s): _____

_____

Abstracting Question

1. How many cassettes were submitted? _____

_____

22

Medicine Section (90281-99607)

Most procedures noninvasive (not entering body)

Contains invasive procedures
Example: 92973, Percutaneous thrombectomy
Many specialized tests
Example: Audiology and biofeedback
Special lightning bolt icon (↗)
- Indicates substances pending FDA (Food and Drug Administration) approval

Immunizations

Often used
Two types of immunizations
- Active and passive
Correct coding includes
- Supply injected
- Administration of injection

Active—Bacteria or Virus

Bacteria that cause disease made nontoxic (toxoid)
- Injected to build immunity
  Small dose active virus injected (vaccine)
- Injected to build immunity
  Example: Poliovirus

Passive Immunization

Does not cause immune response
   Contains antibodies against certain diseases—immune globulins

Immune Globulins (90281-90399)

Identifies immune globulin product
   Example: Botulism antitoxin
   Report administration separately

Immune Globulin Codes Divided by

Type
e.g., rabies, hepatitis B

Method
e.g., intramuscular, intravenous, subcutaneous

Dose
e.g., full dose, minidose

Immunization Administration (90460-90474)

Administration (giving of substance)
- Reported in addition to substance given
- 90460, 90461 Patients through age 18 when counseled regarding immunization
- 90471-90474
- 90471, +90472 = Percutaneous, intradermal, subcutaneous, or intramuscular injection
- 90473, +90474 = Oral or intranasal

Methods of Administration

- Percutaneous
- Intradermal
- Subcutaneous
- Intramuscular
- Intranasal
- Oral

Report Administration for Each Dose— Single or Combination

Example: 10-year-old patient receives 3 separate injections
- 90471 administration tetanus
- 90472 administration rubella
- 90472 administration diphtheria
  OR depending on payer:
- 90471 administration tetanus
- 90472 × 2 administration rubella and diphtheria

Vaccines, Toxoids (Vaccine Product Codes) (90476-90749)

Many codes age or dosage specific

Example: 90702, Diphtheria and tetanus toxoids absorbed (DT), younger than 7 years
Codes for products for single diseases
Example: 90713, Poliovirus vaccine, inactivated (IPV)
Codes for combination diseases

Example: 90700, diphtheria, tetanus toxoids, and acellular pertussis (DTaP)

Some vaccines given on schedule

Example: 90633, 2-dose hepatitis A vaccine

- 1st dose, 1st visit
- 2nd dose, 2nd visit

Caution: There Are Multiple Diphtheria Codes

- 90696-90723 diphtheria and diphtheria with other substances

  Example: 90698, diphtheria, tetanus toxoids, and acellular pertussis (synthetic form of pertussis) (DTaP), *Haemophilus influenzae* type b (HiB), and inactivated poliovirus (IPV) for IM use

> **NOTE**
>
> **Remember**
>
> Third-party payers do not usually require modifier -51 used with Vaccine/Toxoid codes
>
> Rather, depending on payer, list each code multiple times or use times (x) symbol and indicate number

Important Reporting Rule

If vaccine administered during an office visit that was not related to the E/M

- Report E/M service (with modifier -25) + vaccine + administration

  Office visit for vaccine only: Report only vaccine and the administration (no E/M service)

Routine Vaccinations

Influenza

Substance (vaccine) 90653-90668 and 90685-90688

- G0008 HCPCS National Level II for Medicare patients
- 90471/90472

Pneumococcal

Substance (vaccine) 90732

Administration

- G0009 HCPCS National Level II for Medicare
- 90471/90472 administration

Psychiatry (90785-90899)

Psychiatric Diagnostic Evaluation

Involved assessment to identify patient diagnosis and develop treatment plan

  Codes for evaluation (90791) and evaluation with medical service (90792)

Psychotherapy

Therapeutic treatment of psychological disorder or behavior

Service reported with codes 90832-90838

- Time based codes
  - 90832, 90833 (16-37 minutes), 90834, 90836 (38-52 minutes), 90837, 90838 (53 minutes or more)
- Codes subdivided based on if psychotherapy provided in addition to a primary procedure
- Provided to patient only

Other Psychotherapy

- Crisis psychotherapy provides treatment for a patient's experiencing a reaction to a more specific event or situation (90839, 90840)

  Codes 90845-90853 report services for
- Psychoanalysis
- Family, multiple-family, and group psychotherapy

Biofeedback (90901, 90911)

Used to help patients gain control over body processes

Example: Elevated BP (blood pressure) or manage chronic pain

Patient training in biofeedback by professional

- Continues on own

Services often part psychophysiologic (mind/body) therapy

Dialysis (90935-90999)

Cleanses blood

- Temporary (non-ESRD [end-stage renal disease])
- Permanent (ESRD)

Two parts to report ESRD dialysis services

- Physician service
- Hemodialysis procedure

Hemodialysis Service (90935-90940)

Hemodialysis is the procedure

Used for ESRD and non-ESRD

Billed per day for inpatients receiving hemodialysis and also for outpatient non-ESRD

Includes all physician E/M services related to procedure

- Use modifier -25 if separate E/M service provided

Miscellaneous Dialysis Procedures (90945-90947)

Describes other dialysis procedures

  Example: Peritoneal dialysis in which toxins are passively absorbed into dialysis fluid

  Services billed on per-day basis for inpatient ESRD patients

ESRD Physician Services (90951-90970)

Include

- Establishment of dialyzing cycle
- Physician services
- E/M outpatient dialysis visits
- Telephone calls
- Patient management during dialysis

Reported Per Month: 90951-90966

Month is defined as 30 days
  Less than full month of service 90967-90970 per day
  Codes divided by age and number of encounters
  Codes are used to report outpatient dialysis services for
    ESRD patients

Other Diagnosis Procedures (90989-90999)

Patients can receive training in self-dialysis (90989, 90993)
  Codes divided by complete or partial training program

Gastroenterology (91010-91299)

For tests and treatments of esophagus, stomach, and intestine
  Codes usually reported with E/M or consultation service
code
- **Caution:** Many bundled services

Ophthalmology (92002-92499)

Contains E/M "eye" codes
Definitions for new and established patients same as for
  E/M section
Codes are for bilateral services
- If only one eye, use modifier -52 (reduced service)

Special Ophthalmologic Services (92015-92287)

For special evaluations of visual system
  Goes beyond those usually provided in evaluation
  May be reported in addition to basic visual service

Special Otorhinolaryngologic Services (92502-92700)

Special treatments and diagnostic services
  Example: Nasal function tests (rhinomanometry) or
    audiometric tests
  All hearing tests bilateral unless one ear indicated in
    description

Cardiovascular in Medicine Section (See pg. 182 for Details)

Services can be
- Invasive or noninvasive
- Diagnostic or therapeutic
Subheadings
- Therapeutic Services and Procedures
- Cardiography
- Cardiovascular Monitoring Services
- Implantable and Wearable Cardiac Device Evaluations
- Echocardiography
- Cardiac Catheterization
- Intracardiac Electrophysiologic Procedures/Studies
- Peripheral Arterial Disease Rehabilitation
- Noninvasive Physiologic Studies and Procedures

- Other Procedures
- Other Vascular Studies
Home and Outpatient International Normalized Ratio
(INR) Monitoring Services, 93792 and 93793
- Anticoagulants such as warfarin
  - Thins the blood
- By physician or another qualified health care
  professional
- Provided in home or outpatient setting
  - 93792 reports training
  - 93793 reports management, billed once per day

Noninvasive Vascular Diagnostic Studies (93880-93998)

Vascular codes for procedures on noncoronary veins and
arteries

Include
- Patient care
- Supervision and interpretation (S&I)
- Copy of results

Pulmonary (94002-94799)

For ventilation management therapies and diagnostic tests
Includes procedure and interpretation of test results
- Additional E/M service reported separately

Allergy and Clinical Immunology (95004-95199)

Divided into three subheadings
1. Allergy Testing (95004-95071)
2. Ingestion Challenge Testing (95076-95079)
3. Allergen Immunotherapy (95115-95199)

Allergy Testing (95004-95071)

Sensitivity testing using various types of tests with type and
number of tests based on physician's judgment

Example: Percutaneous, intracutaneous, inhalation
Example: Extracts, venoms, biologics, and foods
Medical record will indicate
- Number and type of tests
- Method testing

Ingestion Challenge Testing (95076, 95079)

- Sensitivity to food, drugs, and other substances
- 95076 initial 120 minutes; 95079 each additional 60
  minutes
- Services less than 60 minutes, report E/M code

Allergen Immunotherapy (95115-95199)

Codes divided into three types of services:
1. Injection only
2. Prescription and injection

3. Provision of antigen (substance) only
   Physician service bundled into immunotherapy codes
   If separate E/M service provided, report separately

Neurology and Neuromuscular Procedures (95782-96020)

Contains codes to report tests, such as
- Sleep tests
- Muscle tests (electromyography)
- Range-of-motion measurements
- Electroencephalogram (EEG)
- Electromyography (EMG)
- Analysis and programming of neurostimulators
- Motion analysis
- Functional brain mapping
  Many bundled services
  Services usually provided in addition to E/M service

Medical Genetics and Genetic Counseling Services (96040)

Trained genetic counselors assess risk of genetic defects in offspring

Includes
- Pedigree construction
- Obtaining structured genetic history
- Analysis of risk
- Counseling

Central Nervous System (CNS) Assessments/ Tests (96101-96127)

Used to report
- Psychological tests
- Speech/Language assessments
- Developmental progress assessments
- Thinking/Reasoning examinations
Standardized cognitive performance testing
Codes based on per-hour basis
- Includes written report of results

Health and Behavior Assessment/Intervention (96150-96155)

- Identify psychological behavior, emotional, cognitive, or social factors important to treatment or management of physical health problems

Hydration, Therapeutic, Prophylactic, Diagnostic Injections and Infusions, and Chemotherapy and Other Highly Complex Drug or Highly Complex Biologic Agent Administration (96360-96549)

Infusion: Therapeutic procedure to introduce fluid into body

Hydration: Infusion for purpose of rehydration; includes prepackaged fluid

Injection: Subcutaneous (Sub-Q, SC), intramuscular (IM), intra-arterial (IA), and intravenous (IV)

Codes report the physician work related to the infusion, hydration, or injection
- Affirmation of treatment plan
- Direct supervision of staff
- Significant, separately identifiable E/M is reported with -25

Codes include
- Local anesthesia
- Intravenous start
- Access to indwelling intravenous catheter or port
- Flush at conclusion
- Standard tubing, syringes, and supplies

Multiple drug administrations in same session are reported separately

Use only one initial code to report multiple infusions or injections or combinations
  For the physician, assign initial code based on primary reason for encounter
  The secondary infusion/injection is reported with a subsequent or concurrent code, unless the protocol requires two separate IV sites
  Example: If three different agents were administered in the same session, report one initial code and two additional sequential codes
  Determination of initial code is based on primary reason for encounter
  Some codes are time based, so medical documentation must indicate time infusion begins and ends
  Time is defined as the actual time used to administer the drug/substance

Hydration (96360, 96361)

IV infusion for hydration and includes prepackaged fluid/electrolytes
- 96360 IV infusion for hydration up to 1 hour
- 96361 IV infusion for hydration, each additional hour
  - Report for hydration intervals greater than 30 minutes beyond 1 hour
  - Start infusion time over if a different bag is started
  - Do not report hydration codes when the fluid is used to administer a drug (incidental hydration)
  - Do not report hydration codes for infusion of <30 minutes

Therapeutic, Prophylactic, and Diagnostic Injections and Infusions (Excludes Chemotherapy and Other Highly Complex Drug or Highly Complex Biologic Agent Administration) (96365-96379)

Types of drug administration
- Therapeutic
- Prophylactic
- Diagnostic

Codes divided by administration method
- Subcutaneous
- Intramuscular
- Intra-arterial
- Intravenous push
A push is defined as when a health care professional is needed to administer the drug/substance and monitor the patient for an infusion that takes 15 minutes or less to administer

Also report the substance administered

96365-96368 report therapeutic, prophylactic, or diagnostic IV infusions, other than hydration and chemotherapy
- Typically require direct physician supervision
- Special consideration for preparing, dosing, or disposing
- Trained staff who administer infusion
- Monitoring of vital signs during infusion

Chemotherapy and Other Highly Complex Drug or Highly Complex Biologic Agent Administration (96401-96549)

Represents only preparation and administration of chemotherapy
- If separate E/M service provided, report E/M code + -25
Report all drugs/substances separately
Codes are not limited to patients with diagnosis of cancer
Codes also include infusion of antineoplastic agents, monoclonal antibody agents, and biological response modifiers for treatment of noncancer diagnoses
Chemical can be administered (injected) into
- Lesion
- Vein
- Tissue
- Muscle
- Artery
- Cavity
- Nerve
Intravenously injected chemicals: Two methods of delivery of chemical
1. IV push quickly delivers substance/medication into vein (15 minutes or less)
2. IV infusion delivers over longer period of time
Codes often divided by time the infusion/injection procedure takes

Example: 96413 chemotherapy administration, intravenous, infusion up to 1 hour

Report the initial code that represents the main reason why the patient was being treated, even though it might not be the first drug/substance infused

Example: Patient received 1 hour of hydration first, then 2 hours of chemotherapy intravenously. Code the initial chemotherapy infusion 96413 for the first hour of chemo, 96415 for the second hour, then code 96360 for the hydration

Special supplies (e.g., special needles) reported separately using 99070 or HCPCS National Level II code

Report any intra-arterial catheter placement with 36620-36640

Injections with chemotherapy

- Report separately any analgesic or antiemetic (for vomiting)
- Given before or after chemotherapy

> **NOTE**
>
> Use code J0881 to report injection of darbepoetin alfa and J0885 to report injection of epoetin alfa

Photodynamic Therapy (96567-96574)

Used in addition to bronchoscopy or endoscopy codes
Injected agent remains in premalignant cells longer than normal cells
- After agent dissipates from normal cells, patient exposed to laser light
- Agent absorbs light
- Light produces oxygen and premalignant cells destroyed

Special Dermatologic Procedures (96900-96999)

Usually specialized procedures provided on consultation basis
- Separate E/M consultation code would then be appropriate
Treatment of skin conditions:
Actinotherapy—with ultraviolet light
Photochemotherapy—with light-sensitive chemicals and light rays

Physical Medicine & Rehabilitation (97010-97799)

Used by physicians and therapists to report a variety of services

Treatments

Traction
Modalities
Electrical stimulation (used to help heal fractures)
Therapeutic procedures
Gait training
Functional activities

Patient Training

Codes often have time components
Example: 97761 reports prosthetic training, extremity(ies), each 15 minutes

Active Wound Care Management (97597-97610)

Debridement

Debridement without anesthesia with removal of devitalized tissue by different techniques, such as water pressure, sharp selective debridement with scissors, scalpel, and forceps
97597 and 97598 include total surface area of all wounds

Codes based on centimeters treated

Nonselective debridement (97602): Healthy tissue removed along with necrotic tissue, with wet-to-moist dressings, enzymatic or abrasive methods

Negative pressure wound therapy (NPWT) (97605, 97606)

- Vacuuming of drainage and tissue from wound
  - Then negative pressure draws the edges of the wound together
- Application of topical medications/ointments
- Assessment of wound
- Directions to patient on continued care of wound
- Each code for ongoing care reported on per-session basis

Osteopathic and Chiropractic Services (98925-98943)

Both inpatient and outpatient settings

Physician services bundled into codes

Codes divided by body area

Education and Training for Patient Self-Management (98960-98962)

- Use of standardized curriculum for education to individual or group for management of illness

Non–Face-to-Face Nonphysician Services (98966-98969)

Reports nonphysician E/M services using telephone/Internet

Established patient, family member of the patient, or a guardian

98966-98968 telephone E/M services

98969 online E/M services

To report physician services, see 99441-99443

Special Services, Procedures, and Reports (99000-99091)

Handling and conveyance of laboratory specimens

- 99000-99002

  Postoperative follow-up visits included in surgical package
- 99024

  Office visits after posted hours or in locations other than office
- 99050-99060

  Supplies and materials
- 99070

  Hospital mandated on-call services
- 99026, 99027

Moderate (Conscious) Sedation (99151-99157)

Type of sedation in which the patient can respond to verbal commands

When sedation is provided by same physician performing procedure, report with 99151-99153

- Second physician provides sedation, report with 99155-99157

  Included in service is:
- Patient assessment
- IV establishment
- Administration of agent
- Maintenance of sedation
- Monitoring of vital signs
- Recovery

  Codes divided based on patient age (under 5, 5 and over) and time (15 minutes and each 15 minutes over)

PRACTICE EXERCISE 22.1 CARDIAC CATHETERIZATION

CARDIAC CATHETERIZATION REPORT
LOCATION: Inpatient, Hospital
PATIENT: Wade Land
REFERRING PHYSICIAN: James Noonar, MD
CARDIOLOGIST: Marvin Elhart, MD
INDICATION: Unstable angina.
PROCEDURE: Right iliofemoral angiography, left heart catheterization, selective coronary angiography, and left ventriculography.
COMPLICATIONS: None.
  RESULTS: Hemodynamics: The left ventricular pressure before the LV gram was 133/7 with an LVEDP of 11. After the LV gram it was 130/8 with an LVEDP of 12. The aortic pressure on pullback was 130/59.
  Left Ventriculography: Showed that the left ventricle is normal in size. It was hard to assess segmental wall motion because of the frequency of PVCs; however, the overall left ventricular systolic function was normal. There might be some distal anterior wall hypokinesis.
  Selective Coronary Angiography
1. Right coronary artery: This was a medium-size dominant artery that has mild diffuse atherosclerotic changes. After the PDA there was about 30% narrowing.

2. Left main coronary artery: This has 80-90% eccentric narrowing in the midportion.
3. Left circumflex artery: This was a medium-size artery that has mild atherosclerotic changes proximally. It gave rise to a medium-size bifurcating first obtuse marginal that has 99% proximal narrowing. The inferior of the two branches, which was a smaller size artery, has 90% proximal narrowing.
4. Left anterior descending coronary artery: This was a medium-size artery that has mild diffuse atherosclerotic changes. The first diagonal was a small artery that had 90% proximal narrowing. The second diagonal was a larger artery that has about 60% narrowing in the midportion. Immediately after that diagonal, the left anterior descending artery has about 50% narrowing. There was moderate diffuse disease after that. Please note that the visualization of the diagonals and the left anterior descending artery was rather limited as we tried not to inject in a strong way into the left main.
CONCLUSION
1. Normal overall left ventricular systolic function.
2. Severe left main disease.
3. Severe left circumflex and first diagonal disease.

PRACTICE EXERCISE 22.1 CARDIAC CATHETERIZATION—cont'd

RECOMMENDATIONS
1. Maximum medical treatment.
2. Intra-aortic balloon pump.
3. Consult CT surgery to evaluate the patient for bypass surgery.

CPT Code(s): _____

_____

ICD-10-CM Code(s): _____

_____

Abstracting Questions

1. What are the three categories bundled into the code reported for cardiac catheterization? _____

_____

2. What was the approach for this procedure? _____

3. Was a modifier required on the catheterization code and if a modifier was required, which one would it be? _____

_____

4. For what two procedures were injections provided?

_____

PRACTICE EXERCISE 22.2
SAPHENOUS VEIN MAPPING

RADIOLOGY REPORT
LOCATION: Outpatient, Hospital
PATIENT: Mirta Hubert
ORDERING PHYSICIAN: James Noonar, MD
ATTENDING/ADMIT PHYSICIAN: James Noonar, MD
RADIOLOGIST: Morton Monson, MD
PERSONAL PHYSICIAN: Alma Naraquist, MD
EXAMINATION: Saphenous vein mapping.
    CLINICAL SYMPTOMS: Pre-coronary artery bypass graft; atherosclerotic heart disease of native coronary arteries, chest pain.
    FINDINGS: The left greater saphenous vein was mapped from midthigh through the proximal calf. Measurements above the knee were 1.0×0.92 cm, at the knee 0.73×0.73 cm, and below the knee 0.54×0.54 cm. The multiple branches encountered were not evaluated.

CPT Code(s): _____

_____

ICD-10-CM Code(s): _____

_____

Abstracting Question

1. What type of scan was used for mapping of vessels?

_____

PRACTICE EXERCISE 22.3
VENOUS ULTRASOUND

RADIOLOGY REPORT
LOCATION: Inpatient, Hospital
PATIENT: Dave James
ORDERING PHYS ICIAN: Frank Gaul, MD
ATTENDING/ADMIT PHYSICIAN: Frank Gaul, MD
RADIOLOGIST: Morton Monson, MD
PERSONAL PHYSICIAN: Frank Gaul, MD
EXAMINATION: Bilateral lower extremity venous ultrasound.
CLINICAL SYMPTOMS: Leg pain and swelling. Rule out deep venous thrombosis.
    FINDINGS: This examination was somewhat limited as a result of the patient being recently out of surgery and unable to be moved at all. As visualized, both the right and the left common femoral, superficial femoral, popliteal, and posterior tibial veins are fully compressible and demonstrate the presence of normal spontaneous, phasic, and augmented flow.
    IMPRESSION: No evidence for deep venous thrombosis is seen within either of the lower extremities. Please see above comments.

CPT Code(s): _____

_____

Icd-10-Cm Code(S): _____

_____

Abstracting Question

1. What is a deep venous thrombosis? _____

_____

PRACTICE EXERCISE 22.4
EXTREMITIES ULTRASOUND

RADIOLOGY REPORT
LOCATION: Outpatient, Hospital
PATIENT: Eric Tayes
ORDERING PHYSICIAN: Frank Gaul, MD
ATTENDING/ADMIT PHYSICIAN: Frank Gaul, MD
RADIOLOGIST: Morton Monson, MD
EXAMINATION: Ultrasound of both lower extremities; abdomen ultrasound.
CLINICAL SYMPTOMS: Lower extremity swelling, difficulty breathing.
FINDINGS: Ultrasound examination of the deep venous system of both lower extremities is negative. No evidence of deep venous thrombosis in either lower extremity. The posterior tibial, greater saphenous, and popliteal through the femoral veins are patent and negative for thrombus bilaterally. Normal phasicity.

Abdomen Ultrasound: Diffusely coarsened echotexture of the liver with some nodularity consistent with fatty infiltration. Cirrhotic configuration of the liver. Small calcified granuloma in the spleen. The spleen is otherwise negative. There is ascites in all four quadrants. No bile duct dilatation. No gallbladder wall thickening or cholelithiasis. Small amount of fluid adjacent to the gallbladder is likely related to the ascites. The pancreas is obscured by bowel gas. The abdominal aorta is of normal caliber. The right kidney measures approximately 9 cm in length and shows no evidence of hydronephrosis, calculi, or mass. The left kidney measures approximately 9.9 cm in length and shows no evidence of hydronephrosis, calculi, or mass.

CPT Code(s): _____

_____

ICD-10-CM Code(s): _____

_____

Abstracting Questions

1. How was the scan for the abdomen different than the scan for the extremities? _____

_____

2. How would the "cirrhotic configuration of the liver" diagnosis be reported? _____

_____

PRACTICE EXERCISE 22.5
RENAL DIALYSIS PROGRESS NOTE

RENAL DIALYSIS PROGRESS NOTE
LOCATION: Outpatient, Clinic
PATIENT: Jyl Couts
PHYSICIAN: Ira Avila, MD

The 45-year-old patient presents today for regular monthly visit. She has been slightly tired. She denies any shortness of breath or chest pain. No constipation. The patient complains of some weakness in her legs when she walks to the grocery store.

PHYSICAL EXAMINATION: Her blood pressure at home has been in the 130s/80s. On exam today, her weight is 152.5 pounds. Regular heart rate at 79 per minute. The lungs are clear bilaterally without crackles. No edema in the extremities. Catheter condition is good, and the exit site is clean and dry. No evidence of infection.
IMPRESSION/PLAN

1. The patient is on CAPD, two bag sizes of 1.5% and 2.5%; doing well with that.
2. She is on 4000 units of EPO once a week due to anemia due to end-stage renal disease with hemoglobin of 12. We will continue that at this time.
3. The patient has possibility of claudication. She has history of an aneurysm, which was measured at 6.1 cm on a CT scan done in the transverse section. We will obtain an ultrasound to follow up on her abdominal aortic aneurysm and do ABIs on the lower extremities.
4. The patient requested a handicap permit, and I will hold that for now until we do her studies.

The patient seems to agree with the plan.

CPT Code(s): _____

_____

ICD-10-CM Code(s): _____

_____

Abstracting Questions

1. Does the type of dialysis the patient receives affect code selection? _____

_____

2. What is end-stage renal disease? _____

_____

23
HCPCS Coding

Developed by Centers for Medicare and Medicaid Services (CMS)
- Formerly HCFA
  HCPCS developed in 1983
  CPT did not contain all codes necessary for Medicare services reporting

One of Two Levels of Codes

1. Level I, CPT
2. Level II, HCPCS, also known as national codes

Phased out Level III, Local Codes

Developed by Medicare and other carriers for use at local level
  Varied by locale
  Discontinued October 2002 due to HIPAA code set regulations
  Some codes incorporated into HCPCS Level I and Level II

Level II, National Codes

Codes for wide variety of providers
- Physicians
- Dentists
- Orthodontists
  Codes for wide variety of services
- Specific drugs
- Durable medical equipment (DME)
- Ambulance services

Code book published every January, but codes are added and deleted throughout the year and providers are notified through carrier bulletins

Format

Begins with letter, followed by four digits

Example: E0605, Vaporizer, room type
Each letter represents group codes
Example: "J" codes used to report drugs, J0585, onabotulinumtoxinA, 1 unit

Temporary Codes

Certain letters indicate temporary codes
Example: K0552, Supplies for external drug infusion pump
- K codes are temporary codes

HCPCS National Level II Index

Directs coder to specific codes
  Do not code directly from index
  Reference main portion of text before assigning code
  Alphabetical order

Table of Drugs

Listed by generic name, not brand name

PART 4

ICD-10-CM Coding

24
ICD-10-CM Overview

Introduction

Morbidity (illness)
  Mortality (death)
  CM = Clinical Modification
  PCS = Procedural Coding System
  Provides continuity of data
  World Health Organization's ICD-10 used globally
  The United States develops ICD-10-CM and ICD-10-PCS version
  On January 16, 2009, HHS published a final rule adopting ICD-10-CM and ICD-10-PCS
  • Effective implementation date: October 1, 2015

Uses of ICD-10-CM

Facilitate payment of health services
  Evaluate patients' use of health services
  Fiscal entities track health care costs
  Research
  • Health care quality
  • Future needs
  • Newer cancer center built if patient use warrants
  • Predict health care trends
  • Plan for future health care needs

ICD-10-CM on CMS-1500 (Fig. 24.1)

Diagnoses establish medical necessity
  Services and diagnoses must correlate
  CMS-1500 example (Fig. 24.1)

Ethics

Documentation must support diagnosis and match procedures or service performed

Example:
  • Services provided
  • Diagnosis justifies services
    If in doubt, check it out; don't make assumptions
    Your Job: Translate documentation into ICD-10-CM codes

Format

Diseases, Tabular List
  Diseases, Alphabetic Index

Diseases, Tabular List

Contains alphanumeric codes with descriptions
  A00-Z99 diagnosis codes describe condition
  21 chapters

Diseases, Alphabetic Index

Appears first in book
  Refers coder to alphanumeric code in Volume 1
  Never code directly from Index!

Placeholder

Character "X" is used as a placeholder for future expansion
  Example: T36-T50 range of codes, "X" is placeholder
    • T35.5X1A: Poisoning by, tetracyclines, intentional self-harm, initial encounter

7th Character

Certain categories have 7th character
  Example: T36-T50 range of codes, "A" is 7th character to report initial encounter

• **Figure 24.1** Diagnosis code and service must correlate.

- T36.4X2A: Poisoning by tetracyclines, intentional self-harm, initial encounter

Abbreviations

Symbols, abbreviations, punctuation, and notations
NEC: Not elsewhere classifiable
- No more-specific code exists
- Means "other specified"
NOS: Not otherwise specified
- Unspecified in documentation

Punctuation

[ ] Brackets
Tabular:
- Enclose synonyms, alternative wording, or explanatory phrases
- Helpful, additional information
- Can affect code
- Located in Tabular List A00-Z99
Index: Brackets enclose manifestation codes

( ) Parentheses
Located in Tabular List and Index
- Contain enclosed nonessential modifiers
  Does not affect code

: Colon
Located in Tabular
  Completes statement with one or more modifiers
  Bold type
  Codes and code titles in Tabular

Italicized Type
Located in Tabular
  see
  Located in Index
  see also, see condition, *see also* condition, *omit code*

Includes, Excludes, Use Additional Code
Includes: Conditions included in code
  Excludes1: Condition not coded here
  Excludes2: Not included here code but may be an additional code, when documented
  Use additional code: Assignment of other code(s) as necessary

And/With
And: Means "and/or"
  With: One condition with (in addition to) another condition; "associated with" or "due to"

Code, if Applicable, Any Causal Condition First
May be principal or first-listed diagnosis if no causal condition applicable or known
- If the causal condition is known, then a code for that condition should be sequenced as the principal or first-listed code diagnosis

Alphabetic Index

Nonessential modifiers: Have no effect on code selection
- Enclosed in parentheses
- Clarify diagnosis
  Example: **Ileus** (bowel) (colon) (inhibitory) (intestine) K56.7

Terms

Main terms (bold typeface)
  Subterms
  - Indented two spaces to right
  - Not bold

Cross References in the Index

Directs you: *see, see also, use*
- *"see"* directs you to specific term, must be reference
  Example: Pelade—*see* Alopecia, areata
- *"see also"* directs you to another term for more information, may also be reference
  Example: Pneumopericarditis—*see also* Pericarditis
- *"see condition"* directs you to specific information about assignment of the code
  Example: Vesicourethrorectal—*see* condition
- *"see also condition"* directs you to specific information about assignment of the code
  Example: Abdomen, abdominal—*see also* condition
- *"use"* directs you to the appropriate entry

Notes

Define terms
  Give further coding instructions
  Example: Tabular H00-H59
  - Note: Use an external cause code following the code for the eye condition, if applicable, to identify the cause of the eye condition

Eponyms

Disease or syndromes named for person
  Example: Goldberg-Maxwell syndrome E34.51

Etiology and Manifestation of Disease

Etiology = cause of disease
  Manifestation = symptom
  Combination codes = etiology and manifestation in one code
  Example: E11.341 Type 2 diabetes mellitus with severe nonprolifererative diabetic retinopathy with macular edema

Index to Diseases

Largest part
  First step in coding, locate main term in Index by condition, sign, symptom, or disease—not body area
  Subterms indented two spaces to right
  May have more than one subterm

Table of Neoplasms

Table of Neoplasms (illustrated in Fig. 24.2)
• Located after the Z Index entries

Table of Drugs and Chemicals

Located after the Index of Diseases
  Contains classification of drugs and substances to identify poisoning, adverse effects, and underdosing
  • Adverse effect occurs when substance is taken correctly but patient has a negative reaction to substance
  Condition code for drug found under "Adverse Effect" column
  • Poisoning occurs when substance is incorrectly taken

Example: Amoxicillin prescribed for bronchitis causes rash (adverse effect); or rather than one tablet of prescribed amoxicillin, patient takes four tablets and nausea results (poisoning)

Drug name placed alphabetically on left under heading "Substance" (Fig. 24.3)

First column: "Poisoning, Accidental (Unintentional)" lists code for substance involved if not related to an adverse effect

External cause codes identify how poisoning occurred (V, W, X, Y codes)

Table Headings

Poisoning, Accidental (Unintentional)
  Poisoning, Intentional Self-Harm
  Poisoning, Assault
  Poisoning, Undetermined

	Malignant Primary	Malignant Secondary	Ca in situ	Benign	Uncertain	Unspecified Behavior
bile or biliary (tract)	C24.9	C78.89	D01.5	D13.5	D37.6	D49.0
canaliculi (biliferi) (intrahepatic)	C22.1	C78.7	D01.5	D13.4	D37.6	D49.0
canals, interlobular	C22.1	C78.89	D01.5	D13.4	D37.6	D49.0
duct or passage (common) (cystic) (extrahepatic)	C24.0	C78.89	D01.5	D13.5	D37.6	D49.0
interlobular	C22.1	C78.89	D01.5	D13.4	D37.6	D49.0
intrahepatic	C22.1	C78.7	D01.5	D13.4	D37.6	D49.0
and extrahepatic	C24.8	C78.89	D01.5	D13.5	D37.6	D49.0

• **Figure 24.2** Table of Neoplasms.

	External Cause (T-Code)					
Substance	Poisoning, Accidental (Unintentional)	Poisoning, Intentional Self-Harm	Poisoning, Assault	Poisoning, Undetermined	Adverse Effect	Underdosing
Acetylsulfamethoxypyridazine	T37.0X1	T37.0X2	T37.0X3	T37.0X4	T37.0X5	T37.0X6
Achromycin	T36.4X1	T36.4X2	T36.4X3	T36.4X4	T36.4X5	T36.4X6
ophthalmic preparation	T49.5X1	T49.5X2	T49.5X3	T49.5X4	T49.5X5	T49.5X6
topical NEC	T49.0X1	T49.0X2	T49.0X3	T49.0X4	T49.0X5	T49.0X6
Aciclovir	T37.5X1	T37.5X2	T37.5X3	T37.5X4	T37.5X5	T37.5X6
Acid (corrosive) NEC	T54.2X1	T54.2X2	T54.2X3	T54.2X4	—	—
Acidifying agent NEC	T50.901	T50.902	T50.903	T50.904	T50.905	T50.906
Acipimox	T46.6X1	T46.6X2	T46.6X3	T46.6X4	T46.6X5	T46.6X6
Acitretin	T50.991	T50.992	T50.993	T50.994	T50.995	T50.996
Aclarubicin	T45.1X1	T45.1X2	T45.1X3	T45.1X4	T45.1X5	T45.1X6
Aclatonium napadisilate	T48.1X1	T48.1X2	T48.1X3	T48.1X4	T48.1X5	T48.1X6
Aconite (wild)	T46.991	T46.992	T46.993	T46.994	T46.995	T46.996

• **Figure 24.3** Table of Drugs and Chemicals.

Adverse Effect

Underdosing (never a primary or first-listed code)

V, W, X, Y Codes

External Causes of Injuries and Poisonings

Provides additional information about the nature of the injury/poisoning, locality, activity and status codes

Never principal (inpatient) or first-listed/primary (outpatient) diagnosis

Separate Index to External Causes

Located after Table of Drugs and Chemicals

- Alphabetical listing with main terms in bold
- Subterms indented two spaces to right under main term

A Word of Caution About the Alphabetic Index

Some words in Index do not appear in Tabular—saves space

Exact word may not be in code description in Tabular

- Usually found in Alphabetic Index
- Must locate term in Index and then locate in Tabular
- Additional coding instructions found in Tabular

Tabular List

Major Division

Classification of Diseases and Injuries

- 21 Chapters

Classification of Diseases and Injuries

Main portion of ICD-10-CM

Codes from A00-Z99

Most chapters are body systems

Example:

- Digestive System
- Respiratory System

Divisions of Classification of Diseases and Injuries

Blocks: A group of related conditions

Category: Represents single disease/condition

Subcategory: More specific to etiology, anatomical site and severity

7th character requirement

Available for select codes in Chapters 13, 15, 18, 19, 20

Assign to highest level of specificity, based on documentation

- If 4th to 7th characters exist, do not report a code with fewer characters

---

> **NOTE**
>
> **Remember**
>
> Assign to highest level of specificity, based on documentation

25

Using ICD-10-CM

ICD-10-CM OGCR developed by Cooperating Parties
- American Hospital Association (AHA)
- American Health Information Management Association (AHIMA)
- Centers for Medicare and Medicaid Services (CMS)
- National Center for Health Statistics (NCHS)

General Guidelines

Appendix A of this text contains Evolve Resources to link to the ICD-10-CM OGCR
You must know and follow Guidelines when assigning diagnoses codes
- All certification examinations adhere to the OGCR
In ICD-10-CM the chapter instructions take precedence over the OGCR
- As you review this ICD-10-CM material, locate the information in the OGCR
- In this way, you will become familiar with the location of OGCR content to be able to quickly reference the OGCR during the examination

Steps to Diagnosis Coding

Identify MAIN term(s) in diagnosis
  Locate MAIN term(s) in Index
  Review subterms
  Follow cross-reference instructions (e.g., *see*, *see also*)
  Verify code(s) in Tabular

Remember

Read Tabular notes
  Code to highest specificity
  NEVER CODE FROM INDEX!
  A dot/dash (./-) after a code means additional character(s) required

OGCR Section I.A.9. Other (NEC) and Unspecified (NOS)

NEC = Not elsewhere classifiable
- More specific code does NOT exist
NOS = Not otherwise specified (means "unspecified")

- Available information NOT specific enough
- Use ONLY if more specific code NOT available

OGCR Section I.B.2. Level of Detail in Coding

Assign diagnosis to highest level of specificity
  Do NOT use 3-character code if there is 4-character code
  Do NOT use 4-character code if there is 5, 6, 7 character available

OGCR Section I.B.8. Acute and Chronic Conditions

Exists alone or together
  May be separate or combination codes
  If two codes, code acute first
  Example: Acute (K85.9) and chronic (K86.1) pancreatitis
  Combination code: Both acute and chronic conditions in one code
  Example: K80.46 Calculus of bile duct with acute and chronic cholecystitis without obstruction

OGCR Section I.B.9. Combination Code

Always use combination code to classify two diagnoses or diagnosis with associated complication
  Example: Rubella encephalitis B06.01

OGCR Section I.B.7. Multiple Coding for Single Condition

Etiology (cause)
Manifestation (symptom)
- brackets [ ]
  Example: Disease, heart, amyloid E85.4 [143]

OGCR Section I.B.11. Impending or Threatened Condition

Code any condition described as impending or threatened
- Code the symptoms

OGCR Section I.B.13. Laterality

For bilateral sites, the final character identifies laterality
- Right, left, unspecified
  - M93.271 Osteochondritis dissecans, right ankle and joints of right foot

- M93.272 Osteochondritis dissecans, left ankle and joints of left foot
- If no bilateral code is available and condition is bilateral, assign separate codes for left and right

OGCR Section I.B.14. Documentation for BMI, Depth of Non-Pressure Ulcers, Pressure Ulcer Stages, Coma Scale, and NIH Stroke Scale

Code assignment based on medical documentation

BMI documentation may be from health care provider other than physician, such as dietitian
- Nurse often documents pressure ulcer stages
- Emergency medical technician often documents the coma scale
- Associated diagnosis of obesity must be documented by physician

BMI is assigned as secondary diagnosis only

Selection of Primary/First-Listed Diagnosis

Condition for encounter

Documented

Responsible for services provided

Also list coexisting condition(s) or comorbidity(ies)

OGCR Section II.H. Uncertain Diagnosis

If diagnosis states
- Probable
- Suspected
- Likely
- Questionable
- Possible
- Rule Out

Do not code condition. Code the symptoms
Example: "Cough and fever, probably pneumonia"
Code cough and fever; do NOT code pneumonia

Diagnosis and Services

Diagnosis and procedure MUST correlate

Medical necessity established

No correlation = No reimbursement

OGCR Section I.A.7. Punctuation

Codes in Brackets

Never sequence as first-listed diagnosis

Always sequence in order listed in Index

Example: Chorioretinitis, in (due to) histoplasmosis B39.9 [H32]
- Code first histoplasmosis (B39.9), then chorioretinitis (H32)

OGCR Section II.B. Two or More Interrelated Conditions

When two or more interrelated conditions exist and either could be the principal or first-listed diagnosis, either is sequenced first
Example: Patient with mitral valve stenosis and coronary artery disease (two interrelated conditions)
- Either can be principal diagnosis and sequenced first
- Resource intensiveness affects choice

OGCR Section II.C. Two or More Equal Diagnoses

Either can be sequenced first
Example: Diagnosis of viral gastroenteritis and dehydration

Late Effects (Sequela)

Location in the OGCR: Section I.B.10.

Late effect residual of (remaining from) previous illness/injury
- e.g., Burn that leaves scar

Residual coded first (scar)

Cause (burn) coded second

Late effect codes are not in a separate chapter; rather, throughout Tabular

Reference the term "Late, effect(s)" in the Index; you are directed to "*see* Sequelae"

There is no time limit on developing a residual

There may be more than one residual

Example: Patient has a stroke (I63.9) and develops paralysis on right dominant side (hemiparesis, I69.951) and loss of ability to communicate (aphasia, I69.920)

26
ICD-10-CM Chapters 1-10

Chapter 1, Certain Infectious and Parasitic Diseases

Divided based on etiology (cause of disease)
 Many combination codes
 Example: B37.0 candidiasis stomatitis infection of mouth, which reports both the organism and condition with one code

Multiple Codes

Sequencing must be considered.
- UTI due to Escherichia coli
  - N39.0 (UTI) etiology
  - B96.2- (E. coli) organism (in this order)

Ogcr Section I.C.1.A. Human Immunodeficiency Virus

Code HIV or HIV-related illness ONLY if stated as confirmed in diagnostic statement
- B20 HIV or HIV-related illness
- Z21 Asymptomatic HIV status
- R75 Inconclusive HIV serology

Previously Diagnosed HIV-Related Illness

Code prior diagnosis HIV-related disease B20 (HIV)
 NEVER assign these patients to:
- Z21 (Asymptomatic) or
- R75 (Nonspecific serologic evidence of HIV)

Sequencing

- HIV-related condition code:
  B20 HIV followed by all reported HIV-related conditions
- Unrelated condition for patient with HIV:
  Code unrelated condition(s) followed by B20, then all reported HIV-related conditions

HIV and Pregnancy

This is an exception to HIV sequencing
 During pregnancy, childbirth, or puerperium, code:
- O98.7- (Other specified infections and parasitic diseases)
- Followed by B20 (HIV) and then all code(s) for HIV-related illness(es)

Asymptomatic HIV during pregnancy, childbirth, or puerperium
- O98.7- (Other specified infections and parasitic diseases)
- Z21 (Asymptomatic HIV infection status)
- Reporting asymptomatic HIV varies by state
  - Check the state's reporting laws

Inconclusive Laboratory Test for HIV

R75 (Inconclusive serologic test for HIV)
- Reporting inconclusive laboratory HIV tests varies by state
  - Check the state's reporting laws

HIV Screening

Code Z11.4 (Screening for human immunodeficiency virus [HIV])
- Patient in high-risk group for HIV
- Z72.89 (Other problems related to lifestyle)
  Patients returning for HIV screening results = Z71.7 (HIV counseling)

Caution

Incorrectly applying these HIV coding rules can cause patient hardship
 Insurance claims for patients with HIV usually need patient's written agreement to disclosure

OGCR Section I.C.1.d. Sepsis, Severe Sepsis, and Septic Shock

Sepsis: Assign systemic infection code as first-listed diagnosis when sepsis is present
- Assign a sepsis code as secondary when sepsis develops during encounter
  Septicemia/Sepsis: Usually an A41.9 septicemia code and a R65.- SIRS code (in this order)
- Code the organ system dysfunction by the SIRS (e.g., J96.9, respiratory failure followed by R65.2-)
  Septic Shock: Organ dysfunction associated with severe sepsis
- Code underlying systemic infection (e.g., A41.9) followed by the SIRS code with septic shock (R65.21)

Chapter 2, Neoplasms

Two steps for coding neoplasms
- Incorrectly applying these neoplasm codes can also cause patient hardship
  1. Index: Locate histologic type of neoplasm (e.g., sarcoma, melanoma); review all instructions
  2. Locate code identified (usually in Neoplasm Table in Index) by body site

Neoplasm Table divided into columns:
- Malignant (Primary)
- Malignant (Secondary)
- Ca in situ
- Benign
- Uncertain
- Unspecified Behavior

   Example: Pathology report confirmed diagnosis stated in operative report of primary malignant neoplasm of the bladder neck.
- ICD-10-CM, Neoplasm Table, bladder, neck, under Malignant, Primary column, C67.5
- Reference in the Tabular to ensure accurate assignment. Coded as primary site unless specified as secondary site (metastasis)

Bone	Meninges	Brain
Peritoneum	Diaphragm	Pleura
Heart	Retroperitoneum	Liver
Lymph nodes	Spinal cord	Mediastinum

   Unknown status of neoplasm is always reported with D49.9

OGCR Section I.C.2. Neoplasms

Treatment directed at malignancy: Neoplasm is principal/first-listed diagnosis
- Except for chemotherapy, immunotherapy, or radiotherapy:
  - Therapy (treatment), listed first (Z51.–)
  - Neoplasm, listed second
    Chemotherapy: Z51.11
    Radiotherapy: Z51.0
    Immunotherapy: Z51.12

First-Listed Diagnosis, Neoplasms

Surgical removal of neoplasm and subsequent chemotherapy or radiotherapy
- Code malignancy as principal/first-listed diagnosis
  Surgery to determine extent of malignancy
- Code malignancy as principal/first-listed diagnosis

History and Secondary Metastasis of Neoplasms

Report category Z85, "Personal history of malignant neoplasm," if:
- Neoplasm was previously destroyed, AND
- No longer being treated
  If patient receives treatment for secondary neoplasm (metastasis)

- Secondary neoplasm is principal/first-listed diagnosis
- Even though primary is known

Anemia and Complications With/of Neoplasm

Patient treated for anemia due to neoplasm, code in this order:
- Neoplasm
- D63.0 Anemia in neoplastic disease

Patient treated for dehydration due to neoplasm or therapy, code in this order:
- Dehydration
- Neoplasm

Anemia associated with therapy:
- Adverse effect code
- Anemia
  Neoplasm
  Patient admitted to repair complication of surgery for an intestinal malignancy
- Complication, principal/first-listed diagnosis
- Complication is reason for encounter
- Malignancy, secondary diagnosis

Z Codes and Neoplasms

Patient receiving chemotherapy or radiotherapy after removal of neoplasm code:
- Therapy
- Active neoplasm
  Do NOT report H/O (history of) neoplasm

Chapter 3, Diseases of the Blood and Blood-Forming Organs and Certain Disorders Involving the Immune Mechanism

Includes anemia, blood disorders, coagulation defects
   Often used code: Anemia
   Many different types of anemia:
   - Hereditary hemolytic (D58.9)
   - Iron deficiency (D50.9)
   - Acquired hemolytic (D59.9)
   - Aplastic (D61.9)
   - Other specified (D64.89)
   - Unspecified (D64.9)
   Multiple coding often necessary
   Identify underlying disease condition

Chapter 4, Endocrine, Nutritional, and Metabolic Diseases

Disorders of Other Endocrine Glands

Diabetes Mellitus (E10 or E11) coded frequently
- Combination codes include DM type and complication of affected body system
  Example:
- E11.39 reports Type 2 diabetes mellitus with other diabetic ophthalmic complications

- Often requires two codes
- Z79.4 used in addition to diabetes code to report long-term use of insulin
  Temporary insulin use not coded to Z79.4; only long-term
  If type not indicated, report type 2
  Type 1 diabetic is one who is insulin-dependent
  Patient with type 2 diabetes may receive insulin for periods when diabetes is uncontrolled

Other Metabolic and Immunity Disorders Section

Disorders such as gout and dehydration
  Disorders often have many names
- E05.00 Thyrotoxicosis with diffuse goiter also known as
  - Basedow's disease
  - Graves' disease
  - Hyperthyroidism with goiter

Chapter 5, Mental, Behavioral, and Neurodevelopmental Disorders

Includes codes for:
- Personality disorders
- Stress disorders
- Neuroses
- Psychoses
- Sexual dysfunction, etc.
  Pain disorders related to psychological factors
- Assign F45.42 for pain disorder with related psychological factors (see note following G89, acute or chronic pain)
  Mental and behavioral disorders due to psychoactive substance use
- In remission, F10-F19 with -11, -21
- Psychoactive substance use, abuse, and dependence, one code assigned based on hierarchy (see OGCR, Section I.C.5.b.2.)

Chapter 6, Diseases of Nervous System

Central Nervous System
  Peripheral Nervous System

Pain—Category G89

Acute or chronic pain not elsewhere classified due to:
- Acute pain due to trauma G89.11
- Acute post-thoracotomy pain G89.12
- Central pain syndrome G89.0
- Other acute postoperative pain G89.18
- Neoplasm related pain (acute) (chronic) G89.3
- Chronic pain due to trauma G89.21
- Chronic post-thoracotomy pain G89.22
- Other chronic postprocedural pain G89.28
- Chronic pain syndrome G89.4
  Principal/Primary diagnosis

- When definitive diagnosis not established
- Pain management is reason for encounter/admission

Chapter 7, Diseases of Eye and Adnexa

Does not contain all the eye and adnexa codes
  Example: Traumatic injury to eye and orbit of eye, S05.-
  Hordeolum, infection of sebaceous gland of eyelid (stye)
  Reported on location and type
  Example: Externum, report H00.01- or internum, report H00.02-
  Chalazion, infection of eyelid that forms mass
  Reported based on location
  Entropion = turning inward of eyelid (H02.0–)
  Ectropion = turning outward of eyelid (H02.1–)
  Lacrimal System, category H04
  Reported based on right, left, bilateral, unspecified

Chapter 8, Diseases of Ear and Mastoid Process

Excludes2 indicates other categories for reporting other ear conditions
  Examples: Endocrine, nutritional and metabolic disease (E00-E89)
  H60-H95 reports diseases of:
  - External ear
  - Middle ear
  - Inner ear
  - Mastoid
  - Other
  - Surgical complications NEC

Chapter 9, Diseases of Circulatory System

OGCR Section I.C.9.a. Hypertension

Assign hypertension (arterial, benign, essential, malignant, primary, systemic) to I10

OGCR Section I.C.9.a.1. Hypertension with Heart Disease

Category I11
- Any condition in I50.- or I51.4-I51.9 with hypertension
- Use additional code(s) to specify type(s) of heart failure (I50.-)

OGCR Section I.C.9.a.2. Hypertensive Chronic Kidney Disease

Cause-and-effect relationship assumed in chronic kidney failure with hypertension
  Category I12 Hypertensive chronic kidney disease
  - Includes any condition in N18.- due to hypertension chronic kidney disease

Use additional code to identify stage of chronic kidney disease N18.1-N18.4, N18.9

OGCR Section I.C.9.a.3. Hypertensive Heart and Chronic Kidney Disease

Assign category I13 when both hypertensive chronic kidney disease and hypertensive heart disease stated in diagnosis

Assume cause-and-effect relationship
Includes any condition in I11.- with any condition in I12.- cardiorenal disease; cardiovascular renal disease
- Use additional code from category I50 to identify type of heart failure
- Use additional code to identify stage of chronic kidney disease (N18.1-N18.4, N18.9)

OGCR Section I.C.9.a.4. Hypertensive Cerebrovascular Disease for Secondary Pulmonary Hypertension

Use additional code to identify presence of hypertension (I10-I15)
Code:
- Cerebrovascular disease (I60-I69)
- Type of hypertension (I10-I15)

OGCR Section I.C.9.a.5. Hypertensive Retinopathy

Code:
- Hypertensive retinopathy (H35.0-)
- Type of hypertension (I10-I15)
The sequencing is based on the reason for the encounter.

OGCR Section I.C.9.a.6. Hypertension, Secondary

Hypertension caused by an underlying condition
Code:
- Underlying condition
- Type of hypertension (I15)

OGCR Section I.C.9.a.7. Hypertension, Transient

Transient hypertension: Temporary elevation of BP
Do NOT assign I10-I15, Hypertensive disease
- Hypertension diagnosis NOT established
- Assign either:
  - R03.0, Elevated blood pressure
  - O13.-, Gestational hypertension without significant proteinuria (pregnancy induced)
  - O14.-, Pre-eclampsia, for transient hypertension of pregnancy with significant proteinuria

OGCR Section I.C.9.a.8. Hypertension, Controlled

Hypertension controlled by therapy
- Assign appropriate code from categories I10-I15

OGCR Section I.C.9.a.9. Hypertension, Uncontrolled

Untreated hypertension
Uncontrolled hypertension
Assign appropriate code from categories I10-I15

OGCR Section I.C.9.a.10. Hypertensive Crisis

Documented hypertensive urgency, hypertensive emergency or unspecified hypertensive crisis
Assign code from category I16
Code also any identified hypertensive disease (I10-I15)
Sequencing based on reason for encounter

OGCR Section I.C.9.a.10. Pulmonary Hypertension

Assign code from category I27
Code also associated condition/adverse effect for secondary pulmonary hypertension
Sequencing based on reason for encounter

Chapter 10, Diseases of Respiratory System

Watch for "Use additional code to identify infectious organism"
- Some codes include the specific organism and do not need an additional code
- Respiratory Failure Sequencing
  If the respiratory failure is due to an acute condition, such as MI [myocardial infarction] or acute exacerbation of a chronic condition, such as COPD [chronic obstructive pulmonary disease], sequence the acute condition first
  Example: MI (acute condition) and respiratory failure
- Sequence MI (I21.9) first and respiratory failure (J96.0) second
  If the respiratory failure (acute condition) is due to a chronic nonrespiratory condition (such as myasthenia gravis), sequence the respiratory failure first
  Example: Acute respiratory failure (acute) and myasthenia gravis (chronic)
- Sequence acute respiratory failure (J96.0) first and myasthenia gravis (G70.00) second

Acute Respiratory Infection Section

Frequently assigned codes, such as:
- Common cold (J01.-)
- Sore throat (J02, acute pharyngitis)
- Acute tonsillitis (J03)
- Acute bronchitis (J20-J21), chronic bronchitis (J41-J42)
- Acute upper respiratory infection (J06.9)
- Influenza (J09-J10)
- Pneumonia (J12-J18)
  Read OGCR Section I.C.10.a., or Chapter 10 for specifics on coding COPD and asthma

27

ICD-10-CM Chapters 11-14

Chapter 11, Diseases of Digestive System

Mouth to anus and accessory organs

Extensive subcategories
Cholelithiasis (K80)
Commonly assigned codes
- Ulcers (K25-K28)
  - Gastric (K25)
  - Duodenal (K26)
  - Peptic (K27)
  - Gastrojejunal (K28)
  - Hernias (K40-K46)

Chapter 12, Diseases of Skin and Subcutaneous Tissue

Skin

Epidermis
  Dermis
  Subcutaneous tissue
  Infectious skin/Subcutaneous tissue
  Scar tissue

Accessory Organs

Sweat glands
  Sebaceous glands
  Nails
  Hair and hair follicles
  Other
  Example: Cellulitis of right finger due to *Staphylococcus*,
    report:
    - Cellulitis L03.011
    - Staphylococcus aureus B95.61

Chapter 13, Diseases of Musculoskeletal System and Connective Tissue

Bone
  Bursa
  Cartilage

Fascia
Ligaments
Muscle
Synovia
Tendons

Sections

Infectious arthropathies (joint disease)
  Inflammatory polyarthropathies
  Osteoarthritis
  Other joint disorders
  Dentofacial anomalies
  Systemic connective tissue disorders
  Deforming dorsopathies
  Spondylopathies
  Other dorsopathies
  Disorders of muscle
  Disorders of synovium and tendons
  Other soft tissue disorders
  Disorders of bone density and structure
  Other osteopathies
  Chondropathies
  Other disorders of the musculoskeletal system and connective tissue

Intraoperative and postprocedural complications and disorders of musculoskeletal system, not elsewhere classified
  Biomechanical lesions, not elsewhere classified

Chapter 14, Diseases of Genitourinary System

Commonly assigned codes:
- Urinary tract infection (N39.0)
- Inflammatory diseases of prostate (N41)
- Inflammatory disease of female pelvic organs (N70-N77)
  Stages of chronic kidney disease
- Stage 1: Blood flow through kidney increases, kidney enlarges (N18.1)
- Stage 2: (mild) Small amounts of blood protein (albumin) leak into urine (microalbuminuria) (N18.2)

28

ICD-10-CM Chapters 15-21

Chapter 15, Pregnancy, Childbirth, and the Puerperium

Used only on the **maternal** record
    Admission for pregnancy, complication
- Obstetric complication = first-listed diagnosis
    Chapter 15 codes take precedence over codes from other chapters unless the documentation indicates the condition being treated is not affecting the management of the pregnancy
    The majority of codes in Chapter 15 have a final character indicating the trimester of pregnancy
    7 characters are required on specified codes in Chapter 15

OGCR Section I.C.15.a. General Rules

Not all encounters are pregnancy-related

Example: Pregnant woman, broken ankle; report:
- Broken ankle
- Z33.1 Pregnant state incidental

Must be documented in medical record that condition being treated is not affecting pregnancy
- If NOT documented, assume condition is affecting pregnancy

Trimesters

Trimesters are counted from the first day of the last menstrual period
- 1st trimester: Less than 14 weeks 0 days
- 2nd trimester: 14 weeks 0 days to less than 28 weeks 0 days
- 3rd trimester: 28 weeks 0 days until delivery

OGCR Section I.C.15.b.1. Complications of Pregnancy, Childbirth, and the Puerperium

Chapter 15 codes (O00-O9A)
- Assigned only to mother's medical record
- Not assigned to newborn medical record
    Episodes when no delivery occurs
- Principal diagnosis should correspond to the principal complication of the pregnancy which necessitated the encounter.

OGCR Section I.C.15.b.4, When a delivery occurs
OGCR Section I.C.15.b.5, Outcome of delivery code (Z37) when delivered

OGCR Section I.C.15.b.1.-2. Selection of Principal or First-listed Diagnosis

Routine prenatal visits, no complications:
- Z34, Supervision, normal pregnancy
    Prenatal outpatient visits for high-risk pregnancies
- O09, Supervision of high-risk pregnancy

OGCR Section I.C.15.n.1.-3. Normal Delivery

Normal delivery includes:
- Vaginal delivery
- Minimal or no assistance
- With or without episiotomy
- No fetal manipulation or instrumentation
- Full-term, single, liveborn infant

Postpartum Period

After delivery and continues for 6 weeks

Peripartum Period

Defined as the last month of pregnancy to five months postpartum

Abortions

No identifiable fetus
    500 grams or less
    Less than 22 weeks' gestation
    Codes O00-O08

Abortions With Liveborn Fetus

Attempted abortion results in liveborn fetus
- Category O60 (Early onset of delivery) appropriately Assign Z37 (Outcome of delivery)
    Attempted abortion code also assigned

Chapter 16, Certain Conditions Originating in the Perinatal Period

Birth through 28 days following birth

Conditions Originating in Perinatal Period (P00-P96)
- Perinatal period through 28th day following birth
- Codes can be used after 28th day, if documented that condition originated during perinatal period

Chapter 16 codes are for use on the maternal record
Assign Z38.– as first-listed diagnosis according to type of birth

Use of Codes Z00

Z00.11 Newborn health examination
Suspected of having an abnormal condition
Infant 28 days or less
Excludes1 health check for child over 28 days old (Z00.12-)

Coding Additional Diagnosis

Code conditions that require
- Treatment
- Further investigation
- Additional resource
Prolonged length of stay (LOS)
Implications for future care
Insignificant conditions, signs, symptoms
- Resolve with no treatment
- Need no code
- EVEN IF documented

Prematurity and Fetal Growth Retardation

Codes from categories
- P05 (Slow fetal growth and fetal malnutrition) and
- P07 (Disorders relating to short gestation and low birth-weight NEC)
Not assigned solely on birthweight or gestational age
Use physician's assessment of maturity
Use additional code for weeks of gestation (P07.30, P07.31, P07.32)

Chapter 17, Congenital Malformations, Deformations, and Chromosomal Abnormalities

When a malformation/deformation/or chromosomal abnormality does not have a unique code assignment, assign additional code(s) for any manifestations that may be present.

Codes from Chapter 17 may be used throughout the life of the patient. If a congenital malformation or deformity has been corrected, a personal history code should be used to identify the history of the malformation or deformity.

Chapter 18, Symptoms, Signs, and Abnormal Clinical and Laboratory Findings, Not Elsewhere Classified

Do NOT code a sign or symptom if
- Definitive diagnosis made (symptoms are part of disease)

Used only if no specific diagnosis made
One category requires 7 characters (Coma, R40.2-)

Chapter 19, Injury, Poisoning, and Certain Other Consequences of External Causes

Block Examples

- S00-S09 Injuries to the head
- S10-S19 Injuries to the neck
- S20-S29 Injuries to the thorax
- S30-S39 Injuries to the abdomen, lower back, lumbar spine, pelvis, and external genitals
- S40-S49 Injuries to the shoulder and upper arm
- S50-S59 Injuries to the elbow and forearm
- S60-S69 Injuries to the wrist, hand, and fingers
- S70-S79 Injuries to the hip and thigh
- S80-S89 Injuries to the knee and lower leg
- S90-S99 Injuries to the ankle and foot

When Coding Injuries

- Assign separate codes for each injury unless a combination code is provided, in which case the combination code is assigned
- Multiple injury codes are provided in ICD-10-CM but should not be assigned unless information for a more specific code is not available
- Traumatic injury codes (S00-T14.9) are not assigned for normal, healing surgical wounds or to identify complications of surgical wounds
- Most categories in Chapter 19 have 7th character extensions that are required for each applicable code
Most categories in this chapter have three extensions (with the exception of fractures):

A, initial encounter
D, subsequent encounter
S, sequela

External Cause Codes: Index and Tabular

V, W, X, Y, Z code Index located following the Table of Drugs and Chemicals
Directly before the Tabular
Not in the Index to Disease and Injuries
Codes V, W, X, Y are located in Chapter 20 in the Tabular

Chapter 20, External Causes of Morbidity

Adverse effects of correct medication correctly given and correctly taken

Provide supplemental information
Identify
- Cause of an injury or poisoning
- Intent (unintentional or intentional)
- Place it occurred
- Activity

Chapter 20, General Code Guidelines

Use with any code in Volume 1 in the range of A00.0-T88.9, Z00-Z99

7th character required on most codes to describe the initial encounter, subsequent encounter, or sequela (late effect)

Assign as many external cause codes as necessary
Certain external cause codes are combination codes
Initial encounter
- Use external cause code, if applicable

Table of Drugs and Chemicals

Follows the Neoplasm Table in Index
Alphabetic listing with codes
Do NOT code directly from Table
Always reference Tabular

Late Effects of External Cause

Should be used with late effect of a previous injury/poisoning
Should NOT be used with related current injury code
Report using the external cause code with the 7th character extension "S" for Sequela
These codes should be used with any report of a late effect or sequel resulting from a previous injury

Signs and Symptoms and Definitive Diagnosis

Do NOT code a sign/symptom if definitive diagnosis made
- Symptoms are part of disease
  Use only if no specific diagnosis is made

Burns/Corrosions Classified

According to extent of body surface involved
Burn site NOT specified
Additional data required
Burn—heat
Corrosion—chemical

Category

Category T31.- = % body surface involved and % body surface involved in 3rd-degree burns
Rule of Nines applies
Burn Example: 3rd-degree burn of abdomen (10%) and 2nd-degree burn of left thigh (5%) by hot water, initial encounter
- T21.32XA Burn, abdomen, 3rd degree
- T24.212A Burn, thigh, left, 2nd degree
- T31.11 15% total burn area and 10% 3rd degree
- X12.XXXA Burn by hot liquid

Debridement of Wound, Infection, or Burn

Excisional debridement
- Cut away
- Performed by physician or other health care provider
Nonexcisional procedure
- Shaved or scraped
- Performed by physician or nonphysician

Coding for Multiple Injuries

Separate code for each injury
Most serious injury first

Vessel and Nerve Damage

Code primary injury first
- Use additional code if nerve damage minor
Primary injury = Nerve damage
- Code nerve damage first

Multiple Fractures

Same coding principles as multiple injuries
Code multiple fractures by site
Sequenced by severity

Fractures

Not indicated as closed or open = closed
Same bone fractured AND dislocated:
- Code fracture ONLY (highest level of injury)
- Laterality

Chapter 21, Factors Influencing Health Status and Contact With Health Services

Z Codes

Located after Y99.9 in Tabular
Three characters before decimal (e.g., Z11.8)
Main terms: Contraception, counseling, dialysis, status, examination

Uses of Z Codes

Not sick BUT receives health care (e.g., vaccination)
Services for known disease/injury (e.g., chemotherapy)
A circumstance/problem that influences patient's health BUT NOT current illness/injury
Example: Organ transplant status
Example: Birth status and outcome of delivery (newborn)

Special Note About "History of"

Index to Disease, MAIN term "History"
Entries between "family" and "visual loss Z82.1" = "family history of"
Entries after "family" and after "visual loss Z86.69" = "personal history of"
Draw a line in the Index of your ICD-10-CM coding manual to indicate end of "family history" entries and beginning of "personal history" entries

History Z Codes

Section I.C.21. of the OGCR contains specific guidelines that identify how Z codes can be listed (first, first/additional, additional only)

Categories in Tabular

Z85	Personal history of malignant neoplasm
Z86.59	Personal history of mental and behavioral disorder
Z87.89	Personal history of other specified conditions

Except: Z87.39 Personal history of arthritis, and Z87.79 Personal history of congenital malformations. These conditions are life-long so are not true history codes

Z88	Allergy status to medicinal agents
Z91.89	Other personal risk factors presenting hazards to health
Z80	Family history of primary malignant neoplasm
Z82.8	Family history of certain other disabilities and chronic diseases
Z84.89	Family history of other specified conditions

29

Outpatient Coding

OGCR Section IV, Diagnostic Coding and Reporting Guidelines for Outpatient Services

Part of ICD-10-CM OGCR, Section IV

Guideline A

Use term first-listed diagnosis for outpatient settings

Outpatient surgery: If procedure is not performed due to contraindications, report the reason for the surgery as first-listed diagnosis

Observation stay: Report medical condition as first-listed diagnosis

Patient admitted for outpatient surgery develops complications requiring admission to observation, report reason for admission, followed by codes for complications

Guideline B

Use codes A00.0-T88.9, Z00-Z99 to report diagnosis, symptoms, conditions, problems, complaints, or other reason(s) for visit

Guideline C

Accurate reporting of ICD-10-CM diagnosis codes, documentation should include patient's condition, specific diagnosis(es), symptoms, problems, or reason for encounter

Guideline D

Codes that describe symptoms and signs (rather than diagnoses) are acceptable for outpatient coding

Guideline E

Encounters for circumstances other than a disease or injury are reported with Z00-Z99

Guideline F

Level of detail in coding ICD-10-CM: code to highest number of characters available

Guideline G

First-listed diagnosis is the diagnosis, condition, problem, or other reason for encounter/visit

Guideline H

Uncertain diagnoses are not reported in outpatient settings

Report the condition that is the reason for the encounter, such as symptoms, signs, abnormal test results

Guideline I

Chronic diseases are treated on an ongoing basis

Report the disease each time the disease is treated or managed

Guideline J

Code all documented conditions that coexist

Do not code conditions that were previously treated and no longer exist

Guideline K

Patients receiving diagnostic services only, the first-listed code is the diagnosis, condition, problem, or other reason for encounter that is chiefly responsible for services

Routine laboratory/radiology tests

- When no signs, symptoms, or diagnoses are available, report Z01.89
- When test is to evaluate sign, symptom, or diagnosis, report both the V code and a code to report the reason for the test

    Report any confirmed or definitive diagnosis(es) documented in the test result interpretation

- Do not code signs and symptoms as additional diagnoses

Guideline L

Patients receiving therapeutic services only, sequence first the diagnosis, condition, problem, or reason for encounter chiefly responsible for service

- Report other diagnosis(es), such as chronic conditions, as secondary diagnosis(es)

Guideline M

Patients receiving preoperative evaluations only

- Report a code from subcategory Z01.81 as first-listed diagnosis

- Report condition that prompted surgery as secondary diagnosis
- Code also any findings related to pre operative evaluation

Guideline N

Ambulatory surgery: Report the diagnosis for which the surgery was performed

Report the postoperative diagnosis if different from pre-operative diagnosis

Guideline O

See OGCR, Section I.C.15

Routine prenatal visits, no complications:
- Z34, Supervision, normal first pregnancy

Prenatal outpatient visits for high-risk pregnancies
- O09, Supervision of high-risk pregnancy

Guideline P

Encounters for general medical examinations, with or without abnormal findings, report Z00.0-

If examination results in abnormal finding, report as first-listed diagnosis a code for general medical examination with abnormal findings
- Secondary code to report the abnormal finding

Guideline Q

Encounters for routine health screening, see OGCR, Section I.C.21

PART 5

Coding Challenge

30

Examinations

You have three opportunities to practice taking an examination:

- Pre-Examination (before study)
- Post-Examination (after study)
- Final Examination (at the end of your complete program of study)

For the purposes of this text, two practice exam formats have been developed so you can focus on the exam format that most closely resembles the certification exam you've chosen to take:

- Exam Format A
  Pre-/Post-Examination and Final Examination (150 multiple-choice questions each)
- Exam Format B
  Pre-/Post-Examination and Final Examination (97 multiple-choice and 8 case scenarios each)
  You should have the following manuals:
- 2018 ICD-10-CM (*International Classification of Diseases,* 10th Revision, Clinical Modification)
- 2018 HCPCS (*Healthcare Common Procedure Coding System*)
- 2018 CPT (*Current Procedural Terminology*)
  No other reference material is allowed for any of the practice examinations.
- For all Pre-Examinations, Post-Examinations, and Final Examinations, you will need a computer that has

Internet access and the three coding references listed above (ICD-10-CM, HCPCS, CPT).
- For the Exam Format A: Final Examination, you will also need paper, pencils, and an eraser.
- Each organization's certification examination has different scoring requirements, but as you take the examinations with this text, you should strive for 80% to 90% on the Post-Examination and 70% as a minimum on the Final Examination.

Pre-Examination and Post-Examination

The Pre-Examination is located on the companion Evolve website. The purpose of the Pre-Examination is only to assess your beginning level of knowledge and skill—your starting place. Based on your scores, you can tailor your study to target your weakest areas and increase your scores. Take the Pre-Examination before you begin your studies.

Your score will automatically be calculated for you. A passing score for the examinations in this text requires 70%.

The practice examinations program on Evolve will calculate and retain your scoring information.

Immediately on completion of your study, you should complete the Post-Examination on Evolve. After you are finished, the practice examinations on Evolve will automatically compare your Pre-Examination scores with your

Post-Examination scores and will store your results. By comparing the results of the Pre-Examination and the Post-Examination (the same examination will be taken twice), the electronic program illustrates the improvements you have achieved or the areas that you will need to practice more on before taking the Final Examination.

Rationales for each question are available for review after you complete the Post-Examination. Study the questions for which you did not choose the right response. Did you misread the question, did you not know the material well enough to answer correctly, or did you run out of time? Knowing why you missed a question is an important step toward improving your skill level.

Ideally, you should complete each examination in one sitting; if time does not allow, spread the examination times over several periods. There are no time extensions during an actual examination setting, and learning how to judge the amount of time you should spend on each question is an important part of this learning experience to prepare you for the real certification examination.

Final Examination

If you scored well on all areas of the Post-Examination (80% or higher), you are ready to move on to the Final

Examination, located in Part 5 of the text for Exam Format A, and on the companion Evolve site for Exam Format B.

For Exam Format A, there is an answer sheet on which to place your answers; it is located directly before the examination. Remove your answer sheet from this text, and enter your answer for each of the 150 questions using paper and pencil.

Once you have completed the answer sheet, go to the electronic program on Evolve to enter your answers on the electronic score sheet. The electronic program will then provide you with the answers and compare your scores to illustrate your improvement.

A passing score for the Final Examination is the same as for the Pre/Post-Examination—70%.

If you did not attain a minimum score on each section, you should develop a plan to restudy those particular areas where the examination indicates you are having difficulties. There are rationales for each question in the Final Examination, and you should review that information as well as material in the text. You can take any of the practice examinations again after your additional study.

EXAM FORMAT A: FINAL EXAMINATION ANSWER SHEET

Medical Terminology
1. Ⓐ Ⓑ Ⓒ Ⓓ
2. Ⓐ Ⓑ Ⓒ Ⓓ
3. Ⓐ Ⓑ Ⓒ Ⓓ
4. Ⓐ Ⓑ Ⓒ Ⓓ
5. Ⓐ Ⓑ Ⓒ Ⓓ
6. Ⓐ Ⓑ Ⓒ Ⓓ
7. Ⓐ Ⓑ Ⓒ Ⓓ
8. Ⓐ Ⓑ Ⓒ Ⓓ

Anatomy
9. Ⓐ Ⓑ Ⓒ Ⓓ
10. Ⓐ Ⓑ Ⓒ Ⓓ
11. Ⓐ Ⓑ Ⓒ Ⓓ
12. Ⓐ Ⓑ Ⓒ Ⓓ
13. Ⓐ Ⓑ Ⓒ Ⓓ
14. Ⓐ Ⓑ Ⓒ Ⓓ
15. Ⓐ Ⓑ Ⓒ Ⓓ
16. Ⓐ Ⓑ Ⓒ Ⓓ

ICD-10-CM
17. Ⓐ Ⓑ Ⓒ Ⓓ
18. Ⓐ Ⓑ Ⓒ Ⓓ
19. Ⓐ Ⓑ Ⓒ Ⓓ
20. Ⓐ Ⓑ Ⓒ Ⓓ
21. Ⓐ Ⓑ Ⓒ Ⓓ
22. Ⓐ Ⓑ Ⓒ Ⓓ
23. Ⓐ Ⓑ Ⓒ Ⓓ
24. Ⓐ Ⓑ Ⓒ Ⓓ
25. Ⓐ Ⓑ Ⓒ Ⓓ
26. Ⓐ Ⓑ Ⓒ Ⓓ

HCPCS
27. Ⓐ Ⓑ Ⓒ Ⓓ
28. Ⓐ Ⓑ Ⓒ Ⓓ
29. Ⓐ Ⓑ Ⓒ Ⓓ
30. Ⓐ Ⓑ Ⓒ Ⓓ
31. Ⓐ Ⓑ Ⓒ Ⓓ
32. Ⓐ Ⓑ Ⓒ Ⓓ

Compliance and Regulatory
33. Ⓐ Ⓑ Ⓒ Ⓓ
34. Ⓐ Ⓑ Ⓒ Ⓓ
35. Ⓐ Ⓑ Ⓒ Ⓓ
36. Ⓐ Ⓑ Ⓒ Ⓓ
37. Ⓐ Ⓑ Ⓒ Ⓓ

Coding Guidelines
38. Ⓐ Ⓑ Ⓒ Ⓓ
39. Ⓐ Ⓑ Ⓒ Ⓓ
40. Ⓐ Ⓑ Ⓒ Ⓓ
41. Ⓐ Ⓑ Ⓒ Ⓓ
42. Ⓐ Ⓑ Ⓒ Ⓓ
43. Ⓐ Ⓑ Ⓒ Ⓓ

10000 Integumentary System
44. Ⓐ Ⓑ Ⓒ Ⓓ
45. Ⓐ Ⓑ Ⓒ Ⓓ
46. Ⓐ Ⓑ Ⓒ Ⓓ
47. Ⓐ Ⓑ Ⓒ Ⓓ
48. Ⓐ Ⓑ Ⓒ Ⓓ
49. Ⓐ Ⓑ Ⓒ Ⓓ
50. Ⓐ Ⓑ Ⓒ Ⓓ
51. Ⓐ Ⓑ Ⓒ Ⓓ
52. Ⓐ Ⓑ Ⓒ Ⓓ
53. Ⓐ Ⓑ Ⓒ Ⓓ

20000 Musculoskeletal System
54. Ⓐ Ⓑ Ⓒ Ⓓ
55. Ⓐ Ⓑ Ⓒ Ⓓ
56. Ⓐ Ⓑ Ⓒ Ⓓ
57. Ⓐ Ⓑ Ⓒ Ⓓ
58. Ⓐ Ⓑ Ⓒ Ⓓ
59. Ⓐ Ⓑ Ⓒ Ⓓ
60. Ⓐ Ⓑ Ⓒ Ⓓ
61. Ⓐ Ⓑ Ⓒ Ⓓ
62. Ⓐ Ⓑ Ⓒ Ⓓ
63. Ⓐ Ⓑ Ⓒ Ⓓ

30000 Respiratory and Cardiovascular System
64. Ⓐ Ⓑ Ⓒ Ⓓ
65. Ⓐ Ⓑ Ⓒ Ⓓ
66. Ⓐ Ⓑ Ⓒ Ⓓ
67. Ⓐ Ⓑ Ⓒ Ⓓ
68. Ⓐ Ⓑ Ⓒ Ⓓ
69. Ⓐ Ⓑ Ⓒ Ⓓ
70. Ⓐ Ⓑ Ⓒ Ⓓ
71. Ⓐ Ⓑ Ⓒ Ⓓ
72. Ⓐ Ⓑ Ⓒ Ⓓ
73. Ⓐ Ⓑ Ⓒ Ⓓ

40000 Digestive System
74. Ⓐ Ⓑ Ⓒ Ⓓ
75. Ⓐ Ⓑ Ⓒ Ⓓ
76. Ⓐ Ⓑ Ⓒ Ⓓ
77. Ⓐ Ⓑ Ⓒ Ⓓ
78. Ⓐ Ⓑ Ⓒ Ⓓ
79. Ⓐ Ⓑ Ⓒ Ⓓ
80. Ⓐ Ⓑ Ⓒ Ⓓ
81. Ⓐ Ⓑ Ⓒ Ⓓ
82. Ⓐ Ⓑ Ⓒ Ⓓ
83. Ⓐ Ⓑ Ⓒ Ⓓ

50000 Urinary, Male Genital System, Female Genital System, and Maternity Care and Delivery
84. Ⓐ Ⓑ Ⓒ Ⓓ
85. Ⓐ Ⓑ Ⓒ Ⓓ
86. Ⓐ Ⓑ Ⓒ Ⓓ
87. Ⓐ Ⓑ Ⓒ Ⓓ
88. Ⓐ Ⓑ Ⓒ Ⓓ
89. Ⓐ Ⓑ Ⓒ Ⓓ
90. Ⓐ Ⓑ Ⓒ Ⓓ
91. Ⓐ Ⓑ Ⓒ Ⓓ
92. Ⓐ Ⓑ Ⓒ Ⓓ
93. Ⓐ Ⓑ Ⓒ Ⓓ

60000 Endocrine System, Hemic and Lymphatic System, Nervous System, Eye and Ocular Adnexa, Auditory System
94. Ⓐ Ⓑ Ⓒ Ⓓ
95. Ⓐ Ⓑ Ⓒ Ⓓ
96. Ⓐ Ⓑ Ⓒ Ⓓ
97. Ⓐ Ⓑ Ⓒ Ⓓ
98. Ⓐ Ⓑ Ⓒ Ⓓ
99. Ⓐ Ⓑ Ⓒ Ⓓ
100. Ⓐ Ⓑ Ⓒ Ⓓ
101. Ⓐ Ⓑ Ⓒ Ⓓ
102. Ⓐ Ⓑ Ⓒ Ⓓ
103. Ⓐ Ⓑ Ⓒ Ⓓ

Evaluation and Management (E/M)
104. Ⓐ Ⓑ Ⓒ Ⓓ
105. Ⓐ Ⓑ Ⓒ Ⓓ
106. Ⓐ Ⓑ Ⓒ Ⓓ
107. Ⓐ Ⓑ Ⓒ Ⓓ
108. Ⓐ Ⓑ Ⓒ Ⓓ
109. Ⓐ Ⓑ Ⓒ Ⓓ
110. Ⓐ Ⓑ Ⓒ Ⓓ
111. Ⓐ Ⓑ Ⓒ Ⓓ
112. Ⓐ Ⓑ Ⓒ Ⓓ
113. Ⓐ Ⓑ Ⓒ Ⓓ

Anesthesia
114. Ⓐ Ⓑ Ⓒ Ⓓ
115. Ⓐ Ⓑ Ⓒ Ⓓ
116. Ⓐ Ⓑ Ⓒ Ⓓ
117. Ⓐ Ⓑ Ⓒ Ⓓ
118. Ⓐ Ⓑ Ⓒ Ⓓ
119. Ⓐ Ⓑ Ⓒ Ⓓ
120. Ⓐ Ⓑ Ⓒ Ⓓ
121. Ⓐ Ⓑ Ⓒ Ⓓ

70000 Radiology
122. Ⓐ Ⓑ Ⓒ Ⓓ
123. Ⓐ Ⓑ Ⓒ Ⓓ
124. Ⓐ Ⓑ Ⓒ Ⓓ
125. Ⓐ Ⓑ Ⓒ Ⓓ
126. Ⓐ Ⓑ Ⓒ Ⓓ
127. Ⓐ Ⓑ Ⓒ Ⓓ
128. Ⓐ Ⓑ Ⓒ Ⓓ
129. Ⓐ Ⓑ Ⓒ Ⓓ
130. Ⓐ Ⓑ Ⓒ Ⓓ

80000 Pathology and Laboratory
131. Ⓐ Ⓑ Ⓒ Ⓓ
132. Ⓐ Ⓑ Ⓒ Ⓓ
133. Ⓐ Ⓑ Ⓒ Ⓓ
134. Ⓐ Ⓑ Ⓒ Ⓓ
135. Ⓐ Ⓑ Ⓒ Ⓓ
136. Ⓐ Ⓑ Ⓒ Ⓓ
137. Ⓐ Ⓑ Ⓒ Ⓓ
138. Ⓐ Ⓑ Ⓒ Ⓓ
139. Ⓐ Ⓑ Ⓒ Ⓓ
140. Ⓐ Ⓑ Ⓒ Ⓓ

90000 Medicine
141. Ⓐ Ⓑ Ⓒ Ⓓ
142. Ⓐ Ⓑ Ⓒ Ⓓ
143. Ⓐ Ⓑ Ⓒ Ⓓ
144. Ⓐ Ⓑ Ⓒ Ⓓ
145. Ⓐ Ⓑ Ⓒ Ⓓ
146. Ⓐ Ⓑ Ⓒ Ⓓ
147. Ⓐ Ⓑ Ⓒ Ⓓ
148. Ⓐ Ⓑ Ⓒ Ⓓ
149. Ⓐ Ⓑ Ⓒ Ⓓ
150. Ⓐ Ⓑ Ⓒ Ⓓ

Exam Format A - Final Examination

Direction: Report only the professional component unless specifically directed to do otherwise within the question.

Subject Area: Medical Terminology

1. This term means the surgical removal of the fallopian tube:
   A. ligation
   B. hysterectomy
   C. salpingostomy
   D. salpingectomy

2. This combining form means thirst:
   A. dips/o
   B. acr/o
   C. cortic/o
   D. somat/o

3. This term is also known as a homograft:
   A. autograft
   B. allograft
   C. xenograft
   D. zenograft

4. Which of the following terms means taste?
   A. Meissner
   B. pacinian
   C. gustatory
   D. astrocytes

5. This suffix means removal:
   A. -penia
   B. -ectomy
   C. -itis
   D. -pexy

6. Which of the following terms does NOT describe a receptor of the body?
   A. mechanoreceptor
   B. proprioceptor
   C. thermoreceptor
   D. endoreceptor

7. This term means abnormal thickening of the skin:
   A. ductus
   B. dermatofibroma
   C. dermatitis
   D. pachyderma

8. The term that defines the relaxation phase of the heart-beat is:
   A. systole
   B. sinoatrial
   C. diastole
   D. septa

Subject Area: Anatomy

9. This is the first portion of the small intestine:
   A. jejunum
   B. ileum
   C. duodenum
   D. cecum

10. This is a part of the inner ear:
    A. vestibule
    B. malleus
    C. incus
    D. stapes

11. This is the area behind the cornea:
    A. anterior chamber
    B. choroid layer
    C. ciliary body
    D. fundus

12. Which of the following is a covering of the chamber walls of the heart?
    A. endocardium
    B. myocardium
    C. pericardium
    D. epicardium

13. The shaft of a long bone:
    A. diaphysis
    B. epiphysis
    C. metaphysis
    D. periosteum

14. The act of turning upward, such as the hand turned palm upward:
    A. supination
    B. adduction
    C. pronation
    D. circumduction

15. The middle layer of the skin, also known as the corium or true skin:
    A. epidermis
    B. stratum corneum
    C. dermis
    D. subcutaneous

16. This is the collarbone:
    A. patella
    B. tibia
    C. scapula
    D. clavicle

Subject Area: ICD-10-CM

17. Three-week-old female with obstructive apnea.
    A. P28.3
    B. P28.4
    C. R06.81
    D. G47.33

18. Mild intellectual disabilities due to congenital iodine-deficiency hypothyroidism.
    A. E00.9, F70
    B. E01.8, F70
    C. E03.0, F78
    D. F70, E00.9

19. Admission for hemodialysis because of acute renal failure.
    A. Z49.01, N17.9
    B. N19, Z49.01
    C. N17.9, Z99.2
    D. Z99.2, N17.9
20. Glomerulonephritis due to viral hepatitis.
    A. N05, B19
    B. B19, N00.9
    C. N05.9, B19.9
    D. B19.9, N05.9
21. Initial encounter to repair a laceration of the left hand.
    A. S61.412A
    B. S61.402A, Y93.9
    C. S61.421A
    D. S61.412A, Y93.9
22. Mr. Hallberger is 62 and has multiple problems. I am examining him in the intensive critical care unit. I understand he has fluid overload with acute renal failure and was started on ultrafiltration by the nephrologist on duty. He has an abnormal chest x-ray. He has preexisting type II diabetes mellitus and sepsis. We are left with a patient now who is still sedated and on a ventilator because of acute respiratory failure. Code the diagnoses only.
    A. A42.7, N18.9, J96.00, R60.9, E11.29, R84.9
    B. A42.7, R18.8, J96.00, N17.0, E11.4, R91.8
    C. A41.9, B17.0, J96.00, E11.9, E86.9, R91.8, 99223
    D. A41.9, N17.9, J96.00, E11.9, R91.8
23. Bloody stool.
    A. P54.1
    B. R19.5
    C. K92.1
    D. K62.5
24. A lethargic patient presents with vomiting and severe cramping and the physician determines during the initial encounter that the condition was caused by the ingestion of five tablets of Tylenol with codeine and half a bottle of whiskey.
    A. T40.2X4, T39.1X4, T51.0X4, R53.83, R11.10, R10.9
    B. T40.2X4A, T39.1X4A, R53.82, R11.10, R10.9
    C. T40.2X4A, T39.1X4A, T51.0X4A, R53.83, R11.11, R10.9
    D. T40.2X4A, T39.1X4A, T51.0X4A, R53.83, R11.10, R10.9
25. Initial encounter to treat a fracture of the right patella with abrasion.
    A. S82.001A, S80.211A
    B. S82.001A
    C. S80.211A, S82.001B
    D. S82.001B
26. Sarcoidosis with cardiomyopathy.
    A. D86.89
    B. D86.85
    C. D86.89, I42.9
    D. D85.85, I42.9

Subject Area: HCPCS

27. A patient is issued a 22-inch seat cushion for his wheelchair.
    A. E2601
    B. E0950
    C. E0190
    D. E2602
28. A patient with chronic lumbar pain previously purchased a TENS and now needs replacement batteries.
    A. E1592
    B. A5082
    C. A4772
    D. A4630
29. A patient presents for trimming of 10 dystrophic toenails.
    A. G0127 × 2, L60.3
    B. G0127, G0127 × 9, L60.0
    C. G0127, L60.3
    D. G0127 × 5, G0127 × 5, Q84.6
30. A patient with chronic obstructive pulmonary disease is issued a medically necessary nebulizer with a compressor and humidifier for extensive use with oxygen delivery.
    A. E0570, E0550
    B. E0555, E0571
    C. E0580, E0550
    D. E0575, E0550
31. Which HCPCS modifier indicates the great toe of the right foot?
    A. T1
    B. T3
    C. T4
    D. T5

Subject Area: Practice Management

32. This program was developed by CMS to promote national correct coding methods and to control inappropriate payment of Part B claims and hospital outpatient claims.
    A. NCCI
    B. NFS
    C. HIPAA
    D. MA-PA
33. What is an NPI?
    A. National Payer Incentive
    B. National Provider Identification
    C. National Provider Index
    D. National Payer Identification
34. The RBRVS is a
    A. payment reform implemented in 1992
    B. listing of the customary charge for services
    C. payment list that indicates the prevailing charge in a locality
    D. listing of the physician's individual charges for a service

35. Which of the following is NOT considered fraud or abuse?
 A. Lack of documentation of medical necessity for services reported
 B. Accepting a $20 gift card from a shoe repair representative for each Medicare patient referred to his store
 C. Referring patients to a radiology center in which your physician is a partner
 D. Going to lunch with a pharmaceutical representative

36. This document is a notification to the patient in advance of services rendered that Medicare probably will not pay for those services, in addition to providing the estimated cost for which the patient will be responsible.
 A. Wavier of Liability
 B. Coordination of Benefits
 C. Advanced Beneficiary Notice
 D. UPIN

37. This entity develops and publishes an annual plan that outlines the Medicare monitoring program.
 A. MAC
 B. FI
 C. OIG
 D. CMS

Subject Area: Coding Guidelines

38. Which punctuation mark between codes in the index of the CPT manual indicates a range of codes is available?
 A. period
 B. comma
 C. semicolon
 D. hyphen

39. Which of the following most accurately describes the designation "(Separate procedure)." The procedure is:
 A. Integral to another procedure.
 B. Reported if it is the only procedure performed.
 C. Reported if the procedure is unrelated to a more major procedure performed at the same time at a different site.
 D. All of the above

40. Specific coding guidelines in the CPT manual are located in:
 A. the index.
 B. the introduction.
 C. the beginning of each section.
 D. Appendix A.

41. The symbol that indicates an add-on code in the CPT manual is:
 A. ▲
 B. ●
 C. +
 D. ▶ ◀

42. When you see the symbol ⊘ next to a code in the CPT manual, you know that:
 A. the code is a new code.
 B. the code contains new or revised text.
 C. the code is a modifier −51 exempt code.
 D. FDA approval is pending.

43. The term that indicates this is the type of code for which the full code description can be known only if the common part of the code (the description preceding the semicolon) of a preceding entry is referenced:
 A. stand-alone
 B. indented
 C. independent
 D. add-on

Subject Area: 10000 Integumentary System

44. OPERATIVE REPORT
 OPERATIVE PROCEDURE: Excision of back lesion.
 INDICATIONS FOR SURGERY: The patient has an enlarging lesion on the upper midback.
 FINDINGS AT SURGERY: There was a 5-cm, upper midback lesion.
 OPERATIVE PROCEDURE: With the patient prone, the back was prepped and draped in the usual sterile fashion. The skin and underlying tissues were anesthetized with 30 mL of 1% lidocaine with epinephrine.
 Through a 5-cm transverse skin incision, the lesion was excised. Hemostasis was ensured. The incision was closed using 3-0 Vicryl for the deep layers and running 3-0 Prolene subcuticular stitch with Steri-Strips for the skin.
  The patient was returned to the same-day surgery center in stable postoperative condition. All sponge, needle, and instrument counts were correct. Estimated blood loss is 0 mL.
 PATHOLOGY REPORT LATER INDICATED: Dermatofibroma, skin of back. Assign code(s) for the physician service only.
 A. 11406, 12002, D23.5
 B. 11424, D21.6
 C. 11406, 12032, D23.5
 D. 11606, D04.5

45. What CPT and ICD-10-CM codes would be used to code a subsequent encounter in which a split-thickness skin graft, both thighs to the abdomen, measuring 45 × 21 cm is performed on a patient who has third-degree burns of the abdomen? Documentation stated 20% of the body surface was burned, with 9% third degree. The patient also sustained second-degree burns of the upper back.
 A. 15100 × 2, T21.32XD, T21.24XD, T31.0
 B. 15100, 15101 × 9, T21.32XD, T21.23XD, T31.20
 C. 15100, 15101-51 × 9, T21.32XA, T21.23XA, T31.20
 D. 15100, 15101 × 8, T21.32XD, T21.23XD

46. **EMERGENCY DEPARTMENT REPORT CHIEF COMPLAINT:** Nasal bridge laceration.

SUBJECTIVE: The patient is a 74-year-old male who presents to the emergency department with a laceration to the bridge of his nose. He fell in the bathroom tonight. He recalls the incident. He just sort of lost his balance. He denies any vertigo. He denies any chest pain or shortness of breath. He denies any head pain or neck pain. There was no loss of consciousness. He slipped on a wet floor in the bathroom and lost his balance; that is how it happened. He has not had any blood from the nose or mouth.

PAST MEDICAL HISTORY:

1. Parkinson's
2. Back pain
3. Constipation

MEDICATIONS: See the patient record for a complete list of medications.

ALLERGIES: NKDA.

REVIEW OF SYSTEMS: Per HPI. Otherwise, negative.

PHYSICAL EXAMINATION: The exam showed a 74-year-old male in no acute distress. Examination of the HEAD showed no obvious trauma other than the bridge of the nose, where there is approximately a 1.5- to 2-cm laceration. He had no bony tenderness under this. Pupils were equal, round, and reactive. EARS and NOSE: OROPHARYNX was unremarkable. NECK was soft and supple. HEART was regular. LUNGS were clear but slightly diminished in the bases.

PROCEDURE: The wound was draped in a sterile fashion and anesthetized with 1% Xylocaine with sodium bicarbonate. It was cleansed with sterile saline and then repaired using interrupted 6-0 Ethilon sutures (Dr. Barney Teller, first-year resident, assisted with the suturing).

ASSESSMENT: Nasal bridge laceration, status post-fall.

PLAN: Keep clean. Sutures out in 5 to 7 days. Watch for signs of infection.

A. 12051, S01.21XA, W01.10XA
B. 12011, S01.21XA, W01.10XA
C. 12011, S01.20XA, W01.10XA
D. 12011, 11000, S01.20XA, S01.20XS

47. The patient is brought to surgery for repair of an accidentally inflicted open wound of the left thigh, the total extent measuring approximately 40 × 35 cm.

DESCRIPTION OF PROCEDURE: The legs were prepped with Betadine scrub and solution and then draped in a routine sterile fashion. Split-thickness skin grafts measuring about a 10,000th-inch thick were taken from both thighs, meshed with a 3: 1 ratio mesher, and stapled to the wounds. The donor sites were dressed with scarlet red, and the recipient sites were dressed with Xeroform, Kerlix fluffs, and Kerlix roll, and a few ABD pads were used for absorption.

Estimated blood loss was negligible. The patient tolerated the procedure well and left surgery in good condition.

A. 15120, 15121 × 12, S71.132A
B. 15100, 15101, 11010, S71.132A
C. 15220, 15221 × 13, S71.102A
D. 15100, 15101 × 13, S71.102A

48. What CPT and ICD-10-CM codes would be used to code the destruction by cryosurgery of a malignant lesion on the skin of the female genitalia measuring 1.6 cm?

A. 17272, C51.9
B. 11602, C57.9
C. 11420, C79.82
D. 11622, C51.9

49. **SAME-DAY SURGERY**

DIAGNOSIS: Inverted nipple with mammary duct ectasia, left.

OPERATION: Excision of mass deep to left nipple. With the patient under general anesthesia, a circumareolar incision was made with sharp dissection and carried down into the breast tissue. The nipple complex was raised up using a small retractor. We gently dissected underneath to free up the nipple entirely. Once this was done, we had the nipple fully unfolded, and there was some evident mammary duct ectasia. An area 3 × 4 cm was excised using electrocautery. Hemostasis was maintained with the electrocautery, and then the breast tissue deep to the nipple was reconstructed using sutures of 3-0 chromic. Subcutaneous tissue was closed using 3-0 chromic, and then the skin was closed using 4-0 Vicryl. Steri-Strips were applied. The patient tolerated the procedure well and was returned to the recovery area in stable condition. At the end of the procedure, all sponges and instruments were accounted for.

A. 19120-RT, N60.42
B. 11404-LT, N62
C. 19112, N60.42
D. 19120-LT, N60.42

50. This patient returns today for palliative care to her feet. Her toenails have become elongated and thickened, and she is unable to trim them on her own. She states that she has had no problems and no acute signs of any infection or otherwise to her feet. She returns today strictly for trimming of her toenails.

EXAMINATION: Her pedal pulses are palpable bilaterally. The nails are mycotic, 1 through 4 on the left, and 1 through 3 on the right.

ASSESSMENT: Onychomycosis, 1 through 4 on the left and 1 through 3 on the right.

PLAN: Mild debridement of mycotic nails × 7. This patient is to return to the clinic in 3 to 4 months for follow-up palliative care.

A. 11721 × 7, B35.9
B. 99212, 11721, B35.1
C. 11719, B35.1
D. 11721, B35.1

51. OPERATIVE REPORT

With the patient having had a wire localization performed by radiology, she was taken to the operating room and, under local anesthesia of the left breast, was prepped and draped in a sterile manner. A breast line incision was made through the entry point of the wire, and a core of tissue surrounding the wire (approximately 1 × 2 cm) was removed using electrocautery for hemostasis. The specimen, including the wire, was then submitted to radiology, and the presence of the lesion within the specimen was confirmed. The wound was checked for hemostasis, and this was maintained with electrocautery. The breast tissue was reapproximated using 2-0 and 3-0 chromic. The skin was closed using 4-0 Vicryl in a subcuticular manner. Steri-Strips were applied. The patient tolerated the procedure well and was discharged from the operating room in stable condition. At the end of the procedure, all sponges and instruments were accounted for.

Pathology report later indicated: Benign tissue, breast.

A. 11602-LT, N64
B. 11400-LT, C50.912
C. 19125-LT, D24.2
D. 19125-LT, D24.1

52. What CPT and ICD-10-CM codes would be assigned to report an initial encounter for treatment of a 40 sq cm debridement of an open anterior abdominal laceration, including subcutaneous tissue and muscle, with grit and rubble? The patient fell while speed walking and landed on a sharp rock, injuring the epigastric region of the abdomen.

A. 11000, S31.129A, W01.118A, W45.8A, Y93.01A
B. 11010, S31.622A, W18.39, W45.8
C. 11042, 11045, S31.142A
D. 11043, 11046, S31.122A, W01.118A, W45.8XXA, Y93.01

53. What code(s) is used by the radiologist when performing ultrasound preoperative placement of a needle localization wire of a single lesion of the breast? The patient was diagnosed with adenocarcinoma of the upper outer quadrant of the right breast, primary site.

A. 19285-RT, 19125-RT, C50.511
B. 19125-RT, C50.411
C. 19285-RT, C50.411
D. 19286-RT, C50.511

Subject Area: 20000 Musculoskeletal System

54. A small incision was made over the left proximal tibia, and a traction pin was inserted through the bone to the opposite side. Weights were then affixed to the pins to stabilize the closed tibial fracture temporarily until fracture repair could be performed. Assign codes for the physician service.

A. 20650-LT, S82.102A
B. 20663-LT, S82.162A
C. 20690-LT, S82.302A
D. 20692-LT, S82.302A

55. OPERATIVE REPORT
PREOPERATIVE DIAGNOSIS: Left thigh abscess.
PROCEDURE PERFORMED: Incision and drainage of left thigh abscess.
OPERATIVE NOTE: With the patient under general anesthesia, he was placed in the lithotomy position. The area around the anus was carefully inspected, and we saw no evidence of communication with the perirectal space. This appears to have risen in the crease at the top of the leg, extending from the posterior buttocks region up toward the side of the base of the penis. In any event, the area was prepped and draped in a sterile manner. Then we incised the area in fluctuation. We obtained a lot of very foul-smelling, almost stool-like material (it was not stool, but it was brown and very foul-smelling material). This was not the typical pus one sees with a *Staphylococcus aureus*–type infection. The incision was widened to allow us to probe the cavity fully. Again, I could see no evidence of communication to the rectum, but there was extension down the thigh and extension up into the groin crease. The fascia was darkened from the purulent material. I opened some of the fascia to make sure the underlying muscle was viable. This appeared viable. No gas was present. There was nothing to suggest a necrotizing fasciitis. The patient did have a very extensive inflammation within this abscess cavity. The abscess cavity was irrigated with peroxide and saline and packed with gauze vaginal packing. The patient tolerated the procedure well and was discharged from the operating room in stable condition.

A. 26990-LT, L02.416A
B. 27301-LT, L02.416
C. 27301-LT, L02.416A
D. 27025-LT, L02.416

56. OPERATIVE REPORT
PREOPERATIVE DIAGNOSIS: Compound fracture, left humerus, with possible loss of left radial pulse.
PROCEDURE PERFORMED: Open reduction internal fixation, left compound humerus fracture.
PROCEDURE: While under a general anesthetic, the patient's left arm was prepped with Betadine and draped in sterile fashion. We then created a longitudinal incision over the anterolateral aspect of his left arm and carried the dissection through the subcutaneous tissue. We attempted to identify the lateral intermuscular septum and progressed to the fracture site, which was actually fairly easy to do because there was some significant tearing and rupturing of the biceps and brachialis muscles. These were partial ruptures, but the bone was relatively easy to expose through this. We then identified the fracture site and thoroughly irrigated it with several liters of saline. We also noted that the radial nerve was easily visible, crossing along the posterolateral aspect of the fracture site. It

was intact. We carefully detected it throughout the remainder of the procedure. We then were able to strip the periosteum away from the lateral side of the shaft of the humerus both proximally and distally from the fracture site. We did this just enough to apply a 6-hole plate, which we eventually held in place with six cortical screws. We did attempt to compress the fracture site. Due to some comminution, the fracture was not quite anatomically aligned, but certainly it was felt to be very acceptable.

Once we had applied the plate, we then checked the radial pulse with a Doppler. We found that the radial pulse was present using the Doppler, but not with palpation. We then applied Xeroform dressings to the wounds and the incision. After padding the arm thoroughly, we applied a long-arm splint with the elbow flexed about 75 degrees. He tolerated the procedure well, and the radial pulse was again present on Doppler examination at the end of the procedure.
- **A.** 24515-RT, S42.352A
- **B.** 24500-LT, S42.392B
- **C.** 24515-LT, S42.352B
- **D.** 24505-LT, S42.352B

57. John, an 84-year-old male, tripped while on his morning walk. He stated he was thinking about something else when he inadvertently tripped over the sidewalk curb and fell to his knees. X-ray indicated a fracture of his right patella. With the patient under general anesthesia, the area was opened and extensively irrigated. The left aspect of the patella was severely fragmented, and a portion of the patella was subsequently removed. The remaining patella fragments were wired. The surrounding tissue was repaired, thoroughly irrigated, and closed in the usual manner.
- **A.** 27524-RT, S82.001A, W10.1XXA
- **B.** 27520-RT, S82.001A, W10.1XXA
- **C.** 27524-RT, S82.099A, W19.XXXA
- **D.** 27524-RT, S82.001A, W19.XXXA

58. Libby was thrown from a horse while riding along the side of the road; a truck that honked the horn as it passed her startled her horse. The horse reared up and Libby was thrown to the ground. The medial condyle of her left tibia was fractured and required insertion of multiple pins to stabilize the defect area. A Monticelli multiplane external fixation system was then attached to the pins. Code the placement of the fixation device and diagnosis(es) only.
- **A.** 20661-LT, S82.142A, V80.018A
- **B.** 20692-LT, S82.132A, V80.010A
- **C.** 20692-LT, S82.142A, V80.018A
- **D.** 20690-LT, S82.132A, S82.142A

59. Maryann received a blow to her right tibial shaft while moving a large stuffed chair up a flight of stairs when the person in front of the chair slipped and released his hold on the chair. The full weight of the chair was pushed against her. When she was unable to hold the

chair in place, both she and the chair fell to the landing a dozen steps below. The chair tipped on its side and landed on her tibia. On x-ray, the right tibia shaft was fractured in three places. Screws and pins were placed through the skin to secure the fracture sites.
- **A.** 27750-RT, S82.291A, W20.8XXA
- **B.** 27756-RT, S82.291A, W19.XXXA
- **C.** 27756-RT, S82.201A, W20.8XXA
- **D.** 27750-RT, S82.201A, W20.8XXA

60. The physician applies a Minerva-type fiberglass body cast from the hips to the shoulders and to the head. Before application, a stockinette is stretched over the patient's torso, and further padding of the bony areas with felt padding was done. The patient was diagnosed with Morquio-Brailsford kyphosis. Assign codes for the physician service only.
- **A.** 29040, E76.219, M49.80
- **B.** 29590, M40.10
- **C.** 29025, M49.80, E76.219
- **D.** 29000, M41.20, E76.219

61. Mary tells her physician that she has been having pain in her left wrist for several weeks. The physician examines the area and palpates a ganglion cyst of the tendon sheath. He marks the injection sites, sterilizes the area, and injects corticosteroid into two areas of the left wrist.
- **A.** 20550-LT × 2, M67.422
- **B.** 20551-LT, M67.432A
- **C.** 20551-LT × 2, M67.422A
- **D.** 20612-LT, 20612-59-LT, M67.432

62. Darin was a passenger in an automobile rollover accident and was not wearing a seat belt at the time. He was thrown from the automobile and was pinned under the rear of the overturned vehicle. He sustained craniofacial separation, Le Fort III fracture that required complicated internal and external fixation using an open approach to repair the extensive damage. A halo device was used to hold the head immobile.
- **A.** 21435, 20661
- **B.** 21435
- **C.** 21432
- **D.** 21436, 20661

63. Carl Ostrick, a 21-year-old male, slipped on a patch of ice on his sidewalk while shoveling snow. When he fell, his left hand was wedged under his body and his second carpometacarpal joint was dislocated. After manipulating the joint back into normal alignment, the surgeon on the following day fixed the dislocation by placing a wire through the skin at the tip of the finger and on through the carpometacarpal joint to maintain alignment. Code the subsequent procedure and diagnoses.
- **A.** 26608-F1, S63.052A, W00.0XXA
- **B.** 26650-FA, S63.042D, W19.XXXD
- **C.** 26706-LT, S63.002D, W00.0XXD
- **D.** 26676-LT, S63.052xD, W00.0XXD

64. OPERATIVE PROCEDURE

PREOPERATIVE DIAGNOSIS: 68-year-old male in a coma.

POSTOPERATIVE DIAGNOSIS: 68-year-old male in a coma.

PROCEDURE PERFORMED: Placement of a triple lumen central line in right subclavian vein.

With the usual Betadine scrub to the right subclavian vein area and with a second attempt, the subclavian vein was cannulated and the wire was threaded. The first time the wire did not thread right, and so the attempt was aborted to make sure we had good identification of structures. Once the wire was in place, the needle was removed and a tissue dilator was pushed into position over the wire. Once that was removed, the central lumen catheter was pushed into position at 17 cm and the wire removed. All three ports were flushed. The catheter was sewn into position, and a dressing applied.

A. 36011, R40.20X0
B. 36011, R40.20
C. 36556, R40.20X0
D. 36556, R40.20

65. What CPT and ICD-10-CM codes report a percutaneous insertion of a dual-chamber pacemaker by means of the subclavian vein? The diagnosis is sick sinus syndrome, tachy-brady.

A. 33249, I47.1, I49.5
B. 33217, I49.5
C. 33208, I49.5
D. 33240, I44.0, I47.1

66. OPERATIVE REPORT

PREOPERATIVE DIAGNOSIS: Atelectasis of the left lower lobe.

PROCEDURE PERFORMED: Fiberoptic bronchoscopy with brushings and cell washings.

PROCEDURE: The patient was already sedated, on a ventilator, and intubated; so his bronchoscopy was done through the ET tube. It was passed easily down to the carina. About 2 to 2.5 cm above the carina, we could see the trachea, which appeared good, as was the carina. In the right lung, all segments were patent and entered, and no masses were seen. The left lung, however, had petechial ecchymotic areas scattered throughout the airways. The tissue was friable and swollen, but no mucous plugs were noted, and all the airways were open, just somewhat swollen. No abnormal secretions were noted at all. Brushings were taken as well as washings, including some with Mucomyst to see whether we could get some distal mucous plug, but nothing really significant was returned. The specimens were sent to appropriate cytological and bacteriological studies. The patient tolerated the procedure fairly well.

A. 31622, 31623-51, J98.11
B. 31623, P28.0
C. 31623-LT, J98.11
D. 31624, P28.0

67. OPERATIVE REPORT

PREOPERATIVE DIAGNOSIS:
1. Hypoxia.
2. Pneumothorax.

POSTOPERATIVE DIAGNOSIS:
1. Hypoxia.
2. Pneumothorax.

PROCEDURE: Chest tube placement.

DESCRIPTION OF PROCEDURE: The patient was previously sedated with Versed and paralyzed with Nimbex. Lidocaine was used to numb the incision area in the midlateral left chest at about nipple level. After the lidocaine, an incision was made, and we bluntly dissected to the area of the pleural space, making sure we were superior to the rib. On entrance to the pleural space, there was immediate release of air noted. An 18-gauge chest tube was subsequently placed and sutured to the skin. There were no complications for the procedure, and blood loss was minimal.

DISPOSITION: Follow-up, single-view, chest x-ray showed significant resolution of the pneumothorax except for a small apical pneumothorax that was noted. Code only the operative procedure and diagnosis(es).

A. 32422, R09.02, J93.9
B. 32551, 71045, R09.02, J93.9
C. 32551, J93.9, R09.02
D. 32422, R09.02, J93.0

68. OPERATIVE REPORT

PREOPERATIVE DIAGNOSIS: Atherosclerotic heart disease.

POSTOPERATIVE DIAGNOSIS: Atherosclerotic heart disease.

OPERATIVE PROCEDURE: Coronary bypass grafts × 2 with a single graft from the aorta to the distal left anterior descending and from the aorta to the distal right coronary artery.

PROCEDURE: The patient was brought to the operating room and placed in a supine position. Under general intubation anesthesia, the anterior chest and legs were prepped and draped in the usual manner. A segment of greater saphenous vein was harvested from the left thigh, utilizing the endoscopic vein harvesting technique, and prepared for grafting. The sternum was opened in the usual fashion, and the left internal mammary artery was taken down and prepared for grafting. The flow through the internal mammary artery was very poor. The patient did have a 25-mm difference in arterial pressure between the right and left arms, the right arm being higher. The left internal mammary artery was therefore not used. The pericardium was incised sharply and a pericardial well created. The patient was systemically heparinized and placed on bicaval to aortic cardiopulmonary bypass with the stump in the main pulmonary artery for cardiac decompression. The patient was cooled to 26°C, and on fibrillation an aortic cross-clamp was applied and potassium-rich cold crystalline cardioplegic solution was administered through the aortic root with satisfactory cardiac arrest. Subsequent doses were given down the vein grafts as the anastomoses were completed and via the coronary sinus in a retrograde fashion. Attention was directed to the right coronary artery. The end of the greater saphenous vein was then anastomosed with 7-0 continuous Prolene distally. The remaining graft material was then grafted to the left anterior descending at the junction of the middle and distal third. The aortic cross-clamp was removed after 149 minutes with spontaneous cardioversion. The usual maneuvers to remove air from the left heart were then carried out using transesophageal echocardiographic technique. After all the air was removed and the patient had returned to a satisfactory temperature, he was weaned from cardiopulmonary bypass after 213 minutes utilizing 5 g per kilogram per minute of dopamine. The chest was closed in the usual fashion. A sterile compression dressing was applied, and the patient returned to the surgical intensive care unit in satisfactory condition.

A. 33511, 33517, I70.91

B. 33511, 33508, I25.10

C. 33534, 33508, I25.709

D. 33511, 33517, I25.10

69. **OPERATIVE REPORT:** The patient is in for a bone marrow biopsy. The patient was sterilized by standard procedure. Bone marrow core biopsies were obtained from the left posterior iliac crest with minimal discomfort. At the end of the procedure, the patient denied discomfort, without evidence of complications. The patient has diffuse, large B-cell malignant lymphoma. Assign codes for the physician service only.

A. 20225, C83.00

B. 38221, C83.30

C. 38230, C83.00

D. 38220, C83.30

70. Patient is a 40-year-old male who was involved in a motor vehicle crash. He is having some pulmonary insufficiency.

PROCEDURE: Bronchoscope was inserted through the accessory point on the end of the ET tube and was then advanced through the ET tube. The ET tube came pretty close to the carina. We selectively intubated the right mainstem bronchus with the bronchoscope. There were some secretions here, and these were aspirated. We then advanced this selectively into first the lower and then the middle and upper lobes. Secretions were present, more so in the middle and lower

lobes. No mucous plug was identified. We then went into the left mainstem and looked at the upper and lower lobes. There was really not much in the way of secretions present. We did inject some saline and aspirated this out. We then removed the bronchoscope and put the patient back on the supplemental O_2. We waited a few minutes. The oxygen level actually stayed pretty good during this time. We then reinserted the bronchoscope and went down to the right side again. We aspirated out all secretions and made sure everything was clear. We then removed the bronchoscope and pulled back on the ET tube about 1.5 cm. We then again placed the patient on supplemental oxygenation.

FINDINGS: No mucous plug was identified. Secretions were found mainly in the right lung and were aspirated. The left side looked pretty clear.

A. 31646, J80, V49.9XXA

B. 32654, J98.4, V49.9

C. 31645-50, J80, V49.9XXA

D. 31645-RT, J80, V49.9XXA

71. This 52-year-old male has undergone several attempts at extubation, all of which failed. He also has morbid obesity and significant subcutaneous fat in his neck. The patient is now admitted for a flap tracheostomy and cervical lipectomy. The cervical lipectomy is necessary for adequate exposure and access to the trachea and also to secure tracheotomy tube placement. Assign code(s) for the physician service only.

A. 31610, 15839-51

B. 31610

C. 31610, 15838

D. 31603, 15839-51

72. Connie was brought to the operating room for repair of an acute, traumatic diaphragmatic hernia.

A. 39540, K44.9

B. 39503, K44.0

C. 39541, K44.9

D. 39540, Q79.0

73. This patient returns to the operating room for placement of an additional chest tube for an anterior pneumothorax due to a contusion lung injury. The same physician had just placed a chest tube 4 days earlier.

A. 32551, S27.0XXD

B. 32420, S27.329D

C. 32551-58, S27.329D

D. 32551, S25.419D

Subject Area: 40000 Digestive System

74. What CPT code would you use if the physician performs a pyloroplasty and vagotomy in the same surgical session?

A. 43865

B. 50400

C. 43635

D. 43640

75. This 43-year-old female comes in with a peritonsillar abscess. The patient is brought to same-day surgery and given general anesthetic. On examination of the peritonsillar abscess, an incision was made and fluid was drained. The area was examined again, saline was applied, and then the area was packed with gauze. The patient tolerated the procedure well.

A. 42825, J36
B. 42700, J36
C. 42825, J35.01
D. 42700, J36.00

76. OPERATIVE REPORT
PREOPERATIVE DIAGNOSIS: Abdominal pain.
POSTOPERATIVEDIAGNOSIS: Normalendoscopy.
PROCEDURE: The flexible video therapeutic endoscope was passed without difficulty into the oropharynx. The gastroesophageal junction was seen at 40 cm. Inspection of the esophagus revealed no erythema, ulceration, varices, or other mucosal abnormalities. The stomach was entered and the endoscope advanced to the second duodenum. Inspection of the second duodenum, first duodenum, duodenal bulb, and pylorus revealed no abnormalities. Retroflexion revealed no lesions along the curvature. Inspection of the antrum, body, and fundus of the stomach revealed no abnormalities. The patient tolerated the procedure well. The patient complained of abdominal pain and weight loss.

A. 45378, R10.9, R63.4
B. 43235, R10.9, R63.4
C. 49320, R63.0, R10.9
D. 43255, E66.01, R10.32

77. This 70-year-old male is brought to the operating room for a biopsy of the pancreas. A wedge biopsy is taken and sent to pathology. The report comes back immediately, indicating that primary malignant cells were present in the specimen. The decision was made to perform a total pancreatectomy. Code the operative procedure(s) and diagnosis only.

A. 48100, C78.89
B. 48155, C25.8
C. 48155, 48100-51, C25.9
D. 48155, 48100-51, 88309, C25.9

78. This patient is taken to the operating room from the intensive care unit (ICU). The area of the stoma appears to be necrotic, and on this basis the surgeon indicates that the patient has been taken back to the operating room. The stoma was originally created 4 months ago by her previous surgeon.
PROCEDURE PERFORMED: Revision ileostomy stoma.
OPERATIVE NOTE: With the patient moved onto the operating table, the abdomen was prepped and draped. The segment of bowel that was serving as the ileostomy was freed up. Going in through this large open wound, we were able to identify which segment

of bowel this was. We resected the end of the bowel that was necrotic and freed up enough of the distal small bowel so that we could bring it out through a new stoma that was placed lateral to the original stoma. The stoma was created, the bowel was brought out, and the mucosa was sewn onto the skin. With this accomplished, we appeared to have a viable stoma. The patient tolerated this procedure and was returned to the ICU in stable condition.

A. 44310, K94.00
B. 45136, L03.311
C. 44312, K94.13
D. 44314, K94.03

79. This patient is brought back to the operating room during the postoperative period by the same physician to repair an esophagogastrostomy leak, transthoracic approach, done 2 days ago. The patient is status post-esophagectomy for esophageal cancer and is still undergoing chemotherapy. Code the procedure and the diagnosis for the complication.

A. 43320-78, C15.9
B. 43340-78, Z85.01
C. 43341, K94.33, D49.0
D. 43415-78, K94.33, C15.9

80. The patient was taken to the operating room for a repair of a strangulated inguinal hernia. This hernia was previously repaired 4 months ago.

A. 49521, K40.31
B. 49520, K40.00
C. 49492, K40.90
D. 49521-78, K40.31

81. The physician is using an abdominal approach to perform a proctopexy combined with a sigmoid resection; the patient was diagnosed with colon cancer, primary site sigmoid flexure of the colon.

A. 45540, C18.7
B. 45541, C18.9
C. 45550, C18.7
D. 45345, C19

82. What code would you use to report a rigid proctosigmoidoscopy with removal of two nonadenomatous polyps of the rectum by snare technique?

A. 45320, K62.1
B. 45383, D12.8
C. 45309 × 2, K62.1
D. 45315, K62.1

83. OPERATIVE REPORT
PREOPERATIVE DIAGNOSIS: Leaking from intestinal anastomosis.
POSTOPERATIVE DIAGNOSIS: Leaking from intestinal anastomosis.
PROCEDURE PERFORMED: Proximal ileostomy for diversion of colon. Oversew of right colonic fistula.
OPERATIVE NOTE: This patient was taken back to the operating room from the intensive care unit. She was having acute signs of leakage from an anastomosis

I performed 3 days previously. We took down some of the sutures holding the wound together. We basically exposed all of this patient's intestine. It was evident that she was leaking from the small bowel as well as from the right colon. I thought the only thing we could do would be to repair the right colon. This was done in two layers, and then we freed up enough bowel to try to make an ileostomy proximal to the area of leakage. We were able to do this with great difficulty, and there was only a small amount of bowel to be brought out. We brought this out as an ileostomy stoma, realizing that it was of questionable viability and that it should be watched closely. With that accomplished, we then packed the wound and returned the patient to the intensive care unit.
A. 44310, K91.89
B. 44310-78, K91.89, T85.638A
C. 45136, K91.89
D. 45136-78, K91.89

Subject Area: 50000 Urinary, Male Genital System, Female Genital System, and Maternity Care and Delivery

84. This patient is 35 years old at 36 weeks' gestation. She presents in spontaneous labor. Because of her prior cesarean section, she is taken to the operating room to have a repeat lower-segment transverse cesarean section performed. The patient also desires sterilization, and so a bilateral tubal ligation will also be performed. A single, liveborn infant was the outcome of the delivery.
A. 59510, 58600-51, Z30.2, Z3A.36
B. 59620, 58615-51, O60.14X0, Z37.0, Z38.01, Z3A.36
C. 59514, 58605-51, Z37.0, Z3A.36
D. 59514, 58611, O34.211, O60.14X0, Z37.0, Z30.2, Z3A.36

85. The pediatric physician takes this newborn male to the nursery to perform a clamp circumcision with regional block.
A. 54160, N47.0
B. 54150, Z41.2
C. 54160, Z41.2
D. 54150, N47.0

86. **OPERATIVE REPORT**
PREOPERATIVE DIAGNOSIS: Possible recurrent transitional cell carcinoma of the bladder.
POSTOPERATIVE DIAGNOSIS: No evidence of recurrence.
PROCEDURE PERFORMED: Cystoscopy with multiple bladder biopsies.
PROCEDURE NOTE: The patient was given a general mask anesthetic, prepped, and draped in the lithotomy position. The 21-French cystoscope was passed into the bladder. There was a hyperemic area on the posterior wall of the bladder, and a biopsy was taken. Random biopsies of the bladder were also performed. This area was fulgurated. A total of 7sq cm of bladder was fulgurated. A catheter was left at the end of the procedure. The patient tolerated the procedure well and was transferred to the recovery room in good condition. The pathology report indicated no evidence of recurrence.
A. 52224, N32.89, Z85.51
B. 51020, 52204, Z80.52
C. 52234, Z85.51
D. 52224 × 4, D41.4

87. This 1-year-old boy has a midshaft hypospadias with a very mild degree of chordee. He also has a persistent right hydrocele. The surgeon brought the boy to surgery to perform a right hydrocele repair and one-stage repair of hypospadias with preputial onlay flap.
A. 54322, 55040, Q54.1, N43.3, Q54.4
B. 54322, 55041-51, Q54.1, N43.3
C. 54324, 55060-51, Q54.1, N43.3
D. 54324, 55060, Q54.1, N43.3, Q54.4

88. This gentleman has worsening bilateral hydronephrosis. He did not have much of a post-void residual on bladder scan. He is taken to the operating room to have a bilateral cystoscopy and retrograde pyelogram. The results come back as gross prostatic hyperplasia with urinary retention as the cause of the hydronephrosis.
A. 52005, N40.0
B. 52000, N13.39, N40.1
C. 52005, N40.0, N13.39
D. 52000-50, N13.39, N40.1

89. This patient is a 42-year-old female who has been having prolonged and heavy bleeding during menstruation.
SURGICAL FINDINGS: On pelvic exam under anesthesia, the uterus was normal size and firm. The examination revealed no masses. She had a few small endometrial polyps in the lower uterine segment.
DESCRIPTION OF PROCEDURE: After induction of general anesthesia, the patient was placed in the dorsolithotomy position, after which the perineum and vagina were prepped, the bladder straight catheterized, and the patient draped. After bimanual exam was performed, a weighted speculum was placed in the vagina and the anterior lip of the cervix was grasped with a single tooth tenaculum. An endocervical curettage was then done with a Kevorkian curet. The uterus was then sounded to 8.5 cm. The endocervical canal was dilated to 7 mm with Hegar dilators. A 5.5-mm Olympus hysteroscope was introduced using a distention medium. The cavity was systematically inspected, and the preceding findings noted. The hysteroscope was withdrawn and the cervix further dilated to 10 mm. Polyp forceps was introduced, and a few small polyps were removed. These were sent separately to the lab. Sharp endometrial curettage was then done. The hysteroscope was then reinserted, and the polyps had essentially been removed. The patient tolerated the procedure well and was returned to the recovery room in stable condition. Pathology confirmed benign endometrial polyps.

A. 58558, 57460-51, N92.0, N84.0
B. 58558, N92.0, N84.0
C. 58558, 57558-51, N92.0, N84.0
D. 58558, N92.1, D49.59

90. **OPERATIVE REPORT**
PREOPERATIVE DIAGNOSIS: Missed abortion with fetal demise, 11 weeks.
POSTOPERATIVE DIAGNOSIS: Missed abortion with fetal demise, 11 weeks.
PROCEDURE: Suction D&C.
The patient was prepped and draped in a lithotomy position under general mask anesthesia, and the bladder was straight catheterized; a weighted speculum was placed in the vagina. The anterior lip of the cervix was grasped with a single-tooth tenaculum. The uterus was then sounded to a depth of 8 cm. The cervical os was then serially dilated to allow passage of a size 10 curved suction curette. A size 10 curved suction curette was then used to evacuate the intrauterine contents. Sharp curette was used to gently palpate the uterine wall with negative return of tissue, and the suction curette was again used with negative return of tissue. The tenaculum was removed from the cervix. The speculum was removed from the vagina. All sponges and needles were accounted for at completion of the procedure. The patient left the operating room in apparent good condition having tolerated the procedure well.
A. 59812, O03.9, Z3A.11
B. 59812, O07.39, Z3A.11
C. 59820, O02.1, Z3A.11
D. 59856, O02.1, Z3A.11

91. **OPERATIVE REPORT**
PREOPERATIVE DIAGNOSIS: Right ureteral stricture.
POSTOPERATIVE DIAGNOSIS: Right ureteral stricture.
PROCEDURE PERFORMED: Cystoscopy, right ureteral stent change.
PROCEDURE NOTE: The patient was placed in the lithotomy position after receiving IV sedation. He was prepped and draped in the lithotomy position. The 21-French cystoscope was passed into the bladder, and urine was collected for culture. Inspection of the bladder demonstrated findings consistent with radiation cystitis, which has been previously diagnosed. There is no frank neoplasia. The right ureteral stent was grasped and removed through the urethral meatus; under fluoroscopic control, a guidewire was advanced up the stent, and the stent was exchanged for a 7-French 26-cm stent under fluoroscopic control in the usual fashion. The patient tolerated the procedure well.
A. 51702-LT, N13.5
B. 52005-RT, N30.90
C. 52332-RT, N30.90
D. 52332-RT, N13.5

92. This 41-year-old female presented with a right labial lesion. A biopsy was taken and the results were reported as VIN III, cannot rule out invasion. The decision was therefore made to proceed with wide local excision of the right vulva.
PROCEDURE: The patient was taken to the operating room and general anesthesia was administered. The patient was then prepped and draped in the usual manner in lithotomy position, and the bladder was emptied with a straight catheter. The vulva was then inspected. On the right labium minora at approximately the 11 o'clock position, there was a multifocal lesion. A marking pen was then used to mark out an elliptical incision, leaving a 1-cm border on all sides. The skin ellipse was then excised using a knife. Bleeders were cauterized with electrocautery. A running locked suture of 2-0 Vicryl was then placed in the deeper tissue. The skin was finally reapproximated with 4-0 Vicryl in an interrupted fashion. Good hemostasis was thereby achieved. The patient tolerated this procedure well. There were no complications.
A. 56605, C51.9
B. 56625, D07.1
C. 56620, D07.1
D. 11620, C51.9

93. This 32-year-old female presents with an ectopic pregnancy without intrauterine pregnancy. The physician elects to remove the entire left fallopian tube with the products of conception laparoscopically.
A. 59120, O00.90
B. 59151, O00.90
C. 58943, O00.102
D. 59120, O00.80

Subject Area: 60000 Endocrine System, Hemic and Lymphatic System, Nervous System, Eye and Ocular Adnexa, Auditory System

94. **OPERATIVE REPORT**
PREOPERATIVE DIAGNOSIS: FUO.
PROCEDURE PERFORMED: Lumbar puncture.
DESCRIPTION OF PROCEDURE: The patient was placed in the lateral decubitus position with the left side up. The legs and hips were flexed into the fetal position. The lumbosacral area was sterilely prepped. It was then numbed with 1% Xylocaine. I then placed a 22-gauge spinal needle on the first pass into the intrathecal space between the L4 and L5 spinous processes. The fluid was minimally xanthochromic. I sent the fluid for cell count for differential, protein, glucose, Gram stain, and culture. The patient tolerated the procedure well without apparent complication. The needle was removed at the end of the procedure. The area was cleansed, and a Band-Aid was placed.
A. 62272, R68.12
B. 62268, R50.9
C. 62272, R60.9, R50.9
D. 62270, R50.9

95. **OPERATIVE REPORT**

    PREOPERATIVE DIAGNOSIS: Mechanical ectropion, left lower eye.

    PROCEDURE PERFORMED: Medial tarsorrhaphy, left lower eye.

    In the operating room, after intravenous sedation, the patient was given a total of about 0.5 mL of local infiltrative anesthetic. The skin surfaces on the medial area of the lid, medial to the punctum, were denuded. A bolster had been prepared and double 5-0 silk suture was passed through the bolster, which was passed through the inferior skin and raw lid margin, then through the superior margin, and out through the skin. A superior bolster was then applied. The puncta were probed with wire instrument and found not to be obstructed. The suture was then fully tied and trimmed. Bacitracin ointment was placed on the surface of the skin. The patient left the operating room in stable condition, without complications, having tolerated the procedure well.

    A. 67875-LT, H02.125
    B. 67710-LT, H02.135
    C. 67882-LT, H02.109
    D. 67880-LT, H02.125

96. Marginal laceration involving the left lower eyelid and laceration of the left upper eyelid involving the tarsus. Both required full-thickness repair. Also, there were multiple stellate lacerations above the left eye, totaling 24.2 cm and requiring full-thickness layered repair. Assign code(s) for the physician service only.

    A. 67935-E2, 12017
    B. 67930-E2, 13152-51, 13153
    C. 67935-E2, 67935-E1-51, 12056-51
    D. 67935-E2, 12017-51

97. This 66-year-old male has been diagnosed with a senile cataract of the posterior subcapsular and is scheduled for a cataract extraction by phacoemulsification of the right eye. The physician has taken the patient to the operating room to perform a posterior subcapsular cataract extraction with IOL placement, diffuse of the right eye.

    A. 66982-RT, H25.031
    B. 66984-RT, H25.041
    C. 66983-RT, H25.031
    D. 66830-RT, H25.041

98. **OPERATIVE REPORT**

    PREOPERATIVE DIAGNOSIS: Brain tumor versus abscess.

    PROCEDURE: Craniotomy.

    DESCRIPTION OF PROCEDURE: Under general anesthesia, the patient's head was prepped and draped in the usual manner. It was placed in Mayfield pins. We then proceeded with a craniotomy. An inverted U-shaped incision was made over the posterior right occipital area. The flap was turned down. Three burr holes were made. Having done this, I then localized the tumor through the burr holes and dura. We then made an incision in the dura in an inverted U-shaped fashion. The cortex looked a little swollen but normal. We then used the localizer to locate the cavity. I separated the gyrus and got right into the cavity and saw pus, which was removed. Cultures were taken and sent for pathology report, which came back later describing the presence of clusters of gram-positive cocci, confirming that this was an abscess. We cleaned out the abscessed cavity using irrigation and suction. The bed of the abscessed cavity was cauterized. Then a small piece of Gelfoam was used for hemostasis. Satisfied that it was dry, I closed the dura. I approximated the scalp. A dressing was applied. The patient was discharged to the recovery room.

    A. 61154, G06.0
    B. 61154, D49.6
    C. 61320, G06.0, B96.89
    D. 61150, D49.6

99. This patient is in for a recurrent herniated disc at L5-S1 on the left. The procedure performed is a repeat laminotomy and foraminotomy at the L5-S1 interspace.

    A. 63030-LT, M51.27
    B. 63030-LT, M51.07
    C. 63042-LT, M51.07
    D. 63042-LT, M51.27

100. **OPERATIVE REPORT**

    PREOPERATIVE DIAGNOSIS: Herniated disc L4-5 on the left.

    PROCEDURE PERFORMED: Laminotomy, foraminotomy, removal of herniated disc L4-5 on the left.

    PROCEDURE: Under general anesthesia, the patient was placed in the prone position and the back was prepped and draped in the usual manner. An incision was made in the skin extending through subcutaneous tissue. Lumbodorsal fascia was divided. The erector spinae muscles were bluntly dissected from the lamina of L4-5 on the left. The interspace was localized. I then performed a generous laminotomy and foraminotomy here, and retracted on the nerve root. It was obvious there was a herniated disc. I removed it, entered the space, and removed degenerating material, satisfied that I had decompressed the root well. There were free fragments lying around beneath the nerve root. We removed all of these. I was able to pass a hockey stick down the foramen across the midline, satisfied I had taken out the large fragments from the interspace at L4-5, and decompressed it well. I irrigated the wound well, put a Hemovac drain in the wound, and then closed the wound in layers using double-knotted 0 chromic on the lumbodorsal fascia with Vicryl 2-0 plain, in the subcutaneous tissue, and surgical staples on the skin. A dressing was applied. The patient was discharged to the recovery room.

    A. 63030-LT, M51.26
    B. 63012-LT, M51.46
    C. 63047-LT, M51.9
    D. 63047-LT, 63048-LT, M51.26

101. This patient came in with an obstructed ventriculo-peritoneal shunt. The procedure performed was to be a revision of shunt. After inspecting the shunt system, the entire cerebrospinal fluid shunt system was removed and a similar replacement shunt system was placed. Patient has normal pressure hydrocephalus (NPH).

   A. 62180, T85.890A, G91.0
   B. 62258, T85.890A, G91.2
   C. 62256, T85.890A, G91.1
   D. 62190, T85.890A, G91.2

102. Twist drill for a left frontal ventricular puncture for implanting catheter, layered repair of 8-cm scalp laceration, and repair of multiple facial and eyelid lacerations with an approximate total length of 12 cm. Assign code(s) for the physician service only.

   A. 61020, 12015-51
   B. 61107, 12034-51, 12015-51
   C. 61215, 12015-51
   D. 61107, 12034-51

103. What CPT and ICD-10-CM codes would you assign to report the removal of 30% of the left thyroid lobe, with isthmusectomy? The diagnosis was benign growth of the thyroid.

   A. 60210, D34
   B. 60220, D44.0
   C. 60212, D49.7
   D. 60225, D34, D49.7

Subject Area: Evaluation and Management (E/M)

104. Dr. Black admits a patient with an 8-day history of a low-grade fever, tachycardia, tachypnea, and possible radiologic evidence of basal consolidation of the lung and limited pleural effusion on the left side, per patient as seen at outside clinic several days prior. The patient has also been experiencing swelling of the extremities. The pulse is rapid and thready, as checked by patient on her own during the past couple days. A complete ROS of constitutional factors, ophthalmologic, otolaryngologic, cardiovascular, respiratory, gastrointestinal, genitourinary, musculoskeletal, integumentary, neurologic, psychiatric, endocrine, hematologic, lymphatic, allergic, and immunologic was performed and negative except for the symptoms described above. Past history includes tachycardia and pneumonia. Family history includes heart disease, hypertension, and high cholesterol in both parents. The patient drinks only occasionally and quit smoking 4 years ago. The comprehensive examination was performed and diminished bowel sounds were noted. The physician orders laboratory tests and radiographic studies, including a follow-up chest x-ray as he considers the extensive diagnostic options and the medical decision-making complexity is high for this patient.

   A. 99233, R00.0, R50.9, R06.82, J90, R19.15, Z87.891
   B. 99233, R00.0, I47.9, R06.82, J18.1, J90

   C. 99223, R00.0, R50.9, R06.82
   D. 99223, R50.9, R00.0, R06.82, J90, R19.15, Z87.891, Z82.49

105. Bill, a retired U.S. Air Force pilot, was on observation status 12 hours to assess the outcome of a fall from the back of a parked pickup truck into a gravel pit. History of Present Illness: The patient is a 42-year-old gentleman who works at the local garden shop. He explained that yesterday he fell from his pickup truck as he was loading gravel for a landscaping project. He lost his footing when attempting to climb from the pickup bed and fell approximately four feet and landed on a rock that was protruding from the ground 4 inches, striking his head on the rock. He did not lose consciousness, but was dizzy. He subsequently developed a throbbing headache (8/10) and swelling at the point of impact. The duration of the dizziness was approximately 10 minutes. The headache persisted for 26 hours after the fall. He did take ibuprofen without significant improvement in the pain level. Review of Systems: Constitutional, eyes, ears, nose, throat, lungs, cardiovascular, gastrointestinal, skin, neurologic, lymphatic, and immunologic negative except for HPI statements. PFSH: He is married and has 2 children. He has been working at the garden shop for 4 years. He currently smokes one pack of cigarettes a day and has smoked for 10 years. His father died of heart disease when he was 52. He has one brother with ankylosing spondylitis and one sister who is healthy as far as he knows. His mother died when he was 14 years old. He is currently on no prescribed medications. A comprehensive exam is documented and rendered. The medical decision making is of low complexity.

   The physician discharged Bill from observation that same day after 10 hours, after determining that no further monitoring of his condition was necessary. The physician provided a detailed examination and indicated that the medical decision making was of low complexity.

   A. 99218, R51, W17.89XA
   B. 99234, Z04.2, W17.89XA, Y93.H2
   C. 99217, Z04.2, W17.89XA
   D. 99234, 99217, R51, W17.89A

106. A gynecologist admits an established patient, a 35-year-old female with dysfunctional uterine bleeding, after seeing her in the clinic that day. During the course of the history, the physician notes that the patient has a history of infrequent periods of heavy flow. She has had irregular heavy periods and intermittent spotting for 4 years. The patient has been on a 3-month course of oral contraceptives for symptoms with no relief. The patient states that she has occasional headaches. A complete ROS was performed, consisting of constitutional factors, ophthalmologic, otolaryngologic, cardiovascular, respiratory, gastrointestinal, genitourinary, musculoskeletal, integumentary, neurologic, psychiatric, endocrine, hematologic, lymphatic, allergic, and immunologic which were all negative, except for the symptoms described above. The family history is positive for endometrial cancer, with mother, two aunts, and two sisters who had endometrial cancer. The patient has a personal history of cervical and endometrial polyp removal 3 years prior to admission. The patients states that she does not smoke and only drinks socially. As a part of the comprehensive examination, the physician notes the patient has a large amount of blood in the vault and an enlarged uterus. The prolonged hemorrhaging has resulted in a very thin and friable endometrial lining. The physician orders the patient to be started on intravenous Premarin and orders a full laboratory workup. The medical decision making is of moderate complexity.

A. 99215, 99222, Z87.42, Z80.49
B. 99222, N93.8, Z87.42, Z80.49
C. 99215, 99222, N92.5, Z87.42, Z80.49
D. 99222, N92.1, Z80.49

107. Karra Hendricks, a 37-year-old female, is an established patient who presents to the office with right lower quadrant abdominal pain with fever. The patient states she has had the pain for 3 days. She has taken Tylenol for her fever with some relief. The patient does have occasional diarrhea and headaches. She smokes approximately 5-10 cigarettes a day and drinks socially. The physician performs a detailed examination. The medical decision making is noted to be of a moderate complexity.

A. 99203, R10.31
B. 99213, R10.32, R50.9
C. 99214, R10.31, R50.9
D. 99221, R10.33, R50.9

108. A neurological consultation in the emergency department of the local hospital is requested by the ED physician for a 25-year-old male with suspected closed head trauma. The neurologist saw the patient in the ED. The patient had a loss of consciousness this morning after receiving a blow to the head in a basketball game. He presents to the emergency department with a headache, dizziness, and confusion. During the course of the history, the patient relates that he has been very irritable, confused, and has had a bit of nausea since the incident. All other systems reviewed and are negative: Constitutional, ophthalmologic, otolaryngologic, cardiovascular, respiratory, genitourinary, musculoskeletal, integumentary, psychiatric, endocrine, hematologic, lymphatic, allergic, and immunologic. The patient states that he does have a history of headaches and that both parents have hypertension, also a grandfather with heart disease. He also states that he does drink beer on the weekends and does not smoke. Physical examination reveals the patient to be unsteady and exhibiting difficulty in concentration when stating months in reverse. The pupils dilate unequally (anisocoria). The physician

continues with a complete comprehensive examination involving an extensive review of neurological function. The neurologist orders a stat CT and MRI. The physician suspects a subdural hematoma or an epidural hematoma and the medical decision-making complexity is high. The neurologist admits the patient to the hospital. Assign codes for the neurologist's services only.

A. 99285, R41.82, R42, R51, W22.8XXA, Y93.67
B. 99253, R51, R41.82, R42, W22.8XXA, Y93.67
C. 99255, H57.02, R51, R41.0, R42, W22.8XXA, Y93.67
D. 99245, R51, R41.82, R42, W22.8XXA, Y93.67

109. Dr. Stephanopolis makes subsequent hospital visits to Salanda Ortez, who has been in the hospital for primary viral pneumonia. She was experiencing severe dyspnea, rales, fever, and chest pain for over a week. The patient states that this morning she had nausea and her heart was racing while she was experiencing some dyspnea and SOB. The chest radiography showed patchy bilateral infiltrates and basilar streaking. Sputum microbiology was positive for a secondary bacterial pneumonia. An expanded problem-focused physical examination was performed. The medical decision making complexity was moderate. The patient was given intravenous antibiotic as treatment for the bacterial pneumonia.

A. 99233, R06.02, R50.9, R07.9
B. 99232, J15.9, J12.9
C. 99221, R06.02, R50.9, R07.9
D. 99234, J15.8

110. An obstetrician is requested by Dr. A to provide an office consultation to a 23-year-old female with first-trimester bleeding. The patient presents with a history of brownish discharge and occasional pinkish discharge. During the history, the patient relates that she has had suprapubic pain in the past week and cramping. She states her pain is 8/10. She has felt nausea and has vomited on three occasions. On one occasion, the nausea was accompanied by dizziness and vertigo. All other systems are negative at this time and included: Constitutional factors, ophthalmologic, otolaryngologic, cardiovascular, respiratory, musculoskeletal, integumentary, neurologic, psychiatric, endocrine, hematologic, lymphatic, allergic, and immunologic. The PFSH included patient history of tonsillectomy with family history of breast cancer on her mother's side. The patient does not smoke or drink. The physician conducts a comprehensive examination focused on the chief complaint and related systems. The uterus is found to be soft and involuted. There is cervical motion tenderness and significant abdominal tenderness on palpation. A left pelvic mass is palpated in the left quadrant. The physician orders a pelvic ultrasound, a complete CBC, and differential. Considering the range of possible diagnoses, the medical decision-making complexity is high.

A. 99255, O03.4, R19.00
B. 99242, O20.0, R19.00
C. 99245, O20.9, R19.04
D. 99245, O46.90, R19.04

111. Dr. Martin admits a 65-year-old female patient to the hospital to rule out acute pericarditis following a severe viral infection. The patient has complained of retrosternal, sharp, intermittent pain of 2 days' duration that is reduced by sitting up and leaning forward, accompanied by tachypnea. ROS: She does not currently have chest pain but is complaining of shortness of breath. She states that her legs and feet have been swollen of late. She reports no change in her vision or her hearing, and she has not had a rash. No dyspnea stated. PFSH: She states that she has had an echocardiogram in the past when she complained of chest tightness and her family physician gave her some medication, but she is not certain what it was. She has three adult children, all healthy. Her husband is deceased. She does not smoke or consume alcohol. Her father died at age 69 from congestive heart failure, and her mother died of influenza at 70. Refer to the admission form for a list of current medications. The examination was detailed. The medical decision making was of high complexity.
A. 99236, R07.2, R06.82, R06.02
B. 99223, I30.9, I50.9
C. 99245, I30.9, I50.9
D. 99221, R07.2, R06.82, R06.02

112. A 57-year-old male was sent by his family physician to a urologist for an office consultation due to hematuria. The patient has had bright red blood in his urine sporadically for the past 3 weeks. His family physician gave him a dose of antibiotic therapy for urinary tract infection; however, the symptom still persists. The patient states that he does experience some lower back discomfort when urinating, with no fever, chills, or nausea. The patient is currently taking Lotrel 10/20 for his hypertension, which is stable at this time, and has allergies to Sulfa. The urologist performs a detailed history and physical examination. The urologist recommends a cystoscopy to be scheduled for the following day and discusses the procedure and risks with the patient. The urologist also contacted the family physician with the recommendations and is requested to proceed with the cystoscopy and any further follow-up required. The medical decision making is of moderate complexity. A report was sent to attending physician. Report only the office service.
A. 99243, R31.0, M54.5
B. 99244-57, 52000, R31.9, M54.5
C. 99253, R31.9, M54.5
D. 99221, R31.0, M54.5

113. A 56-year-old established male patient presents to his family physician for a preventive checkup at the local outpatient clinic. The physician conducts a multi-system history and physical examination, and the checkup takes 45 minutes.
A. 99214, Z02.71
B. 99403, Z02.1
C. 99386, Z00.00
D. 99396, Z00.00

Subject Area: Anesthesia

114. Which HCPCS modifier indicates an anesthesia service in which the anesthesiologist medically directs one CRNA?
A. QX
B. QY
C. QZ
D. QK

115. This is the anesthesia formula:
A. B + M + P
B. B + P + M
C. B + T + M
D. B + T + N

116. Anesthesia service for a pneumocentesis for lung aspiration, 32420.
A. 00522
B. 00500
C. 00520
D. 00524

117. If the anesthesia service were provided to a patient who had severe systemic disease, what would the physical status modifier be?
A. P1
B. P2
C. P3
D. P4

118. This type of anesthesia is also known as a nerve block.
A. Local
B. Epidural
C. Regional
D. MAC

119. The anesthesiologist provides anesthesia services for a kidney harvest from a living donor for transplant.
A. 00868
B. 01990
C. 00860
D. 00862

120. Anesthesia service includes the following care:
A. Preoperative, intraoperative
B. Preoperative, intraoperative, postoperative
C. Intraoperative, postoperative
D. Preoperative, postoperative

121. What qualifying circumstances code would be used to identify the administration of anesthesia that is complicated by an emergency condition?
A. 99100
B. 99116
C. 99135
D. 99140

122. **EXAMINATION OF:** Right hip.
DIAGNOSIS: Primary unilateral osteoarthritis right hip.
ONE-VIEW RIGHT HIP: A single frontal view is obtained of the right hip. No previous studies are available for comparison. Right hip arthroplasty is seen. Alignment appears grossly unremarkable on this single view. There are skin staples present. Air is seen in the soft tissues, likely due to recent surgery. There appear to be two drains present. The tip of one overlies the soft tissues superolateral to the greater trochanter. The second one is more inferior. The tip overlies the right proximal femoral prosthesis.
IMPRESSION: Single view of the right hip with findings consistent with recent right total hip arthroplasty.
A. 72100, M16
B. 73501-RT, M16.11
C. 72100-26, M16.1
D. 73501-26-RT, M16.11, Z96.641

123. **EXAMINATION OF:** Cervical spine.
CLINICAL SYMPTOMS: Herniated disc.
FINDINGS: A single spot fluoroscopic film from the operating room is submitted for interpretation. The cervical spine is not well demonstrated above the level of the inferior aspect of C6. There is a metallic surgical plate seen anterior to the cervical spine. The cephalic portion of the plate is at the level of C6 at its superior endplate. That extends in an inferior direction, presumably anterior to C7; however, there is not adequate visualization of C7 to confirm location. Density overlies the C6-7 intervertebral disc space, suggesting the presence of a bone plug in this area; however, again visualization is not adequate in this area. Further evaluation with plain radiographs is recommended.
A. 72100-26, M51.26
B. 72020-26, M50.20
C. 72100-52-26, M50.20
D. 72020-52-26, M51.26

124. This patient undergoes a gallbladder sonogram due to epigastric pain. The report indicates that the visualized portions of the liver are normal. No free fluid noted within Morison's pouch. The gallbladder is identified and is empty. No evidence of wall thickening or surrounding fluid is seen. There is no ductal dilatation. The common hepatic duct and common bile duct measure 0.4 and 0.8 cm, respectively. The common bile duct measurement is at the upper limits of normal.
A. 76700-26, R10.84
B. 76705-26, R10.13
C. 76775-26, R10.33
D. 76705, R10.84

125. **EXAMINATION OF:** Chest.
CLINICAL SYMPTOMS: Pneumonia.
PA AND LATERAL CHEST X-RAY.

CONCLUSION: Ventilation within the lung fields has improved compared with previous study.
A. 71046-26, J15.8
B. 71034, J15.8
C. 71046-26, J18.9
D. 71046, J18.9

126. **EXAMINATION OF:** Abdomen and pelvis.
CLINICAL SYMPTOMS: Ascites.
CT OF ABDOMEN AND PELVIS: Technique: CT of the abdomen and pelvis was performed without oral or IV contrast material per physician request. No previous CT scans for comparison.
FINDINGS: No ascites. Moderate-sized pleural effusion on the right.
A. 74160-26, R18.8
B. 74176-26, J90
C. 74150, J90
D. 74160, R18.8

127. Report the professional component of the following service: This 68-year-old male is seen in Radiation Oncology Department for prostate cancer. The oncologist performs a complex clinical treatment planning, approves a dosimetry calculation, manages a complex isodose plan, and orders treatment devices, which include blocks, special shields, and wedges. He also performs treatment management. The patient had 5 days of radiation treatments for 2 weeks, a total of 10 days of treatment.
A. 77263, 77300-26, 77315-26, 77334, C61
B. 77300, 77315, 77334, 77427 × 2, C61
C. 77263, 77300-26, 77315-26, 77334-26, 77427 × 2, C61
D. 77263, 77427 × 2, C61

128. This 69-year-old female is in for a magnetic resonance examination of the brain because of new seizure activity. After imaging without contrast, contrast was administered and further sequences were performed. Examination results indicated no apparent neoplasm or vascular malformation.
A. 70543-26, R56.00
B. 70543-26, R56.9
C. 70553-26, R56.9
D. 70553, G40.909

129. **EXAMINATION OF:** Brain.
CLINICAL FINDING: Acute onset, severe headache.
COMPUTED TOMOGRAPHY OF THE BRAIN was performed without contrast material.
FINDINGS: There is blood within the third ventricle. The lateral ventricles show mild dilatation with small amounts of blood.
IMPRESSION: Acute nontraumatic subarachnoid hemorrhage.
A. 70460-26, R51
B. 70250, R51
C. 70450-26, I60.9
D. 70450-26, R51

130. This patient is suffering from primary lung cancer and is in for a follow-up CT scan of the thorax with contrast material. Code the physician component only.
    A. 71250-26, C78.00
    B. 71260, C34.90
    C. 71260-26, C34.90
    D. 71270-26, D49.1

Subject Area: 80000 Pathology and Laboratory

131. This 69-year-old female presents to the laboratory after her physician ordered quantitative and qualitative assays for troponin to assist in the diagnosis of her chief complaint of acute onset of chest pain.
    A. 84484, 80299, R07.2
    B. 84512, 84484, 80299, R07.89
    C. 84484, 84512, R07.9
    D. 84484, 84512, R07.89

132. **Report the global service.**
    CLINICAL HISTORY: Mass, left atrium.
    SPECIMEN RECEIVED: Left atrium.
    GROSS DESCRIPTION: The specimen is labeled with patient's name and "left atrial myxoma" and consists of a 4 × 4 × 2-cm ovoid mass with a partially calcified hemorrhagic white-tan tissue.
    INTRAOPERATIVE FROZEN SECTION DIAGNOSIS: Myxoma
    MICROSCOPIC DESCRIPTION: Sections show a well-circumscribed mass consisting of fibromyxoid tissue showing numerous vascular channels. Areas of superficial ulceration and chronic inflammatory infiltrate are noted. Areas of calcification are also present.
    DIAGNOSIS: Myxoma, benign, left atrium.
    A. 88305, D49.89
    B. 88307-26, 88331-26, D15.1
    C. 88307, 88331-26, D15.1
    D. 88305, D15.1

133. This 34-year-old established female patient is in for her yearly physical and lab. The physician orders a comprehensive metabolic panel, hemogram automated and manual differential WBC count (CBC), and a thyroid-stimulating hormone. Code the lab only.
    A. 99395, 80050
    B. 80050-52
    C. 80069, 80050
    D. 80050

134. **CLINICAL HISTORY:** Necrotic soleus muscle, right leg.
    SPECIMEN RECEIVED: Soleus muscle, right leg.
    GROSS DESCRIPTION: Submitted in formalin, labeled with the patient's name and "soleus muscle right leg," are multiple irregular fragments of tan, gray, brown soft tissue measuring 8 × 8 × 2.5 cm in aggregate. Multiple representative fragments are submitted in four cassettes.
    MICROSCOPIC DESCRIPTION: The slides show multiple sections of skeletal muscle showing severe coagulative and liquefactive necrosis. Patchy neutrophilic infiltrates are present within the necrotic tissue.
    DIAGNOSIS: Soft tissue, soleus muscle, right leg debridement; necrosis and patchy acute inflammation, skeletal muscle—infective myositis.
    A. 88305-26, M60.003
    B. 88304-26, M60.61
    C. 88307-26, I96
    D. 88304-26, M62.561

135. This patient is in for a kidney biopsy (50200) because a mass was identified by ultrasound. The specimen is sent to pathology for gross and microscopic examination. Report the technical and professional components for this service. The results are pending.
    A. 88305-26, N28.89
    B. 88307-26, N28.9
    C. 88307, N28.89
    D. 88305, N28.89

136. This patient presented to the laboratory yesterday to have blood drawn for a creatine measurement. The results came back at higher than normal levels; therefore, the patient was asked to return to the laboratory today for a repeat creatine blood test before the nephrologist is consulted. Report the second day of test only.
    A. 82540 × 2, R79.89
    B. 82550, R79.89
    C. 82550, R94.4
    D. 82540, R79.89

137. Code a pregnancy test, urine.
    A. 84702
    B. 84703
    C. 81025
    D. 84702 × 2

138. This is a patient with atrial fibrillation who comes to the clinic laboratory routinely for a quantitative digoxin level. This test was performed today.
    A. 80101, 80102, I50.9
    B. 81001, Z51.81, Z79.899, I49.01
    C. 80162, Z51.81, Z79.899, I48.91
    D. 80162, I48.91

139. What CPT code would you use to report a bilirubin, total (transcutaneous)?
    A. 82252
    B. 82247
    C. 82248
    D. 88720

140. **CLINICAL HISTORY:** Boil, left groin.
    SPECIMEN RECEIVED: Necrotic fascia left groin and leg (anterior and posterior).
    GROSS DESCRIPTION: The specimen is labeled with the patient's name and "fascia left groin and leg" and consists of multiple segments of skin and soft tissue measuring up to 30 cm in greatest dimension. The skin is unremarkable, with the soft tissue being hemorrhagic and friable and foul smelling.

MICROSCOPIC DESCRIPTION: Sections of skin and soft tissue show coagulative necrosis with neutrophilic exudates.

DIAGNOSIS: Skin and soft tissue, left groin and leg, anterior and posterior showing coagulative necrosis and acute inflammation.
A. 88304, L02.92
B. 88305-26, I96
C. 88304-26, I96, L02.224
D. 88305, L03.314

Subject Area: 90000 Medicine

141. What CPT code would be used to code the technical aspect of an evaluation of swallowing by video recording using a flexible endoscope?
A. 92611
B. 92612
C. 92610
D. 92613

142. The patient presented for a spontaneous nystagmus test that included gaze, fixation, and recording and used vertical electrodes. Assign code(s) for the physician service only.
A. 92541
B. 92547
C. 92541, 92544, 92547
D. 92541, 92547

143. How would you report a screening hearing test in which no abnormalities are reported?
A. 92551, Z13.5
B. 92555, Z01.10
C. 92553, Z01.10
D. 92620, Z13.5

144. This 40-year-old patient who is a type II diabetic is seen in an inpatient setting for psychotherapy. The doctor spends 50 minutes face-to-face with the patient. The patient is seen for depression.
A. 90818, F32.9, E11.69
B. 90817, F32.9, E11.69
C. 90818, F32.9, E11.9
D. 90817, F32.9, E11.9

145. A patient presents for a pleural cavity chemotherapy session with 10 mg doxorubicin HCl that requires a thoracentesis to be performed.
A. 96446, J9000
B. 96440, 32421, J9000
C. 96440, J9000
D. 96446, 32421, J9000

146. What CPT code would be used to report a home visit to care for the mechanical ventilation of a respiratory patient?
A. 99503
B. 99504
C. 99505
D. 99509

147. Which code would be used to report an EEG (electroencephalogram) provided during carotid surgery?
A. 95816
B. 95819
C. 95822
D. 95955

148. **INDICATION:** Pulmonary hypertension secondary to newly diagnosed acute myocardial infarction.
PROCEDURE PERFORMED: Insertion of Swan-Ganz catheter.
DESCRIPTION OF PROCEDURE: The right internal jugular and subclavian area was prepped with antiseptic solution. Sterile drapes were applied. Under usual sterile precautions, the right internal jugular vein was cannulated. A 9-French introducer was inserted, and a 7-French Swan-Ganz catheter was inserted without difficulty. Right atrial pressures were 2 to 3, right ventricular pressures 24/0, and pulmonary artery 26/9 with a wedge pressure of 5. This is a Trendelenburg position. The patient tolerated the procedure well.
A. 93451, 93503-51, I21.9
B. 93454, I27.20
C. 93503, 93452, I27.20
D. 93503, I27.20, I21.9

149. **DIALYSIS INPATIENT NOTE:** This 24-year-old male patient is on continuous ambulatory peritoneal dialysis (CAPD) using 1.5% dialysate. He drains more than 600 mL. He is tolerating dialysis well. He continues to have some abdominal pain, but his abdomen is not distended. He has some diarrhea. His abdomen does not look like acute abdomen. His vitals, other than blood pressure in the 190s over 100s, are fine. He is afebrile.

At this time, I will continue with 1.5% dialysate. Because of diarrhea, I am going to check stool for white cells, culture. Next we will see what the primary physician says today. His HIDA scan was normal. The patient suffers from ESRD and has had 6 encounters this month. Code this service.
A. 90947, 90960, N18.6, R19.7, Z99.2
B. 90945, N18.6, R19.7, Z99.2
C. 90960, N18.6, Z99.2
D. 90945, N18.6

150. **DIAGNOSIS:** Atrial flutter.
PROCEDURE PERFORMED: Electrical cardioversion.
DESCRIPTION OF PROCEDURE: The patient was sedated with Versed and morphine. She was given a total of 5 mg of Versed. She was cardioverted with 50 joules into sinus tachycardia. The patient was given a 20-mg Cardizem IV push. Her heart rate went down to the 110s, and she was definitely in sinus tachycardia.
CONCLUSION: Successful electrical cardioversion of atrial flutter into sinus tachycardia.
A. 92961, I49.1
B. 92960, I48.92
C. 92960, 92973, I48.92
D. 92960, R00.0

Figure Credits

1-1 ©Elsevier Collection

1-2 ©Elsevier Collection

4-4 ©Elsevier Collection

7-3 From Kumar V, Abbas AK, Aster JC: *Robbins and Cotran Pathologic Basis of Disease*, ed 9, Philadelphia, 2015, Saunders.

8-3 ©Elsevier Collection

8-7 From Damjanov I: *Pathology for the Health Professions*, ed 5, St. Louis, 2017, Elsevier.

8-8 From Kissane JM, editor: *Anderson's Pathology*, ed 9, St. Louis, 1990, Mosby.

11-1 ©Elsevier Collection

11-2 From Canale ST, Beaty JH: *Campbell's Operative Orthopaedics*, ed 11, Philadelphia, 2008, Mosby.

11-3 From Patton KT, Thibodeau GA: *Anatomy & Physiology*, ed 8, St. Louis, 2013, Mosby.

13-2 From Yanoff M, Duker J, eds: *Ophthalmology*, ed 4, St. Louis, 2014, Saunders.

14-1 Courtesy U.S. Department of Health and Human Services, Centers for Medicare and Medicaid Services.

14-2 From *Federal Register*, January 17, 2017, Vol. 82, No 10, Rules and Regulations.

14-3 Courtesy U.S. Department of Health and Human Services, Centers for Medicare and Medicaid Services.

15-1 Courtesy U.S. Department of Health and Human Services, Centers for Medicare and Medicaid Services.

16-3 Courtesy U.S. Department of Health and Human Services, Centers for Medicare and Medicaid Services.

18-1 Courtesy U.S. Department of Health and Human Services, Centers for Medicare and Medicaid Services.

24-2 From Buck CJ: *2018 ICD-10-CM Hospital Professional Edition*, St. Louis, 2018, Elsevier.

24-3 From Buck CJ: *2018 ICD-10-CM Hospital Professional Edition*, St. Louis, 2018, Elsevier.

Part 5 Final Exam answer sheet Copyright © 2018, Elsevier Inc. All rights reserved.

Appendix A

Resources

The most current coding guidelines and code system updates are posted to the Evolve website at ***http://evolve.elsevier.com/Buck/physicianexam.***

Once registered for your free Evolve resources (using the access code provided on the inside front cover of this text), go to the ***Course Content*** section and click ***Resources*** to reference the following:

Exam Review

Exam Format A
Exam Format B

Mobile Quick Quizzes

Parts 1, 3, and 4

Coding Tips and Links

GEMs Files
ICD-10-CM Official Guidelines for Coding and Reporting

1995 Guidelines for E/M Services
1997 Documentation Guidelines for Evaluation and Management Services
CPT Updates
ICD-10-CM Updates
HCPCS Updates
Study Tips
Weblinks

Content Updates—Student

Some of the CPT code descriptions for physician services include physician extender services. Physician extenders, such as nurse practitioners, physician assistants, and nurse anesthetists, etc., provide medical services typically performed by a physician. Within this educational material the term "physician" may include "and other qualified health care professionals" depending on the code. Refer to the official CPT® code descriptions and guidelines to determine codes that are appropriate to report services provided by non-physician practitioners.

Appendix B

Answers

Chapter 1—Integumentary System

Anatomy and Terminology Quiz

1. c
2. d
3. a
4. b
5. d
6. c
7. d
8. b
9. c
10. c

Pathophysiology Quiz

1. c
2. c
3. a
4. d
5. b
6. c
7. d
8. b
9. d
10. a

Chapter 2—Musculoskeletal System

Anatomy and Terminology Quiz

1. b
2. c
3. a
4. c
5. a
6. d
7. b
8. d
9. a
10. c

Pathophysiology Quiz

1. d
2. c

3. b
4. a
5. d
6. d
7. a
8. c
9. b
10. d

Chapter 3—Respiratory System

Anatomy and Terminology Quiz

1. b
2. d
3. c
4. a
5. a
6. c
7. c
8. b
9. d
10. d

Pathophysiology Quiz

1. b
2. a
3. d
4. d
5. d
6. a
7. c
8. b
9. a
10. c

Chapter 4—Cardiovascular System

Anatomy and Terminology Quiz

1. d
2. a
3. c
4. a
5. d
6. b
7. d

8. a
9. d
10. d

Pathophysiology Quiz

1. b
2. c
3. c
4. c
5. d
6. a
7. c
8. c
9. a
10. d

Chapter 5—Female Genital System and Pregnancy

Anatomy and Terminology Quiz

1. d
2. a
3. a
4. b
5. c
6. a
7. b
8. b
9. c
10. d

Pathophysiology Quiz

1. b
2. d
3. a
4. c
5. b
6. a
7. a
8. c
9. b
10. c

Chapter 6—Male Genital System

Anatomy and Terminology Quiz

1. c
2. a
3. d
4. b
5. a
6. a
7. a
8. d
9. d
10. b

Pathophysiology Quiz

1. a
2. b
3. d
4. a
5. c
6. b
7. d
8. b
9. a
10. b

Chapter 7—Urinary System

Anatomy and Terminology Quiz

1. c
2. d
3. a
4. c
5. b
6. d
7. c
8. b
9. d
10. a

Pathophysiology Quiz

1. c
2. d
3. d
4. c
5. b
6. c
7. a or c
8. c
9. b
10. c

Chapter 8—Digestive System

Anatomy and Terminology Quiz

1. b
2. d
3. d
4. b
5. c
6. b
7. a
8. c
9. a
10. b

Pathophysiology Quiz

1. c
2. a
3. d

4. b
5. a
6. c
7. a
8. c
9. a
10. a

Chapter 9—Mediastinum and Diaphragm

Anatomy and Terminology Quiz

1. a
2. b
3. d
4. c
5. c
6. b
7. a
8. b
9. a
10. d

Chapter 10—Hemic and Lymphatic System

Anatomy and Terminology Quiz

1. b
2. d
3. a
4. d
5. c
6. c
7. a
8. d
9. b
10. d

Pathophysiology Quiz

1. c
2. a
3. b
4. d
5. b
6. b
7. a
8. a
9. c
10. b

Chapter 11—Endocrine System

Anatomy and Terminology Quiz

1. c
2. d
3. b
4. a

5. d
6. a
7. d
8. a
9. b
10. d

Pathophysiology Quiz

1. a
2. b
3. c
4. a
5. d
6. b
7. a
8. d
9. a
10. c

Chapter 12—Nervous System

Anatomy and Terminology Quiz

1. b
2. a
3. a
4. b
5. b
6. c
7. a
8. d
9. b
10. a

Pathophysiology Quiz

1. a
2. c
3. b
4. d
5. a
6. b
7. a
8. b
9. b
10. c

Chapter 13—Senses

Anatomy and Terminology Quiz

1. d
2. d
3. a
4. a
5. a
6. b
7. c
8. b

9. d
10. a

Pathophysiology Quiz

1. d
2. b
3. c
4. a
5. b
6. a
7. a
8. a
9. b
10. b

PART 2 QUIZ ANSWERS

Chapter 14—Reimbursement Issues

Reimbursement Quiz

1. b
2. a
3. c
4. b
5. d
6. a
7. a
8. b
9. d
10. b

PART 3 PRACTICE EXERCISE ANSWERS AND RATIONALES

Chapter 16—Evaluation and Management (E/M) Section

Practice Exercise 16.1

Professional Service: 99232 (Evaluation and Management, Hospital)

ICD-10-CM: N17.9 (Failure, renal, acute), **I12.9** (Hypertension, kidney, with stage I through stage IV chronic kidney disease), **N18.9** (Failure, renal, chronic), **E86.9** (Depletion, volume NOS), **I73.9** (Disease, peripheral, vascular [occlusive])

Rationale: The service in this inpatient progress note is reported with 99232 because it describes an expanded problem-focused history and examination. The patient has two stable chronic conditions (hypertension and peripheral vascular disease) and acute-on-chronic renal failure that is improving; therefore, the medical decision making is of moderate complexity.

The patient has acute renal failure (N17.9) and chronic renal failure (N18.9), but according to ICD-10-CM Section I.C.9.a.2 of the *Official Guidelines for Coding and Reporting*, the coder is to assign a code from the I12 category to report hypertensive kidney disease, when a hypertensive patient has a condition that is classifiable to N18. You are to assume a cause-and-effect relationship and classify the chronic renal failure with hypertension as hypertensive renal disease (I12.9 and N18.9). The acute renal failure category N17 is not included in the Guideline to assume a cause-and-effect relationship. The acute renal failure would be reported because when you reference the Excludes note following I12, the coder is directed to assign N17.x for acute renal failure. Note that according to ICD-10-CM, Section I.B.8. of the Guidelines, when there is both an acute and chronic condition present, the acute condition is reported first.

The patient also has volume depletion (E86.9), which is reported because the condition contributes to the patient's renal status. The peripheral vascular disease (I73.9) is reported because it was important enough for the physician to mention it in the impression section of the report.

Practice Exercise 16.2

Professional Service: 99214 (Evaluation and Management, Office and Other Outpatient)

ICD-10-CM: A08.4 (Gastroenteritis, viral NEC)

Rationale: Code 99214 reports an office visit for an established patient. The note is titled as a follow-up clinic visit. The patient is established with this provider. The history is expanded problem focused and the examination is detailed. The medical decision making is moderate because there are possibly two new problems—gastroenteritis and possible otitis media. Prescription drugs were given—making this a moderate medical decision making. Only two components of history, exam, and medical decision making are required for an established visit.

The diagnosis is viral gastroenteritis reported with A08.4, and because the otitis media was stated as possible, that diagnosis would not be reported.

Practice Exercise 16.3

Professional Service: 99284 (Evaluation and Management Emergency Department)

ICD-10-CM: R11.2 (Vomiting, with nausea), **E86.0** (Dehydration), **C15.9** (Neoplasm, esophagus, Malignant Primary), **C79.51** (Neoplasm, bones, Malignant Secondary), **C78.89** (Neoplasm, stomach, Malignant Secondary)

Rationale: This was a level 4 emergency department service and included a detailed history, comprehensive examination, and moderate decision making level of complexity.

The first-listed diagnosis is the primary reason the patient presented to the emergency department—vomiting and nausea, reported with R11.2. The dehydration was noted in the assessment and was treated and would be reported with E86.0. The underlying condition that is causing these symptoms is the primary malignant neoplasm of the esophagus and is reported with C15.9. She has severe pain due to the metastases being treated with morphine. Assign the codes for these conditions because they were treated. Metastases included bones (C79.51) and stomach (C78.89).

Practice Exercise 16.4

Professional Service: 99391 (Preventive Medicine, Established Patient)

ICD-10-CM: Z00.129 (Examination, child [over 28 days old])

Rationale: This is a routine checkup for an established infant and is considered preventive medicine. When choosing a code from this category, the age of the infant or child and whether the patient is new or established determines the code choice. Code 99391 is assigned for a newborn until 1 year of age.

The diagnosis is a routine health check reported with Z00.129. Note the slightly different terms to locate the correct code. If the infant were seen for a routine health check with abnormal findings or a specific complaint, then report Z00.121 followed by the appropriate code(s) for the abnormal findings.

Practice Exercise 16.5

Professional Service: 99469 (Critical Care Services, Neonatal, Subsequent)

ICD-10-CM: P07.17 (Low birth weight, 1750-1999 grams), **P07.31** (Preterm infant, newborn, with gestation of, 28-31 weeks), **P22.0** (Hyaline, membrane), **P59.9** (Jaundice, newborn), **Q25.0** (Patent ductus arteriosus or Botallo)

Rationale: When a critically ill newborn 30 days of age or less is either born or brought to the hospital and placed in the Neonatal Critical Care Unit, the initial care day is coded with 99468; each additional day is coded with 99469, as long as the baby is considered critically ill.

The diagnosis is preterm infant with a body weight of 1716 kg. Code P07.17 reports the low birth weight between 1750-1999 grams. The preterm gestation is reported with P07.31. The hyaline membrane is reported P22.0. Referencing hyperbilirubinemia of neonate directs the coder to "*see* Jaundice, newborn." The report does not state that the jaundice is due to preterm delivery (P59.0); therefore, the jaundice is reported with code P59.9. This patient also has patent ductus arteriosus (Q25.0). There is mention of some type of pulmonary valve disorder which could be associated with Noonan syndrome; however, that has not been verified and we do not know what the pulmonary valve disorder is.

Chapter 17—Anesthesia Section

Practice Exercise 17.1

Professional Service: 00840-QK-P2 (Anesthesia, Abdomen, Intraperitoneal), **99100** (Anesthesia, Special Circumstances, Extreme Age)

Rationale: The surgical procedure is an abdominal procedure in which the anesthesia is reported with 00840.

HCPCS modifier -QK indicates the anesthesiologist was medically directing two to four concurrent cases. 99100 is added to indicate age over 70, which is a qualifying circumstance that may impact the anesthesia service. -P2 indicates a patient with a mild systemic disease (hypertension).

Practice Exercise 17.2

Professional Service: 00400-AA-QS-P1 (Anesthesia, Integumentary System, Anterior Trunk)

Rationale: The service is an anesthesia service for a procedure to the breast reported with 00400. -AA indicates that the anesthesiologist personally performed the anesthesia service. -P1 indicates a normal healthy patient. This was a monitored anesthesia case (MAC) as noted by modifier -QS.

Practice Exercise 17.3

Professional Service: 00790-QK-P2 (Anesthesia, Abdomen, Intraperitoneal)

Rationale: The service is an abdominal anesthesia service for a procedure of the upper abdomen, reported with 00790. Modifier -QK is added to indicate the anesthesiologist was supervising more than one procedure at the same time. -P2 indicates a patient with a mild systemic disease.

Practice Exercise 17.4

Professional Service: 00902-AA-P3 (Anesthesia, Anus)

Rationale: The service is anesthesia for a procedure of the anus in which a spinal was administered and reported with 00902. -AA indicates that the anesthesiologist personally performed the anesthesia service.

Practice Exercise 17.5

Professional Service: 00211-AA-P5 (Anesthesia, Brain)

Rationale: The service was anesthesia for an intercranial hematoma reported with 00211. -AA indicates that the anesthesiologist personally performed the anesthesia service. -P5 indicates that the patient is not expected to survive without this procedure.

Chapter 18—CPT/HCPCS Level I Modifiers

Practice Exercise 18.1

Professional Service: 49060-78-52 (Drainage, Abscess, Retroperitoneal), **11005-78-51** (Debridement, Skin, Subcutaneous Tissue, Infected)

ICD-10-CM: T81.4XXD (Infection, postoperative wound), **K65.4** (Necrosis, fat, peritoneum), **I96** (Necrosis, skin or subcutaneous tissue), **K63.2** (Fistula, abdominal wall)

Rationale: The primary procedure was drainage of an abdominal abscess reported with 49060. Modifier -78 is added to indicate an unplanned return to the operating room. Modifier -52 (reduced services) is added to indicate that the abdomen was already open and it was packed and left open. This patient had debridement (11005) of an abdominal wound, which was necrotic. Modifier -51 is added to 11005 to indicate multiple procedures were performed. Modifier -78 is also added.

This is a life-threatening condition that required extensive debridement of the skin, fat, and the area behind the abdominal contents. The diagnoses codes are: T81.4XXD reports the postoperative wound infection, K65.4 reports fat necrosis of abdominal wall, I96 reports the necrosis of the skin, and K63.2 reports the fistula of the abdominal wall between the abdominal cavity and the retroperitoneal area. The ICD-10-CM complication code (T81.4XXD) includes the seventh character of "D," indicating a subsequent encounter.

Practice Exercise 18.2

Professional Service: 11404-58 (Excision, Skin, Lesion, Benign)

ICD-10-CM: D23.61 (Neoplasm, skin, arm, Benign)

Rationale: The procedure was re-excision of a benign lesion that measured 1 cm in diameter; the original procedure had 0.5-cm margins. This left a 2-cm incision that the surgeon now re-excised with a 1-cm margin. The total measurement for the re-excision is 4 cm. Modifier -58 is added to indicate that the patient was returned to the operating room during the postoperative period of the first procedure in part two of a two-part procedure.

The pathology report states fibrosis and granulation tissue, and there was no evidence of the Spitz nevus. In cases such as this, when there is excision of additional skin margins, it is acceptable to report the original diagnosis, which in this case is the Spitz nevus, a benign lesion, and reported with D23.61.

Practice Exercise 18.3

Professional Service: 93306-26 (Echocardiography, Transthoracic)

ICD-10-CM: I07.1 (Insufficiency, tricuspid), **I48.91** (Fibrillation, atrial or auricular [established]), **I51.9** (Dysfunction, ventricular)

Rationale: This patient had an echocardiogram and the key to correctly reporting an echocardiogram is to identify whether it was performed transthoracic or transesophageal, and if it was a complete study or follow-up/limited study. The service in this case was a two-dimensional with M-mode recording complete echo—93306 for the real-time image and documentation. Code 93306 includes spectral and color flow Doppler; therefore, 93320 and 93325 are not reported separately. You would add modifier -26 because you are reporting only the physician portion of the procedure.

The patient has valvular disease, and the report indicates the specific type of valvular disease. In this case, tricuspid insufficiency (I07.1), atrial fibrillation (I48.91), and ventricular dysfunction (I51.9).

Practice Exercise 18.4

Professional Service: 99214-24 (Evaluation and Management, Office and Other Outpatient)

ICD-10-CM: O34.32 (Pregnancy, complicated by, incompetent, cervix), **Z87.51** (History personal [of], obstetric complications, pre-term labor)

Rationale: This is an office visit service in which a decision was made to proceed with surgery. Modifier -57 is not assigned as the global period for 59320 (Cerclage, Cervix, Vaginal) has a 0-day global period. Use modifier -24 to indicate that this service is totally separate from the obstetric global package for a complication of the pregnancy. The examination includes a detailed history and examination, together with medical decision making complexity of a moderate level, reported with 99214.

The diagnosis is incompetent cervix, which is an abnormal cervix with a tendency to dilate prematurely in one who is pregnant, reported with O34.32. Note that ICD-10-CM includes the trimester, which was determined based on the opening statement that patient is 19 weeks 3 days gestation (second trimester). The history of pre-term labor was a factor in the decision to proceed, code Z87.51 is also reported.

Practice Exercise 18.5

Professional Service: 30520 (Septoplasty), **31267-51-50** (Antrostomy, Sinus, Maxillary), **31288-51-50** (Sphenoidotomy, Excision with Nasal/Sinus Endoscopy), **31255-51-50** (Ethmoidectomy, Endoscopic), **30930-51-50** (Turbinate, Fracture, Therapeutic)

ICD-10-CM: J34.2 (Deviation, septum), **J33.9** (Polyp, nasal), **J33.8** (Polyp, sinus), **J32.4** (Pansinusitis), **J34.3** (Hypertrophy, nasal, turbine)

Rationale: The services are listed in the Procedures Performed section of the report and are supported within the body of the report as: (1) bilateral endoscopic total ethmoidectomy, 31255-50-51; (2) bilateral endoscopic maxillary antrostomy with removal of polyps from maxillary sinus, 31267-50-51; (3) bilateral endoscopic sphenoidotomy, 31288-50-51; (4) septoplasty, 30520; and (5) bilateral inferior turbinate outfracture, 30930-50-51. Note that all procedures except the primary procedure, septoplasty, have modifier -50 to indicate bilateral procedures and modifier -51 to indicate multiple procedures.

The diagnoses are listed in the Postoperative Diagnosis section of the report as: (1) septal deviation, J34.2; (2) bilateral sinonasal polyposis, J33.9 (nasal) and (3) J33.8 (sinus); (4) pansinusitis, J32.4, (5) bilateral inferior turbinate hypertrophy, J34.3; and nasal obstruction. The nasal obstruction is not reported because it is caused by the septal deviation.

Chapter 19—Surgery Section

Practice Exercise 19.1

Professional Service: 11312 (Lesion, Skin, Shaving)

ICD-10-CM: D23.39 (Neoplasm, skin, cheek, Benign)

Rationale: The procedure is a shave excision of a lesion on the cheek that measures 1.6 cm. When reporting lesion removal, first identify the technique used. Shaving involves transverse incision or horizontal slicing and does not involve a full-thickness (through the dermis) excision. The excision codes involve full-thickness excision and generally require suture closure. Also identify the body area on which the lesion is located, the size of the lesion, and whether the lesion is benign or malignant. Note that in the case of shavings, the nature (benign or malignant) does not influence the selection of the CPT code.

In this case, the lesion shaved was benign, as indicated by the pathology report and reported with D23.39.

Practice Exercise 19.2

Professional Service: 19120-RT (Breast, Excision, Lesion)
 ICD-10-CM: C50.011 (Neoplasm, breast, female, nipple, Malignant Primary)
 Rationale: This patient presents for excision of a tumor of the right breast (19120-RT). The tumor is submitted for frozen section, which is an analysis performed by the pathologist during the procedure (intraoperatively).

The results of the frozen section were carcinoma of the right breast nipple (C50.011).

Practice Exercise 19.3

Professional Service: 15574-F7 (Pedicle Flap, Formation), **15120-51** (Split, Grafts)
 ICD-10-CM: S68.622A (Amputation, traumatic, finger, transphalangeal, partial, middle), **W31.9XXA** (External Cause Index, Contact with, machinery)
 Rationale: While working on machinery, this patient amputated the tip of her middle finger. A flap was formed from the ulnar aspect of the hand to place over the defect of the right middle finger (15574-F7). Modifier -F7 indicates the middle finger of the right hand. The split-thickness graft is reported with 15120 with modifier -51.

The diagnosis is traumatic amputation of the finger reported with S68.622A. Note that the ICD-10-CM code descriptions specify a traumatic, partial (tip) amputation of each specific finger of the right and left hand. The external cause code W31.9xxA is reported to indicate the injury was sustained while working on machinery. The seventh character "A" indicates the initial encounter for the injury.

Practice Exercise 19.4

Professional Service: 12002-F7 (Closure)
 ICD-10-CM: S61.212A (Laceration, finger[s], middle, right), **W45.8XXA** (External Cause Index, Contact [accidental] with, arrow, not thrown, projected or falling)
 Rationale: The patient presents with multiple lacerations of the finger that total 6 cm for which simple repair is performed (12002). Modifier -F7 is added to indicate the middle right finger.

Code S61.212A reports a laceration of the right finger. S61.212A reports the specific finger and laterality (side) and includes the seventh character of "A," to indicate the initial encounter. An external cause code (W45.8XXA) is reported to indicate how the finger was injured (due to arrow).

Practice Exercise 19.5

Professional Service: 11005-58 (Debridement, Skin, Subcutaneous Tissue, Infected)
 ICD-10-CM: K65.4 (Necrosis, fat, abdominal wall), **I96** (Necrosis, skin or subcutaneous tissue NEC), **T81.83XD** (Fistula, postoperative, persistent)
 Rationale: The patient returns to the operating room for additional debridement of the abdominal wound (11005). Modifier -58 indicates returning to the operating room for a related procedure by the same physician during the postoperative period.

The diagnoses are necrosis of the abdominal wall fat (K65.4), necrosis of the skin/subcutaneous tissue (I96), and postoperative fistula (T81.83XD). The complication code (T81.83XD) includes the seventh character of "D," indicating a subsequent encounter.

Practice Exercise 19.6

Professional Service: 20610-LT (Injection, Joint)
 ICD-10-CM: M75.52 (Bursitis, shoulder)
 Rationale: This is an injection into the shoulder without guidance, which is considered a major joint. The main code 20600 states arthrocentesis, aspiration, and/or injection small joint. This was an injection, so the area is correct, but the small joints are listed in parentheses after 20600 as fingers and toes. The indented codes that follow 20600 indicate shoulder, as included in 20610.

In the ICD-10-CM Index, under bursitis, subacromial instructs the coder to *see* bursitis, shoulder. There is no specific reporting for the different structures within the shoulder. Report code M75.52, which is bursitis of the left shoulder.

Practice Exercise 19.7

Professional Service: 29898-RT (Arthroscopy, Surgical, Ankle)
 ICD-10-CM: M19.071 (Osteoarthritis, ankle), **M25.771** (Osteophyte, ankle), **M79.9** (Disorder, soft tissue, ankle)
 Rationale: The service is an arthroplasty of the right ankle by means of a scope, not an open surgical procedure as would be reported with 27700-27703. The arthroscopic procedures are located in the Endoscopy/Arthroscopy category of codes (29800-29999). When locating the service in the index of the CPT, the main term *Arthroplasty* directs the coder to the incisional procedures. The main term *Arthroscopy* directs the coder to the correct surgical and diagnostic arthroscopic procedure codes. Codes 29894-29898 are the correct range, and the code to report the services in this case is 29898, with modifier -RT to indicate right.

The first diagnosis in the Postoperative Diagnoses section of the report is osteoarthritic change of the ankle. ICD-10-CM code M19.071 includes the sixth character "1," indicating right side.

The second postoperative diagnosis is osteophytic spurring. In ICD-10-CM reference in the Index, Osteophyte, ankle M25.77-. The sixth character "1" indicates the right side.

The third postoperative diagnosis is impinging soft tissue, but when referencing the Index of the ICD-10-CM, the only entry under impingement is of the soft tissue between the teeth. With no more specific entry, the coder would reference a general term, such as "Disorder, soft tissue." In ICD-10-CM, referencing "Disorder, soft tissue, ankle" leads to code M79.9.

Practice Exercise 19.8

Professional Service: 25210-LT (Carpal Bone, Excision), **25310-51-LT** (Tendon, Transfer, Wrist)

ICD-10-CM: M18.12 (Osteoarthritis, primary, hand joint, first carpometacarpal joint)

Rationale: This is an arthroplasty of the patient's carpometacarpal joint. The trapezium, one of the carpal bones, was removed in pieces (25210). The flexor carpi radialis (FCR) tendon was transferred to the site and threaded through bone. This was harvested through two incisions at the distal wrist and in the forearm. The report states that the underlying FCR tendon was preserved and later it was cut at the floor of the thumb and transferred through the hole at the base of the first metatarsal and pinned to the second metatarsal (25310). The report is difficult to read because it appears that the "harvested" FCR is removed; however, it is just separated and the proximal end was left intact. Code 25447 involves the insertion of a prosthesis; therefore, it is not correct. Modifier -LT is appended to both procedures to indicate the procedure was performed on the left wrist. Modifier -51 indicates 25210 is a second procedure during the same session.

The patient has degenerative arthritis. For ICD-10-CM the coder is directed to "see osteoarthritis." Code M18.12 reports localized osteoarthritis, as indicated by the reporting of the specific joint, carpometacarpal (hand).

Practice Exercise 19.9

Professional Service: 27355-RT (Excision, Cyst, Femur)

ICD-10-CM: D16.21 (Neoplasm, bone, femur, right side, Benign)

Rationale: This is an excision of a bone tumor of the femur. You would not use code 27328 because this code reports a procedure of the muscle of the thigh, and the tumor in this case was in the bone, reported with 27355, with -RT to indicate the right leg.

The diagnosis is a benign neoplasm (per the pathology report) of the long bone (D16.21). The femur, or thigh bone, is the longest bone in the leg. It would not be correct to report D16.31 because this is for the short bones of the leg, such as the tibia or fibula.

Practice Exercise 19.10

Professional Service: 27327-LT (Excision, Tumor, Knee)

ICD-10-CM: D21.22 (Neoplasm, connective tissue, knee, Benign)

Rationale: This mass is in the subcutaneous tissue of the patient's knee, reported with 27327, with -LT added to

indicate left side. You would not use code 27328 because this code is for deeper than subcutaneous.

The pathology report indicated a benign mass of the bursa, and when referencing "Neoplasm" in the Index of the ICD-10-CM, subterm *bursa,* the coder is directed to the subterm *connective tissue.* D21.22 reports a benign tumor of the connective tissue of the knee. The fifth character of "2" designates the left knee.

Practice Exercise 19.11

Professional Service: 36217-RT (Insertion, Catheter, Brachiocephalic Artery), **36216-59-LT** (Insertion, Catheter, Brachiocephalic Artery), **36215-59-LT** (Insertion, Catheter, Brachiocephalic Artery)

ICD-10-CM: I61.1 (Hemorrhage, intracranial [nontraumatic], intracerebral, hemisphere, cortical [superficial])

Rationale: You were given instructions to assign the codes for the catheterizations only. When reporting catheterizations of the carotid and peripheral arteries, carotids in this case, you need to know where the catheter tip is being placed. The arteries are listed by family and by order—the deeper the vessel, the higher the order. In this case, the third-order vessel is reported first (right internal carotid artery), the second-order vessel is reported second (left vertebral artery), and the first-order vessel (left common carotid artery) is reported last. Modifier -59 is added to 36215 and 36216 to indicate the catheterizations are in different families than 36217. Modifiers -RT and -LT indicate right or left vessels.

The procedure is being performed because the patient has an intracranial hemorrhage, reported with I61.1. The temporal lobe is a cerebral lobe which is noted under I61.1 in the ICD-10-CM Tabular; therefore, the reference in the Index is Hemorrhage, intracranial, intracerebral, hemisphere, cortical, I61.1.

Practice Exercise 19.12

Professional Service: 36580 (Vein, Catheterization, Replacement)

ICD-10-CM: Z49.01 (Preparatory care for subsequent treatment NEC, for dialysis), **N18.6** (Disease, renal, end stage [ESRD])

Rationale: The service is a venous catheter replacement by means of a percutaneous approach reported with 36580.

In ICD-10-CM, first locate dependence on dialysis and then reference the notes in the Tabular under Z99.2, Excludes to locate the adjustment code Z49.01. The code description for Z49.01 includes removal or replacement of the dialysis catheter. This is also found in the Index under "Preparatory care for subsequent treatment NEC, for dialysis." The diagnosis is stated as end-stage renal failure and reported with N18.6.

Practice Exercise 19.13

Professional Service: 36558 (Insertion, Catheter, Venous), **77001-26** (Fluoroscopy, Venous Access Device), **99152, 99153** (Sedation, Moderate)

ICD-10-CM: C34.90 (Neoplasm, lung, lobe NEC, Malignant Primary)

Rationale: The service was the placement of a Port-a-Cath, which is a catheter that is inserted into a large central vein, such as the jugular in this case, with a pump attached to the other end of the catheter. The small pump (about the size of three silver dollars stacked) is a port or reservoir implanted under the skin. The pump is used to infuse various substances by means of a reservoir. The substance is infused over time. In this case, the pump is being used for chemotherapy administration, and the insertion is reported with 36558. Codes 36555 and 36556 report temporary pump or port placement, 36557 and 36558 report a port or pump that is level with the skin by placing it under the skin. Codes 36560 and 36561 report ports or pumps that extend outside the skin and are not often used.

The physician fluoroscopic guidance service is reported with 77001. Modifier -26 is added to indicate that only the professional component of the service is being provided. Conscious sedation was provided as indicated in the report and was assigned code 99144 (30 minutes) and 99145 (15 minutes) because the patient was over age 5 and the sedation lasted 45 minutes.

The diagnosis is stated as primary lung cancer, reported with C34.90.

Practice Exercise 19.14

Professional Service: 36217-RT (Catheterization, Thoracic Artery), **36218-RT** (Catheterization, Thoracic Artery), **36215-51-LT** (Catheterization, Thoracic Artery)
  ICD-10-CM: I65.23 (Occlusion, artery, carotid)
  Rationale: 36200 (Insertion, Catheter, Aorta) is bundled into 36217-RT (Catheterization, Thoracic Artery), which reports the selective catheterization of the RT vertebral artery. 36218-RT (Catheterization, Thoracic Artery) reports the selective catheterization of the right common carotid artery, which is a second order; therefore, the add-on code is assigned for the additional second or third order in the same family.

36215-51-LT (Catheterization, Thoracic Artery) reports the selective catheterization of the left carotid artery. Modifier -51 is placed to indicate an additional procedure.

The Clinical Symptoms section of the report indicates carotid artery stenosis, and the Impression statement in the third item (30-40% diameter narrowing of the carotid bulb on right) and the fourth item (complete occlusion of the left internal carotid artery) support stenosis of the carotid artery, reported with I65.23. Further, ICD-10-CM 5th character of "3" indicates both carotid arteries have stenosis/occlusion.

Practice Exercise 19.15

Professional Service: 36247-RT (Catheterization, Legs), **37211** (Transcatheter Therapy, Infusion), **75710-59-26-RT** (Angiography, Leg Artery)
  ICD-10-CM: T82.392A (Complication, extremity artery [bypass] graft, mechanical, obstruction, femoral artery), **I74.3** (Thrombosis, thrombotic, leg, arterial)
  Rationale: The service is a selective catheter placement of the arterial system of the second order for a diagnostic right

extremity angiogram (36246-RT, 75710-59-26-RT) followed by catheter placement for infusion of tissue plasminogen activator (tPA). The catheters are placed in the common femoral through the Gore-Tex graft (36247) to below the knee. A coaxial system is one in which catheters are placed into the vessel on each side of the clot to release tPA to dissolve/lyse the clot. 36247 replaces 36246 as it is the highest order. The tPA is a thrombolytic drug used for arterial thrombotic occlusion. The infusion (37211) has a radiology component included. Modifier -59 is required on the diagnostic extremity angiogram to indicate that it was completely separate from the thrombolytic procedure. The patient returns in the morning so that the interventional radiologist can determine the extent to which the procedure was successful.

The reason for the service is a complication due to a Gore-Tex graft that is reported with T82.392A. Note that ICD-10-CM code includes seventh character "A" to indicate the first encounter for this condition. The patient has a complete occlusion of the peripheral artery of the lower extremity, reported with I74.3.

Practice Exercise 19.16

Professional Service: 43752 (Placement, Orogastric Tube)
  ICD-10-CM: K31.84 (Gastroparesis)
  Rationale: The service is placement of an orogastric tube (43752), known as CORFLO placement. The tube is placed to ensure that the patient receives proper nutrition. The KUB (kidneys, ureter, bladder) would be reported separately by the radiologist.

The patient has gastroparesis (K31.84).

Practice Exercise 19.17

Professional Service: 49440 (Gastrostomy Tube, Placement, Percutaneous, Nonendoscopic), **49446-51** (Gastrostomy Tube, Conversion to Gastrojejunostomy Tube), **76942-26** (Ultrasound, Guidance, Needle Biopsy)
  ICD-10-CM: E46 (Malnutrition)
  Rationale: This patient required placement of a feeding tube for nutritional support. Code 49440 is assigned to report the percutaneous placement of the feeding tube. The notes following 49440 state, "For conversion to a gastrojejunostomy tube at the time of initial gastrostomy tube placement, use 49440 in conjunction with 49446," which is the second procedure. Modifier -51 is appended to the second procedure, 49446-51. Ultrasound guidance 76942-26 was used to locate the edge of the liver to assist with needle placement for the catheter. Modifier -26 is added to indicate that only the professional service was provided. The fluoroscopic guidance is included in codes 49440 and 49446 and is not reported separately.

This procedure was performed because the patient is malnourished, E46.

Practice Exercise 19.18

Professional Service: 49000-78 (Laparotomy, Exploration)
  ICD-10-CM: N99.72 (Complication, intraoperative, puncture or laceration [accidental], genitourinary organ or structure, during procedure on other organ)

Rationale: This patient had a laparoscopy the day before this procedure. After discharge, the patient presents to the emergency department with abdominal pain and is taken to the operating room where she was found to have a large amount of urine in her peritoneal cavity. During her previous surgery the urinary bladder had been punctured. Report 49000 for the exploratory laparotomy because this is the portion of the service that Dr. Martinez performed. Add modifier -78 to indicate the return to the operating room for a related procedure during the postoperative period. The cystorrhaphy (51860) was performed by Dr. Smithson, who dictated the note separately for the cystorrhaphy and intestinal adhesiolysis (44005).

The postoperative complication of the puncture of the urinary bladder is reported with N99.72.

Practice Exercise 19.19

Professional Service: 44640-22 (Repair, Intestines, Small, Fistula), **44120-51** (Excision, Intestines, Small)

ICD-10-CM: K63.2 (Fistula, intestine)

Rationale: A fistula is an abnormal communication between two epithelialized surfaces. An intestinal fistula is an abnormal anatomic connection between a part (or multiple parts) of the intestinal lumen and the lumen of another epithelialized structure or the skin. The goal of the procedure was to restore the continuity of the gastrointestinal tract and restore function to the other involved structures. There were multiple intestinal fistulas repaired and reported with 44640. The report stated that the procedure took significantly more time than would typically be required, which directs the assignment of modifier -22, increased procedural service.

The colon is the large intestine and the small bowel is the small intestine. The small intestine was resected and reported with 44120 with modifier -51 to indicate multiple procedures.

The diagnosis is K63.2 (fistula of the intestine).

Practice Exercise 19.20

Professional Service: 43117-62 (Esophagectomy, Partial), **47100** (Biopsy, Liver), **47000-59-53-51** (Biopsy, Liver), **44015** (Jejunostomy, Insertion, Catheter)

ICD-10-CM: K22.711 (Barrett's esophagus, with dysplasia, high grade), **D18.03** (Hemangioma, intra-abdominal)

Rationale: The report states that a wedge biopsy (47100) was performed on a liver mass on the right lobe of the liver. The pathology report was returned with a diagnosis of hemangioma, which is a benign neoplasm.

The report states that if the cancer has not spread to the liver, an esophagogastrectomy using the Ivor-Lewis technique (43117, partial esophagectomy) will be performed. Dr. White is a co-surgeon with Dr. Sanchez because Dr. White performed the mobilization of the stomach and the pyloroplasty for the abdominal portion of the procedure and closed the abdomen. Dr. Sanchez then performed a thoracotomy for the remainder of the procedure. Co-surgery refers to a single surgical procedure that requires the skill of two surgeons of different specialties to perform parts of the same procedure. It could be that the two surgeons perform different procedures, in which case it is not co-surgery. Co-surgery has been performed if the procedure performed is part of and would be reported using a single surgical code. Each surgeon dictates his part of the procedure and reports 43117-62. Modifier -62 is appended for co-surgeon and each surgeon will be paid 62.5% of the procedure. Dr. White also performed the jejunostomy (44015). Code 44015 is an add-on code when the jejunostomy is performed during another procedure; therefore, modifier -51 is not reported.

Before the open biopsy, the physician attempted to perform a percutaneous biopsy of a lesion on the liver (47000), which was terminated after the start of the procedure because the patient was unable to hold his breath. Since the lesion was very close to the diaphragm, the surgeon elected to discontinue the procedure and take the patient to the operating room. An open wedge biopsy of the liver was performed and is reported with 47100, which is an add-on code when performed with another open procedure. Modifier -59 is required because 47000 is mutually exclusive of 47100. Since 47000 was performed earlier than the abdominal procedure, modifier -59 denotes that the percutaneous biopsy was performed at a different session than 47100. The surgeon elected to terminate the procedure; therefore, modifier -52 (reduced procedure) is also added to 47000-59-52. The liver biopsy was a staged procedure in that a frozen section was performed to rule out metastasis to the liver. The frozen section showed hemangioma. Had the FS showed metastasis, the procedure would have been cancelled.

Code K22.711 is reported for Barrett's syndrome, as is stated in the Postoperative Diagnosis section of the report. Code D18.03 (Hemangioma, intra-abdominal structures) is reported for the liver biopsy because this is indicated in the pathology report. You would not report C15.9 (Malignant neoplasm of the esophagus) because it states possible malignancy and you cannot report possible or rule-out conditions.

Practice Exercise 19.21

Professional Service: 50280-RT (Excision, Cyst, Kidney)

ICD-10-CM: N28.1 (Cyst, kidney [acquired])

Rationale: The procedure was the excision of a cyst on the right kidney, which is reported with 50280. Modifier -RT is added to indicate that the procedure was on the right side.

The diagnosis is stated in the Postoperative Diagnosis section of the report as renal cyst, reported with N28.1.

Practice Exercise 19.22

Professional Service: 50541-RT (Kidney, Cyst, Ablation)

ICD-10-CM: N28.1 (Cyst, kidney [acquired])

Rationale: This service was a laparoscopic cyst removal reported with 50541 with modifier -RT to indicate the right side. The biopsy is included in the ablation code and is not reported separately.

The diagnosis is cyst of the kidney (N28.1) and is confirmed by the pathology report.

Practice Exercise 19.23

Professional Service: 58150 (Hysterectomy, Abdominal, Total)

ICD-10-CM: N92.0 (Menorrhagia [primary]), **D25.9** (Fibroid, uterus)

Rationale: This patient had a total abdominal hysterectomy with bilateral removal of tubes and ovaries. The report indicates this was an open abdominal approach (58150).

Code N92.0 is assigned to report menorrhagia and is listed as the first diagnosis in the Preoperative Diagnoses section of the report. The leiomyomas are listed as the second diagnosis in the Preoperative Diagnoses section and are reported with D25.9. When referencing the Index of the ICD-10-CM under "Fibroid, uterus," the coder is directed to D25.9.

Practice Exercise 19.24

Professional Service: 59515 (Cesarean Delivery, Postpartum Care)

ICD-10-CM: O45.93 (Pregnancy, complicated by, premature separation of placenta, unspecified), **O60.14X0** (Pregnancy, complicated by, preterm labor third trimester, with third trimester preterm delivery), **Z37.0** (Outcome of delivery, single, liveborn)

Rationale: This patient presents for an emergency cesarean section in which the OB surgeon will then follow the patient postpartum (59515).

Code O45.93 reports the premature separation of the placenta for unspecified reasons (i.e., coagulation defect in mother), occurring in the third trimester. The onset of preterm labor complicating pregnancy is reported with O60.14X0. The seventh character "0" denotes single gestation. The outcome of delivery is reported on the mother's record with Z37.0 for single liveborn.

Practice Exercise 19.25

Professional Service: 56630-RT (Vulvectomy, Radical)

ICD-10-CM: D07.1 (Neoplasm, labium, majus, Ca in situ)

Rationale: The vulvectomy, radical/partial is the excision of a portion of the labia, reported with 56630. We are not told the size of the lesion, only that it was located at the 11 o'clock position of the right labia majora and that a 1 cm margin was taken on all sides. Even a 1 cm margin on two sides would lead to an area of 2 cm (based on size of lesion and the narrowest margin × 2). A partial radical vulvectomy involves removal of less than 80% of the vulvar area and a radical procedure involves removal of the skin and deep subcutaneous tissue. The report does indicate that "running locked suture of 2-0 Vicryl was then placed in the deeper tissues." This is correctly coded with 56630. It would not be appropriate to use the excision of malignant lesions codes (11620-11626) and the intermediate repair codes (12041-12047) because deeper tissue was involved. Modifier -RT indicates the vulvectomy was performed on the right only.

The lesion, which was sent to pathology, was returned with a diagnosis of Neoplasia III, which is carcinoma in situ of the labia majora, reported with D07.1.

The ICD-10-CM Neoplasm Table for "Neoplasm, labia [skin], majora, Ca in situ" indicates D07.0. When you reference the Tabular, you will see Carcinoma in situ of endometrium. The correct code is D07.1 (Carcinoma in situ of vulva). The Tabular lists severe dysplasia of vulva, which is noted in the Postoperative Diagnosis of the report.

Practice Exercise 19.26

Professional Service: 61313-RT (Craniotomy, Surgery)

ICD-10-CM: I61.1 (Hemorrhage, intracranial [nontraumatic], intracerebral, hemisphere, cortical [superficial])

Rationale: This patient had a craniotomy for evacuation of an intracerebral hematoma (supratentorial), 61313. Modifier -RT indicates the surgery was performed on the right temporal lobe. If this procedure was infratentorial, it would be much more extensive, and the physician service would be reported with infratentorial codes.

The diagnosis is stated as a nontraumatic intracerebral hematoma of the right temporal lobe, reported with I61.1. In the ICD-10-CM Index, Hematoma, brain (traumatic), nontraumatic, refers you to "*see* Hemorrhage, intracranial."

Practice Exercise 19.27

Professional Service: 61154-RT (Burr Hole, Skull, Drainage, Hematoma)

ICD-10-CM: I62.01 (Hemorrhage, intracranial [nontraumatic], subdural [nontraumatic], acute)

Rationale: This patient had a nontraumatic subdural hematoma drained through burr holes, which were drilled into the frontal and posterior parietal areas of the right cranium (61154). Code 61154 represents evacuation and/or drainage of either a subdural (under the dura) or extradural (on top of the dura) hematoma. This was a unilateral procedure, so the modifier -RT is appended to indicate the right side.

The diagnosis is stated as a nontraumatic subacute subdural hematoma, reported with I60.9.

Practice Exercise 19.28

Professional Service: 64721-LT (Carpal Tunnel Syndrome, Decompression)

ICD-10-CM: G56.02 (Syndrome, carpal tunnel)

Rationale: Carpal tunnel release is performed on this patient (64721), in which the physician decompresses the median nerve by freeing the nerve inside the carpal tunnel of the wrist. Modifier -LT indicates the procedure was performed on the left wrist.

The diagnosis is stated as carpal tunnel syndrome, reported with G56.02. Note the fifth character "2" indicates the left side.

Practice Exercise 19.29

Professional Service: 63709-78 (Repair, Spinal Cord, Cerebrospinal Fluid Leak)

ICD-10-CM: G97.82 (Pseudomeningocele, postprocedural [spinal])

Rationale: A pseudomeningocele is an abnormal collection of cerebrospinal fluid (CSF) without a membrane (dura) surrounding it. A leak in the dura causes the CSF to build in the extradural space or the tissues. This leak was a complication of a previous procedure. The previous incision was reopened. Repair of pseudomeningocele is performed on this patient for whom the physician repairs an opening in the dura with a fat graft which was taken from the same area; therefore, it is included in the procedure. After the repair the surgeon noticed another leak, and he performed a partial hemilaminectomy of L5 on the left and closed the leak. A hemilaminectomy involves removing lamina and part of the spinal process (63709). Code 63709 describes this procedure as it states repair of pseudomeningocele, with laminectomy. Had the surgeon stopped after the repair of the first leak, you would have reported 63707 for a repair of a pseudomeningocele without laminectomy. Modifier -78 indicates that the patient has returned to the operating room for a related procedure during the postoperative period.

The diagnosis is postprocedural spinal pseudomeningocele (G97.82).

Practice Exercise 19.30

Professional Service: 63047 (Laminectomy, with Facetectomy), **63048 x 2** (Laminectomy, with Facetectomy)

ICD-10-CM: M48.061 (Stenosis, spinal, lumbar region), **M43.16** (Spondylolisthesis, lumbar region)

Rationale: This patient had a bilateral laminectomy with foraminotomy for spinal stenosis that was indicated on an MRI. The first segment is reported with 63047; each additional segment is reported with 63048 (this code is submitted times the number of segments involved, in this case, two). The additional segments are L4 and L5. Modifier -50 is not reported because the description in the CPT for these codes states unilateral or bilateral. Code 63048 is an add-on code; therefore, modifier -51 is not required.

The diagnosis is stated as spinal stenosis, reported with M48.061, and grade 1 spondylolisthesis of L4-5 level, reported with M43.16.

Chapter 20—Radiology Section

Practice Exercise 20.1

Professional Service: 70450-26 (CT Scan, without Contrast, Head)

ICD-10-CM: R41.82 (Alteration [of], Altered, mental status)

Rationale: This is stated as a noncontrast CT scan of the head (70450). Modifier -26 is appended to indicate the physician portion only.

Code R41.82 indicates an altered mental status.

Practice Exercise 20.2

Professional Service: 76705-26 (Ultrasound, Abdomen)

ICD-10-CM: E80.6 (Disorder, bilirubin excretion)

Rationale: This is an ultrasound of the gallbladder, which is an organ located in the right upper abdomen. The physician states that it is a limited ultrasound. Code 76705 specifies that this code is for a single organ ultrasound. You would not use code 76700 because this code describes a complete ultrasound.

The indication for the ultrasound was elevation of the patient's bilirubin (E80.6).

Practice Exercise 20.3

Professional Service: 78452-26 (Stress Tests, Myocardial Perfusion Imaging)

ICD-10-CM: R07.9 (Pain, chest), **I25.10** (Disease, heart, ischemic, atherosclerotic), **Z95.2** (Status, organ replacement, by artificial or mechanical device or prosthesis of, heart, valve)

Rationale: This report is the professional radiologic component of a Cardiolite stress test reported by the radiologist. Modifier -26 would be added to the codes indicating the radiologist's portion of the procedure. Code 78452 reports the SPECT imaging portion of the stress test with multiple studies. Although the stress study and at rest study were performed on separate days, 78452 is reported only once. Note that the code range 78451-78454 contains imaging codes that require careful reading to ensure the correct code has been assigned.

The reason for the encounter was chest pain (R07.9). The report indicates that the patient has arteriosclerotic coronary artery disease (I25.10) and that he has had an aortic and mitral valve replacement (Z95.2). These diagnoses are reported as they may be related to the cause of the chest pain.

Practice Exercise 20.4

Professional Service: 76506-26 (Echoencephalography, Intracranial)

ICD-10-CM: P07.17 (Low birthweight, 1750-1999 grams), **P07.30** (Preterm, newborn, infant)

Rationale: The service was an ultrasound of the head (76506) to examine the brain. The radiology technologist performs the ultrasound to detect intracranial abnormalities, determine ventricular size, and define cerebral contents. The examination (76506) includes all the various imaging methods performed, such as B-scan, A-scan, and real-time. Modifier -26 indicates the professional component.

The diagnosis is preterm newborn with body weight between 1750 and 1999 grams (P07.17). Patient indicated to be preterm; however, gestational weeks not specified, code P07.30 is correctly reported.

Practice Exercise 20.5

Professional Service: 74455-26 (Urethrocystography)

ICD-10-CM: Q62.0 (Hydronephrosis, congenital)

Rationale: Voiding cystourethrogram (74455) is a radiologic examination of the urethra and bladder to evaluate the voiding function. Modifier -26 indicates the professional component.

The clinical symptoms and diagnosis for this examination indicate congenital hydronephrosis (Q62.0).

Chapter 21—Pathology and Laboratory Section

Practice Exercise 21.1

Professional Service: 88304 (Pathology, Surgical, Gross and Micro Exam, Level III)

ICD-10-CM: M51.26 (Displacement, intervertebral disc, lumbar region)

Rationale: Intervertebral disc is listed in the 88304 code description. This includes any intervertebral disc, whether lumbar, thoracic, sacral, or cervical. When reporting this code for payment of service, a word of caution is that 88304 does not mean level 4 pathology; it means level 3 pathology. There is no CPT code 88303. The pathologic findings are fragments of fibrocartilage, consistent with herniated disc L3-4.

When referencing the Index in the ICD-10-CM under the term "Hernia disc," the coder is directed to "*see Displacement intervertebral disc.*" Reference "Displacement" in the Index with the subterm "*intervertebral disc, lumbar*" directs the coder to M51.26.

Practice Exercise 21.2

Professional Service: 88307 (Pathology, Surgical, Gross and Micro Exam, Level V)

ICD-10-CM: N80.0 (Adenomyosis), **N83.01** (Cyst, follicular [ovarian]), **D25.1** (Leiomyoma, uterus, intramural), **N87.9** (Dysplasia, cervix)

Rationale: The specimen taken in this case was the uterus, fallopian tubes, and ovaries. Code 88305 would initially seem to be the right code because it reports the uterus, fallopian tubes, and ovaries, which is the case here. However, under uterus in the description for 88305, it states "for prolapse," which was not stated in this case. Code 88307 states uterus, with or without tubes and ovaries, other than neoplastic/prolapse, which is correct.

This patient had a total hysterectomy due to menorrhagia. The pathology report indicates more definitive diagnoses of adenomyosis (N80.0) and follicular cyst (N83.01), so the menorrhagia would not be reported. Dysplasia of the cervix is reported with N87.9. The proliferating endometrium is included in N80.0 and not reported separately. Also reported are multiple intramural leiomyomata (D25.1).

Practice Exercise 21.3

Professional Service: 88307 (Pathology, Surgical, Gross and Micro Exam, Level V)

ICD-10-CM: O41.143 (Placentitis)

Rationale: This is a pathologic examination of a third-trimester placenta. The description for 88307 states "placenta, third trimester." Third trimester is the last 3 months of a woman's pregnancy. This woman is 31 weeks pregnant. You would not report 88305 because the code description states "placenta, other than third trimester." There was one specimen, as the umbilical cord is attached to the placenta. There is only one report describing the placenta and the umbilical cord; therefore, only one unit is reported for 88307.

The diagnosis is mild early placentitis reported with ICD-10-CM code O41.1430. The 6th character indicates the third trimester. The seventh character "0" indicates single gestation and multiple gestations where the fetus is unspecified. You would not report code O45.93, which reports placental abruption, because the code description states possible abruption, and in the findings no abruption was seen. Remember, although this is an inpatient, you are reporting the professional services of the physician and you cannot report possible or rule-out diagnoses; only facility coders report possible or rule-out diagnoses.

Practice Exercise 21.4

Professional Service: 88304 (Pathology, Surgical, Gross and Micro Exam, Level III)

ICD-10-CM: M48.02 (Stenosis, spinal, cervical region)

Rationale: Listed under the code description for 88304 is intervertebral disc.

Code M48.02 reports stenosis of the cervical spine.

Practice Exercise 21.5

Professional Service: 88304 (Pathology, Surgical, Gross and Micro Exam, Level III)

ICD-10-CM: I61.9 (Hemorrhage, intracranial, intracerebral [nontraumatic])

Rationale: Listed in the code description for 88304 is hematoma; this is the only code that lists hematoma. Nowhere in the description of the code does it state cerebral hematoma. Even though this hematoma was located in the patient's brain, you would still report 88304 because the specimen was the hematoma, not brain tissue.

In the ICD-10-CM Index, referencing "Hematoma, brain, non-traumatic" indicated I61.9 and also directs the coder to "*see Hemorrhage, brain,*" which in turn lists "*see Hemorrhage, intracranial, intracerebral,*" reported with I61.9. Although intracerebral hemorrhage is not specifically stated, review of ICD-10-CM category I61 reveals terms *intracerebral* and *cerebral* can be used interchangeably.

Chapter 22—Medicine Section

Practice Exercise 22.1

Professional Service: 93458-26 (Catheterization, Cardiac, Left Heart, with Ventriculography)

ICD-10-CM: I25.110 (Arteriosclerosis, coronary [artery], native vessel, with angina pectoris, unstable)

Rationale: This patient is having a left heart catheterization (LHC) and coronary artery angiography. The placement of the catheter into the left side of the heart and the injection of contrast and the selective catheterization of the coronary arteries followed by the injection of contrast is reported with 93458. All components of the cardiac catheterization (placement, injection, imaging) are reported with 93458. Modifier -26 is added to indicate only the physician portion of this procedure is being reported.

ICD-10-CM code I25.110 reports the coronary artery disease and includes the unstable angina in one combination code.

Practice Exercise 22.2

Professional Service: 93971-26-LT (Duplex Scan, Venous Studies, Extremity)

ICD-10-CM: Z01.810 (Examination, pre-procedural, cardiovascular), **I25.811** (Arteriosclerosis, coronary [artery], native coronary artery), **R07.9** (Pain, chest)

Rationale: This patient is in need of a bypass procedure on his heart. Before this can be performed, the lower extremity veins need to be mapped to see whether they can be used as bypass grafts. You would not code 93970 because this is for a complete bilateral study and the service was a unilateral service. It states specifically in the note that only the left side was assessed, so you would use code 93971, which is for just one side. You would then add -26 to indicate that only the professional component was provided and -LT to indicate the left side.

The patient has atherosclerotic heart disease of the native coronary arteries (I25.811) and chest pain (R07.9). Z01.810 (Examination, preoperative, cardiovascular) indicates that this is a preoperative examination to assess the veins in the lower extremities before the patient's bypass procedure.

Practice Exercise 22.3

Professional Service: 93971-26 (Duplex Scan, Venous Studies, Extremity)

ICD-10-CM: M79.606 (Pain, limb, lower), **M79.89** (Swelling, leg)

Rationale: This is an ultrasound on the veins of the leg that is performed as a diagnostic test to rule out deep vein thrombosis. The procedure in this report was performed bilaterally and is reported with 93970; however, the ultrasound was a limited study, so rather than 93970, you would report 93971 because that code description indicates a unilateral or limited study. Modifier -26 is assigned to indicate that only the professional component is being reported.

Outpatient coders do not report rule out diagnoses, rather, you report the presenting symptoms, which in this case are leg pain (729.5) and leg swelling (729.81). Note that the ICD-10-CM code for leg pain could be more specific if the portion of the leg, such as thigh or calf, had been

documented. The ICD-10-CM code also could specify the side, left or right. Although bilateral is implied by the study of both legs, bilateral leg pain is not stated in the medical documentation. Studies are often completed on both limbs for comparison purposes.

Practice Exercise 22.4

Professional Service: 93970-26 (Duplex Scan, Venous Studies, Extremity), **76700-26** (Ultrasound, Abdomen)

ICD-10-CM: M79.89 (Swelling, leg), **R06.9** (Abnormal/abnormality/abnormalities, breathing), **R18.8** (Ascites [abdominal])

Rationale: Code 93970 reports the ultrasound of both legs that was performed to diagnose deep vein thrombosis (DVT). Modifier -26 is added to indicate that only the professional component of the service is being reported. An ultrasound of the abdomen was performed (76700) and modifier -26 is added to indicate the professional component of the service. The ultrasound included the liver, spleen, bile ducts, gallbladder, pancreas, kidneys, and abdominal aorta, which is a complete examination reported with 76700.

The diagnosis is M79.89 (swelling of the legs to rule out DVT) and R06.8 (difficulty breathing). The ascites was diagnosed and is reported with R18.8. The ICD-10-CM code for leg pain could be more specific if the portion of the leg, such as thigh or calf, had been documented, as well as the side, left or right; though bilateral is implied, it is not stated. Further, the difficulty breathing is classified as an abnormality of breathing in the Index. When referencing the Index of the ICD-10-CM under the main term "Breathing, labored," the coder is directed to "*see* Hyperventilation." You must then review the codes in the R06 range to determine the most appropriate code.

Practice Exercise 22.5

Professional Service: 90966 (Dialysis, End Stage Renal Disease)

ICD-10-CM: N18.6 (Disease, renal, end stage [ESRD]), **D63.1** (Anemia, in, end stage renal disease)

Rationale: This patient is on home peritoneal dialysis and presents for a monthly checkup. The patient's age is not stated. Usually peritoneal dialysis is performed by the patient at his/her home. The patient is over 20 years of age. The code for the office evaluation is 90966 (Dialysis, End Stage Renal Disease). Although 90945 reports a physician evaluation of a patient one time during dialysis, this would not be the correct code to report because the patient is not receiving dialysis at the time of this visit.

The patient is receiving dialysis for end-stage renal disease N18.6. Code D63.1 is also reported for the anemia in end-stage renal disease because the physician is managing this condition.

Medical Terminology

ablation	removal or destruction by cutting, chemicals, or electrocautery
abortion	termination of pregnancy
absence	without
actinotherapy	treatment of acne using ultraviolet rays
adenoidectomy	removal of adenoids
adipose	fatty
adrenals	glands, located at the top of the kidneys, that produce steroid hormones
albinism	lack of color pigment
allograft	homograft, same species graft
alopecia	condition in which hair falls out
amniocentesis	percutaneous aspiration of amniotic fluid
amniotic sac	sac containing the fetus and amniotic fluid
A-mode	one-dimensional ultrasonic display reflecting the time it takes a sound wave to reach a structure and reflect back; maps the structure's outline
anastomosis	surgical connection of two tubular structures, such as two pieces of the intestine
aneurysm	abnormal dilation of vessels, usually an artery
angina	sudden pain
angiography	radiography of the blood vessels
angioplasty	procedure in a vessel to dilate the vessel opening
anhidrosis	deficiency of sweat
anomaloscope	instrument used to test color vision
anoscopy	procedure that uses a scope to examine the anus
antepartum	before childbirth
anterior (ventral)	in front of
anterior segment	those parts of the eye in the front of and including the lens (cornea, iris, ciliary body, aqueous humor)
anteroposterior	from front to back
antigen	a substance that produces a specific response
aortography	radiographic recording of the aorta
apex cardiography	recording of the movement of the chest wall over the end of the heart
aphakia	absence of the lens of the eye
apicectomy	excision of a portion of the temporal bone
apnea	cessation of breathing
arthrocentesis	injection and/or aspiration of joint
arthrodesis	surgical immobilization of joint
arthrography	radiography of joint
arthroplasty	reshaping or reconstruction of joint
arthroscopy	use of scope to view inside joint
arthrotomy	incision into a joint
articular	pertains to joint
asphyxia	lack of oxygen
aspiration	use of a needle and a syringe to withdraw fluid
assignment	Medicare's payment for the service, which participating physicians agree to accept as payment in full
asthma	shortage of breath caused by contraction of bronchi
astigmatism	condition in which the refractive surfaces of the eye are unequal
atelectasis	incomplete expansion of lung, collapse

atherectomy	removal of plaque by percutaneous method
atrophy	wasting away
audiometry	hearing test
aural atresia	congenital absence of the external auditory canal
auscultation	listening to sounds within the body
autograft	from patient's own body
avulsion	ripping or tearing away of part either surgically or accidentally
axillary nodes	lymph nodes located in the armpit
bacilli	plural of bacillus, a rod-shaped bacterium
barium enema	radiographic contrast medium
beneficiary	person who benefits from health or life insurance
bifocal	two focuses in eyeglasses, one usually for close work and the other for improvement of distance vision
bilaminate skin	skin substitute usually made of silicone-covered nylon mesh
bilateral	occurring on two sides
biliary	refers to gallbladder, bile, or bile duct
bilobectomy	surgical removal of two lobes of a lung
biofeedback	process of giving a person self-information
biometry	application of a statistical measure to a biologic fact
biopsy	removal of a small piece of living tissue for diagnostic purposes
block	frozen piece of a sample
brachytherapy	therapy using radioactive sources that are placed inside the body
bronchiole	smaller division of bronchial tree
bronchography	radiographic recording of the lungs
bronchoplasty	surgical repair of the bronchi
bronchoscopy	inspection of the bronchial tree using a bronchoscope
B-scan	two-dimensional display of tissues and organs
bulbocavernosus	muscle that constricts the vagina in a female and the urethra in a male
bulbourethral	gland with duct leading to the urethra
bundle of His	muscular cardiac fibers that provide the heart rhythm to the ventricles; blockage of this rhythm produces heart block
bundled codes	one code that represents a package of services
bunion	hallux valgus, abnormal increase in size of metatarsal head that results in displacement of the great toe
burr	drill used to create an entry into the cranium
bursa	fluid-filled sac that absorbs friction
bursitis	inflammation of bursa (joint sac)
bypass	to go around
calcaneal	pertaining to the heel bone
calculus	concretion of mineral salts, also called a stone
calycoplasty	surgical reconstruction of a recess of the renal pelvis
calyx	recess of the renal pelvis
cancellous	lattice-type structure, usually of bone
cardiopulmonary	refers to the heart and lungs
cardiopulmonary bypass	blood bypasses the heart through a heart-lung machine
cardioversion	electrical shock to the heart to restore normal rhythm
carotid body	located on each side of the common carotid artery, often a site of tumor
cartilage	connective tissue
cataract	opaque covering on or in the lens
catheter	tube placed into the body to put fluid in or take fluid out
caudal	same as inferior; away from the head, or the lower part of the body
causalgia	burning pain
cauterization	destruction of tissue by the use of cautery
cavernosa	connection between the cavity of the penis and a vein
cavernosography	radiographic recording of a cavity, e.g., the pulmonary cavity or the main part of the penis
cavernosometry	measurement of the pressure in a cavity, e.g., the penis
central nervous system	brain and spinal cord

cervical	pertaining to the neck or to the cervix of the uterus
cervix uteri	rounded, cone-shaped neck of the uterus
cesarean	surgical opening through abdominal wall for delivery
cholangiography	radiographic recording of the bile ducts
cholangiopancreatography	radiographic recording of the biliary system or pancreas
cholecystectomy	surgical removal of the gallbladder
cholecystoenterostomy	creation of a connection between the gallbladder and intestine
cholecystography	radiographic recording of the gallbladder
cholesteatoma	tumor that forms in middle ear
chondral	referring to the cartilage
chordee	condition resulting in the penis being bent downward
chorionic villus sampling	CVS, biopsy of the outermost part of the placenta
circumflex	a coronary artery that circles the heart
Cloquet's node	also called a gland; it is the highest of the deep groin lymph nodes
closed fracture repair	not surgically opened with/without manipulation and with/without traction
closed treatment	fracture site that is not surgically opened and visualized
coccyx	caudal extremity of vertebral column
collagen	protein substance of skin
Colles' fracture	fracture at lower end of radius that displaces the bone posteriorly
colonoscopy	fiberscopic examination of the entire colon that may include part of the terminal ileum
colostomy	artificial opening between the colon and the abdominal wall
component	part
computed axial tomography	CAT or CT, procedure by which selected planes of tissue are pinpointed through computer enhancement, and images may be reconstructed by analysis of variance in absorption of the tissue
conjunctiva	the lining of the eyelids and the covering of anterior sclera
contraction	drawn together
contralateral	opposite side
cordectomy	surgical removal of the vocal cord(s)
cordocentesis	procedure to obtain a fetal blood sample; also called a percutaneous umbilical blood sampling
corneosclera	cornea and sclera of the eye
corpectomy	removal of vertebrae
corpora cavernosa	the two cavities of the penis
corpus uteri	uterus
crackle	abnormal sound when breathing (heard on auscultation)
craniectomy	permanent, partial removal of skull
craniotomy	opening of the skull
cranium	that part of the skeleton that encloses the brain
curettage	scraping of a cavity using a spoon-shaped instrument
curette	spoon-shaped instrument used to scrape a cavity
cutdown	incision into a vessel for placement of a catheter
cyanosis	bluish discoloration
cystocele	herniation of the bladder into the vagina
cystography	radiographic recording of the urinary bladder
cystolithectomy	removal of a calculus (stone) from the urinary bladder
cystolithotomy	cystolithectomy
cystometrogram	CMG, measurement of the pressures and capacity of the urinary bladder
cystoplasty	surgical reconstruction of the bladder
cystorrhaphy	suture of the bladder
cystoscopy	use of a scope to view the bladder
cystostomy	surgical creation of an opening into the bladder
cystotomy	incision into the bladder
cystourethroplasty	surgical reconstruction of the bladder and urethra
cystourethroscopy	use of a scope to view the bladder and urethra
dacryocystography	radiographic recording of the lacrimal sac or tear duct sac
dacryostenosis	narrowing of the lacrimal duct
debridement	cleansing of or removal of dead tissue from a wound

deductible	amount the patient is liable for before the payer begins to pay for covered services
delayed flap	pedicle of skin with blood supply that is separated from origin over time
delivery	childbirth
dermabrasion	planing of the skin by means of sander, brush, or sandpaper
dermatologist	physician who treats conditions of the skin
dermatoplasty	surgical repair of skin
dialysis	filtration of blood
dilation	expansion
discectomy	removal of a vertebral disc
discography	radiographic recording of an intervertebral joint
dislocation	placement in a location other than the original location
distal	farther from the point of attachment or origin
diverticulum	protrusion in the wall of an organ
Doppler	ultrasonic measure of blood movement
dosimetry	scientific calculation of radiation emitted from various radioactive sources
drainage	free flow or withdrawal of fluids from a wound or cavity
duodenography	radiographic recording of the duodenum or first part of the small intestine
dysphagia	difficulty swallowing
dysphonia	speech impairment
dyspnea	shortness of breath, difficult breathing
dysuria	painful urination
echocardiography	radiographic recording of the heart or heart walls or surrounding tissues
echoencephalography	ultrasound of the brain
echography	ultrasound procedure in which sound waves are bounced off an internal organ and the resulting image is recorded
ectopic	pregnancy outside the uterus (i.e., in the fallopian tube)
edema	swelling due to abnormal fluid collection in the tissue spaces
elective surgery	nonemergency procedure
electrocardiogram	ECG, written record of the electrical action of the heart
electrocautery	cauterization by means of heated instrument
electrocochleography	test to measure the eighth cranial nerve (hearing test)
electrode	lead attached to a generator that carries the electrical current from the generator to the atria or ventricles
electroencephalogram	EEG, written record of the electrical action of the brain
electromyogram	EMG, written record of the electrical activity of the skeletal muscles
electronic claim submission	claims prepared and submitted via a computer
electronic signature	identification system of a computer
electro-oculogram	EOG, written record of the electrical activity of the eye
electrophysiology	study of the electrical system of the heart, including the study of arrhythmias
embolectomy	removal of blockage (embolism) from vessel
emphysema	air accumulated in organ or tissue
encephalography	radiographic recording of the subarachnoid space and ventricles of the brain
endarterectomy	incision into an artery to remove the inner lining so as to eliminate disease or blockage
endomyocardial	pertaining to the inner and middle layers of the heart
endopyelotomy	procedure involving the bladder and ureters, including the insertion of a stent into the renal pelvis
endoscopy	inspection of body organs or cavities using a lighted scope that may be inserted through an existing opening or through a small incision
enterolysis	releasing of adhesions of intestine
enucleation	removal of an organ or organs from a body cavity
epicardial	over the heart
epidermolysis	loosening of the epidermis
epidermomycosis	superficial fungal infection
epididymectomy	surgical removal of the epididymis
epididymis	tube located at the top of the testes that stores sperm
epididymography	radiographic recording of the epididymis
epididymovasostomy	creation of a new connection between the vas deferens and epididymis

epiglottidectomy	excision of the covering of the larynx
episclera	connective covering of the sclera
epistaxis	nosebleed
epithelium	surface covering of internal and external organs of the body
erythema	redness of skin
escharotomy	surgical incision into necrotic (dead) tissue
eventration	protrusion of the bowel through an opening in the abdomen
evisceration	pulling the viscera outside of the body through an incision
evocative	tests that are administered to evoke a predetermined response
exenteration	removal of an organ all in one piece
exophthalmos	protrusion of the eyeball
exostosis	bony growth
exstrophy	condition in which an organ is turned inside out
extracorporeal	occurring outside of the body
false aneurysm	sac of clotted blood that has completely destroyed the vessel and is being contained by the tissue that surrounds the vessel
fasciectomy	removal of a band of fibrous tissue
Federal Register	official publication of all "Presidential Documents," "Rules and Regulations," "Proposed Rules," and "Notices"; government-instituted national changes are published in the *Federal Register*
fee schedule	services and payment allowed for each service
femoral	pertaining to the bone from the pelvis to knee
fenestration	creation of a new opening in the inner wall of the middle ear
fissure	cleft or groove
fistula	abnormal opening from one area to another area or to the outside of the body
fluoroscopy	procedure for viewing the interior of the body using x-rays and projecting the image onto a television screen
fracture	break in a bone
free full-thickness graft	graft of epidermis and dermis that is completely removed from donor area
fulguration	use of electrical current to destroy tissue
fundoplasty	repair of the bottom of the bladder
furuncle	nodule in the skin caused by *Staphylococci* entering through hair follicle
ganglion	knot
gastrointestinal	pertaining to the stomach and intestine
gastroplasty	operation on the stomach for repair or reconfiguration
gastrostomy	artificial opening between the stomach and the abdominal wall
gatekeeper	a physician who manages a patient's access to health care
glaucoma	eye diseases that are characterized by an increase of intraocular pressure
globe	eyeball
glottis	true vocal cords
gonioscopy	use of a scope to examine the angles of the eye
Group Practice Model	an organization of physicians who contract with a Health Maintenance Organization to provide services to the enrollees of the HMO
grouper	computer used to input the principal diagnosis and other critical information about a patient and then provide the correct DRG code
Health Maintenance Organization	HMO, a health care delivery system in which an enrollee is assigned a primary care physician who manages all the health care needs of the enrollee
hematoma	mass of blood that forms outside the vessel
hemodialysis	cleansing of the blood outside of the body
hemolysis	breakdown of red blood cells
hemoptysis	bloody sputum
hepatography	radiographic recording of the liver
hernia	organ or tissue protruding through the wall or cavity that usually contains it
histology	study of structure of tissue and cells
homograft	allograft, same species graft
hormone	chemical substance produced by the body's endocrine glands
hydrocele	sac of fluid
hyperopia	farsightedness, eyeball is too short from front to back

hypogastric	lowest middle abdominal area
hyposensitization	decreased sensitivity
hypothermia	low body temperature; sometimes induced during surgical procedures
hypoxemia	low level of oxygen in the blood
hypoxia	low level of oxygen in the tissue
hysterectomy	surgical removal of the uterus
hysterorrhaphy	suturing of the uterus
hysterosalpingography	radiographic recording of the uterine cavity and fallopian tubes
hysteroscopy	visualization of the canal and cavity of the uterus using a scope placed through the vagina
ichthyosis	skin disorder characterized by scaling
ileostomy	artificial opening between the ileum and the abdominal wall
ilium	portion of hip
imbrication	overlapping
immunotherapy	therapy to increase immunity
implantable defibrillator	surgically placed device that directs an electrical shock to the heart to restore rhythm
incarcerated	regarding hernias, a constricted, irreducible hernia that may cause obstruction of an intestine
incise	to cut into
Individual Practice Association	IPA, an organization of physicians who provide services for a set fee; Health Maintenance Organizations often contract with the IPA for services to their enrollees
inferior	away from the head or the lower part of the body; also known as caudalingual
inguinofemoral	referring to the groin and thigh
inofemoral	referring to the groin and thigh
internal/external fixation	application of pins, wires, and/or screws placed externally or internally to immobilize a body part
intracardiac	inside the heart
intramural	within the organ wall
intramuscular	into a muscle
intrauterine	inside the uterus
intravenous	into a vein
intravenous pyelography	IVP, radiographic recording of the urinary system
introitus	opening or entrance to the vagina from the uterus
intubation	insertion of a tube
intussusception	slipping of one part of the intestine into another part
invasive	entering the body, breaking skin
iontophoresis	introduction of ions into the body
ischemia	deficient blood supply due to obstruction of the circulatory system
island pedicle flap	contains a single artery and vein that remain attached to origin temporarily or permanently
isthmus	connection of two regions or structures
isthmus, thyroid	tissue connection between right and left thyroid lobes
isthmusectomy	surgical removal of the isthmus
jaundice	a condition in which excessive bilirubin causes the skin and whites of the eyes to appear yellowish
jejunostomy	artificial opening between the jejunum and the abdominal wall
joint	the place at which two bones attach
jugular nodes	lymph nodes located next to the large vein in the neck
keloid	a fibrous growth that forms at the site of a scar
keratomalacia	softening of the cornea associated with a deficiency of vitamin A
keratoplasty	surgical repair of the cornea
ketones	compounds that are carbon-based by-products of fatty acid metabolism; excess ketone bodies in urine may indicate diabetes mellitus
kidney	organs that filter blood and balance the levels of water, salt, and minerals in the blood
kidney stones	formations of minerals and salt that may form in the urine
Kock pouch	surgical creation of a urinary bladder from a segment of the ileum
kyphosis	humpback
labyrinth	inner connecting cavities, such as the internal ear
labyrinthitis	inner ear inflammation
lacrimal	related to tears
lamina	flat plate

laminectomy	surgical excision of the lamina
laparoscopy	exploration of the abdomen and pelvic cavities using a scope placed through a small incision in the abdominal wall
laryngeal web	congenital abnormality of connective tissue between the vocal cords
laryngectomy	surgical removal of the larynx
laryngography	radiographic recording of the larynx
laryngoplasty	surgical repair of the larynx
laryngoscope	fiberoptic scope used to view the inside of the larynx
laryngoscopy	direct visualization and examination of the interior of larynx with a laryngoscope
laryngotomy	incision into the larynx
lateral	away from the midline of the body (to the side)
lavage	washing out
leukoderma	depigmentation of skin
leukoplakia	white patch on mucous membrane
ligament	fibrous band of tissue that connects cartilage or bone
ligation	binding or tying off, as in constricting the blood flow of a vessel or binding fallopian tubes for sterilization
lipocyte	fat cell
lipoma	fatty tumor
lithotomy	incision into an organ or a duct for the purpose of removing a stone
lithotripsy	crushing of a stone by sound waves or force
lobectomy	surgical excision of lobe of the lung
lordosis	anterior curve of spine
lumbodynia	pain in the lumbar area
lunate	one of the wrist (carpal) bones
lymph node	station along the lymphatic system
lymphadenectomy	excision of a lymph node or nodes
lymphadenitis	inflammation of a lymph node
lymphangiography	radiographic recording of the lymphatic vessels and nodes
lymphangiotomy	incision into a lymphatic vessel
lysis	releasing
magnetic resonance imaging	MRI, procedure that uses nonionizing radiation to view the body in a cross-sectional view
Major Diagnostic Categories	MDC, the division of all principal diagnoses into 25 mutually exclusive principal diagnosis areas within the DRG system
mammography	radiographic recording of the breasts
Managed Care Organization	MCO, a group that is responsible for the health care services offered to an enrolled group of persons
manipulation	movement by hand
manipulation or reduction	alignment of a fracture or joint dislocation to its normal position
mastoidectomy	removal of the mastoid bone
Maximum Actual Allowable Charge	MAAC, limitation on the total amount that can be charged by physicians who are not participants in Medicare
meatotomy	surgical enlargement of the opening of the urinary meatus
medial	toward the midline of the body
Medical Volume Performance Standards	MVPS, government's estimate of how much growth is appropriate for nationwide physician expenditures paid by the Part B Medicare program
Medicare Economic Index	MEI, government mandated index that ties increases in the Medicare prevailing charges to economic indicators
Medicare Fee Schedule	MFS, schedule that listed the allowable charges for Medicare services; was replaced by the Medicare reasonable charge payment system
Medicare Risk HMO	a Medicare-funded alternative to the standard Medicare supplemental coverage
melanin	dark pigment of skin
melanoma	tumor of epidermis, malignant and black in color
Ménière's disease	condition that causes dizziness, ringing in the ears, and deafness
M-mode	one-dimensional display of movement of structures
modality	treatment method

Mohs surgery or Mohs micrographic surgery	removal of skin cancer in layers by a surgeon who also acts as pathologist during surgery
monofocal	eyeglasses with one vision correction
multipara	more than one pregnancy
muscle	organ of contraction for movement
muscle flap	transfer of muscle from origin to recipient site
myasthenia gravis	syndrome characterized by muscle weakness
myelography	radiographic recording of the subarachnoid space of the spine
myopia	nearsightedness, eyeball too long from front to back
myringotomy	incision into tympanic membrane
nasal button	synthetic circular disk used to cover a hole in the nasal septum
nasopharyngoscopy	use of a scope to visualize the nose and pharynx
National Provider Identifier	NPI, a 10-digit number assigned to a physician by Medicare
nephrectomy, paraperitoneal	kidney transplant
nephrocutaneous fistula	a channel from the kidney to the skin
nephrolithotomy	removal of a kidney stone through an incision made into the kidney
nephrorrhaphy	suturing of the kidney
nephrostolithotomy	creation of an artificial channel to the kidney
nephrostolithotomy, percutaneous	procedure to establish an artificial channel between the skin and the kidney
nephrostomy	creation of a channel into the renal pelvis of the kidney
nephrostomy, percutaneous	creation of a channel from the skin to the renal pelvis
nephrotomy	incision into the kidney
neurovascular flap	contains artery, vein, and nerve
noninvasive	not entering the body, not breaking skin
nuclear cardiology	diagnostic specialty that uses radiologic procedures to aid in diagnosis of cardiologic conditions
nystagmus	rapid involuntary eye movements
ocular adnexa	orbit, extraocular muscles, and eyelid
olecranon	elbow bone
Omnibus Budget Reconciliation Act of 1989	OBRA, act that established new rules for Medicare reimbursement
oophorectomy	surgical removal of the ovary(ies)
opacification	area that has become opaque (milky)
open fracture repair	surgical opening (incision) over or remote opening as access to a fracture site
open treatment	fracture site that is surgically opened and visualized
ophthalmodynamometry	test of the blood pressure of the eye
ophthalmology	body of knowledge regarding the eyes
ophthalmoscopy	examination of the interior of the eye by means of a scope, also known as fundoscopy
optokinetic	movement of the eyes to objects moving in the visual field
orchiectomy	castration; removal of the testes
orchiopexy	surgical procedure to release undescended testes and fixate them within the scrotum
order	shows subordination of one thing to another; family or class
orthopnea	difficulty in breathing, needing to be in erect position to breathe
orthoptic	corrective; in the correct place
osteoarthritis	degenerative condition of articular cartilage
osteoclast	absorbs or removes bone
osteotomy	cutting into bone
otitis media	noninfectious inflammation of the middle ear; serous otitis media produces liquid drainage (not purulent) and suppurative otitis media produces purulent (pus) matter
otoscope	instrument used to examine the internal and external ear
oviduct	fallopian tube
papilledema	swelling of the optic disc (papilla)
paraesophageal hiatal hernia	hernia that is near the esophagus
parathyroid	produces a hormone to mobilize calcium from the bones to the blood

paronychia	infection around nail
Part A	Medicare's Hospital Insurance; covers hospital/facility care
Part B	Medicare's Supplemental Medical Insurance; covers physician services and durable medical equipment that are not paid for under Part A
participating provider program	Medicare providers who have agreed in advance to accept assignment on all Medicare claims, now termed Quality Improvement Organizations (QIO)
patella	knee cap
pedicle	growth attached with a stem
Peer Review Organizations	PROs, groups established to review hospital admission and care
pelviolithotomy	pyeloplasty
penoscrotal	referring to the penis and scrotum
percussion	tapping with sharp blows as a diagnostic technique
percutaneous	through the skin
percutaneous fracture repair	repair of a fracture by means of pins and wires inserted through the fracture site
percutaneous skeletal fixation	considered neither open nor closed; the fracture is not visualized, but fixation is placed across the fracture site under x-ray imaging
pericardiocentesis	procedure in which a surgeon withdraws fluid from the pericardial space by means of a needle inserted percutaneously
pericardium	membranous sac enclosing heart and ends of great vessels
perineum	area between the vulva and anus; also known as the pelvic floor
peripheral nerves	12 pairs of cranial nerves, 31 pairs of spinal nerves, and autonomic nervous system; connects peripheral receptors to the brain and spinal cord
peritoneal	within the lining of the abdominal cavity
peritoneoscopy	visualization of the abdominal cavity using one scope placed through a small incision in the abdominal wall and another scope placed in the vagina
pharyngolaryngectomy	surgical removal of the pharynx and larynx
phlebotomy	cutting into a vein
phonocardiogram	recording of heart sounds
photochemotherapy	treatment by means of drugs that react to ultraviolet radiation or sunlight
physics	scientific study of energy
pilosebaceous	pertains to hair follicles and sebaceous glands
placenta	a structure that connects the fetus and mother during pregnancy
plethysmography	determining the changes in volume of an organ part or body
pleura	covers the lungs and lines the thoracic cavity
pleurectomy	surgical excision of the pleura
pleuritis	inflammation of the pleura
pneumonocentesis	surgical puncturing of a lung to withdraw fluid
pneumonolysis	surgical separation of the lung from the chest wall to allow the lung to collapse
pneumonostomy	surgical procedure in which the chest cavity is exposed and the lung is incised
pneumonotomy	incision of the lung
pneumoplethysmography	determining the changes in the volume of the lung
posterior (dorsal)	in back of
posterior segment	those parts of the eye behind the lens
posteroanterior	from back to front
postpartum	after childbirth
Preferred Provider Organization	PPO, a group of providers who form a network and who have agreed to provide services to enrollees at a discounted rate
priapism	painful condition in which the penis is constantly erect
primary care physician	PCP, physician who oversees a patient's care within a managed care organization
primary diagnosis	chief complaint of a patient in outpatient setting
primipara	first pregnancy
prior approval	also known as a prior authorization, the payer's approval of care
proctosigmoidoscopy	fiberscopic examination of the sigmoid colon and rectum
Professional Standards Review Organization	PSRO, voluntary physicians' organization designed to monitor the necessity of hospital admissions, treatment costs, and medical records of hospitals
prognosis	probable outcome of an illness

prostatotomy	incision into the prostate
Provider Identification Number	PIN, assigned to physicians by payers for use in claims submission
pyelography	radiographic recording of the kidneys, renal pelvis, ureters, and bladder
qualitative	measuring the presence or absence of
Quality Improvement Organizations	QIO, consists of a national network of 53 entities that work with consumers, physicians, hospitals, and caregivers to refine care delivery systems
quantitative	measuring the presence or absence of and the amount of
rad	radiation-absorbed dose, the energy deposited in patient's tissues
radiation oncology	branch of medicine concerned with the application of radiation to a tumor site for treatment (destruction) of cancerous tumors
radiograph	film on which an image is produced through exposure to x-radiation
radiologist	physician who specializes in the use of radioactive materials in the diagnosis and treatment of disease and illness
radiology	branch of medicine concerned with the use of radioactive substances for diagnosis and therapy
rales	coarse sounds on inspiration, also known as crackles (heard on auscultation)
real time	two-dimensional display of both the structures and the motion of tissues and organs, with the length of time also recorded as part of the study
reduction	replacement to normal position
Relative Value Unit	RVU, unit value that has been assigned for each service
Resource-Based Relative Value Scale	RBRVS, scale designed to decrease Medicare expenditures, redistribute physician payment, and ensure quality health care at reasonable rates
resource intensity	refers to the relative volume and type of diagnostic, therapeutic, and bed services used in the management of a particular illness
retrograde	moving backward or against the usual direction of flow
rhinoplasty	surgical repair of nose
rhinorrhea	nasal mucous discharge
salpingectomy	surgical removal of the uterine tube
salpingostomy	creation of a fistula into the uterine tube
scan	mapping of emissions of radioactive substances after they have been introduced into the body; the density can determine normal or abnormal conditions
sclera	outer covering of the eye
scoliosis	lateral curve of the spine
sebaceous gland	secretes sebum
seborrhea	excess sebum secretion
sebum	oily substance
section	slice of a frozen block
segmentectomy	surgical removal of a portion of a lung
septoplasty	surgical repair of the nasal septum
serum	blood from which the fibrinogen has been removed
severity of illness	refers to the levels of loss of function and mortality that may be experienced by patients with a particular disease
shunt	an artificial passage
sialography	radiographic recording of the salivary duct and branches
sialolithotomy	surgical removal of a stone of the salivary gland or duct
sinography	radiographic recording of the sinus or sinus tract
sinusotomy	surgical incision into a sinus
skeletal traction	application of pressure to the bone by means of pins and/or wires inserted into the bone
skin traction	application of pressure to the bone by means of tape applied to the skin
skull	entire skeletal framework of the head
somatic nerve	sensory or motor nerve
specimen	sample of tissue or fluid
spirometry	measurement of breathing capacity
splenectomy	excision of the spleen
splenography	radiographic recording of the spleen
splenoportography	radiographic procedure to allow visualization of the splenic and portal veins of the spleen
split-thickness graft	all epidermis and some of dermis

spondylitis	inflammation of vertebrae
Staff Model	a Health Maintenance Organization that directly employs the physicians who provide services to enrollees
steatoma	fat mass in sebaceous gland
stem cell	immature blood cell
stereotaxis	method of identifying a specific area or point in the brain
strabismus	extraocular muscle deviation resulting in unequal visual axes
stratified	layered
stratum (strata)	layer
subcutaneous	tissue below the dermis, primarily fat cells that insulate the body
subluxation	partial dislocation
subungual	beneath the nail
superior	toward the head or the upper part of the body; also known as cephalic
supination	supine position
supine	lying on the back
Swan-Ganz catheter	a catheter that measures pressure in the heart
sympathetic nerve	part of the peripheral nervous system that controls automatic body function and nerves activated under stress
symphysis	natural junction
synchondrosis	union between two bones (connected by cartilage)
tachypnea	quick, shallow breathing
tarsorrhaphy	suturing together of the eyelids
Tax Equity and Fiscal Responsibility Act	TEFRA, act that contains language to reward cost-conscious health care providers
tendon	attaches a muscle to a bone
tenodesis	suturing of a tendon to a bone
tenorrhaphy	suture repair of tendon
thermogram	written record of temperature variation
third-party payer	insurance company or entity that is liable for another's health care services
thoracentesis	surgical puncture of the thoracic cavity, usually using a needle, to remove fluids
thoracic duct	collection and distribution point for lymph, and the largest lymph vessel located in the chest
thoracoplasty	surgical procedure that removes rib(s) and thereby allows the collapse of a lung
thoracoscopy	use of a lighted endoscope to view the pleural spaces and thoracic cavity or to perform surgical procedures
thoracostomy	incision into the chest wall and insertion of a chest tube
thoracotomy	surgical incision into the chest wall
thromboendarterectomy	procedure to remove plaque or clot formations from a vessel by percutaneous method
thymectomy	surgical removal of the thymus
thymus	gland that produces hormones important to the immune response
thyroglossal duct	connection between the thyroid and the tongue
thyroid	part of the endocrine system that produces hormones that regulate metabolism
thyroidectomy	surgical removal of the thyroid
tinnitus	ringing in the ears
titer	measure of a laboratory analysis
tocolysis	repression of uterine contractions
tomography	procedure that allows viewing of a single plane of the body by blurring out all but that particular level
tonography	recording of changes in intraocular pressure in response to sustained pressure on the eyeball
tonometry	measurement of pressure or tension
total pneumonectomy	surgical removal of an entire lung
tracheostomy	creation of an opening into trachea
tracheotomy	incision into trachea
traction	application of pressure to maintain normal alignment
transcutaneous	entering by way of the skin
transesophageal echocardiogram	TEE, echocardiogram performed by placing a probe down the esophagus and sending out sound waves to obtain images of the heart and its movement
transmastoid	creates an opening in the mastoid for drainage antrostomy

transplantation	grafting of tissue from one source to another
transseptal	through the septum
transtracheal	across the trachea
transureteroureterostomy	surgical connection of one ureter to the other ureter
transurethral resection of prostate	TURP, procedure performed through the urethra by means of a cystoscopy to remove part or all of the prostate
transvenous	through a vein
transvesical ureterolithotomy	removal of a ureter stone (calculus) through the bladder
trephination	surgical removal of a disc of bone
trocar needle	needle with a tube on the end; used to puncture and withdraw fluid from a cavity
tubercle	lesion caused by infection of tuberculosis
tumescence	state of being swollen
tunica vaginalis	covering of the testes
tympanolysis	freeing of adhesions of the tympanic membrane
tympanometry	test of the inner ear using air pressure
tympanostomy	insertion of ventilation tube into tympanum
ultrasound	technique using sound waves to determine the density of the outline of tissue
unbundling	reporting with multiple codes that can be reported with one code
unilateral	occurring on one side
uptake	absorption of a radioactive substance by body tissues; recorded for diagnostic purposes in conditions such as thyroid disease
ureterectomy	surgical removal of a ureter, either totally or partially
ureterocolon	pertaining to the ureter and colon
ureterocutaneous fistula	channel from the ureter to exterior skin
ureteroenterostomy	creation of a connection between the intestine and the ureter
ureterolithotomy	removal of a stone from the ureter
ureterolysis	freeing of adhesions of the ureter
ureteroneocystostomy	surgical connection of the ureter to a new site on the bladder
ureteropyelography	ureter and bladder radiography
ureterotomy	incision into the ureter
urethrocystography	radiography of the bladder and urethra
urethromeatoplasty	surgical repair of the urethra and meatus
urethropexy	fixation of the urethra by means of surgery
urethroplasty	surgical repair of the urethra
urethrorrhaphy	suturing of the urethra
urethroscopy	use of a scope to view the urethra
urography	same as pyelography; radiographic recording of the kidneys, renal pelvis, ureters, and bladder
uveal	vascular tissue of the choroid, ciliary body, and iris
varices	varicose veins
varicocele	swelling of a scrotal vein
vas deferens	tube that carries sperm from the epididymis to the urethra
vasectomy	removal of segment of vas deferens
vasogram	recording of the flow in the vas deferens
vasotomy	incision in the vas deferens
vasorrhaphy	suturing of the vas deferens
vasovasostomy	reversal of a vasectomy
vectorcardiogram	VCG, continuous recording of electrical direction and magnitude of the heart
venography	radiographic recording of the veins and tributaries
vertebrectomy	removal of vertebra
vertigo	dizziness
vesicostomy	surgical creation of a connection of the viscera of the bladder to the skin
vesicovaginal fistula	creation of a tube between the vagina and the bladder
vesiculectomy	excision of the seminal vesicle
vesiculography	radiographic recording of the seminal vesicles
vesiculotomy	incision into the seminal vesicle
viscera	an organ in one of the large cavities of the body

volvulus	twisted section of the intestine
vomer	flat bones of the nasal septum
xanthoma	tumor composed of cells containing lipid material, yellow in color
xenograft	different species graft
xeroderma	dry, discolored, scaly skin
xeroradiography	photoelectric process of radiographs

Appendix D

Combining Forms

abdomin/o	abdomen	celi/o	abdomen
acetabul/o	hip socket	cephal/o	head
acr/o	height/extremities	cerebell/o	cerebellum
aden/o	in relationship to a gland	cerebr/o	cerebrum
adenoid/o	adenoids	cervic/o	neck/cervix
adip/o	fat	chol/e	gall/bile
adren/o, adrenal/o	adrenal gland	cholangio/o	bile duct
albin/o	white	cholecyst/o	gallbladder
albumin/o	albumin	choledoch/o	common bile duct
alveol/o	alveolus	cholester/o	cholesterol
ambly/o	dim	chondr/o	cartilage
amni/o	amnion	chori/o	chorion
an/o	anus	clavic/o, clavicul/o	clavicle (collar bone)
andr/o	male	col/o	colon
andren/o	adrenal gland	colp/o	vagina
andrenal/o	adrenal gland	coni/o	dust
angi/o	vessel	conjunctiv/o	conjunctiva
ankyl/o	bent, fused	cor/o, core/o	pupil
aort/o	aorta	corne/o	cornea
aponeur/o	tendon type	coron/o	heart
appendic/o	appendix	cortic/o	cortex
aque/o	water	cost/o	rib
arche/o	first	crani/o	cranium (skull)
arter/o, arteri/o	artery	crin/o	secrete
arthr/o	joint	crypt/o	hidden
atel/o	incomplete	culd/o	cul-de-sac
ather/o	plaque	cutane/o	skin
atri/o	atrium	cyan/o	blue
audi/o	hearing	cycl/o	ciliary body
aut/o	self	cyst/o	bladder
axill/o	armpit	dacry/o	tear
azot/o	urea	dacryocyst/o	pertaining to the lacrimal sac
balan/o	glans penis	dent/i	tooth
bi/o	life	derm/o, dermat/o	skin
bil/i	bile	diaphragmat/o	diaphragm
bilirubin/o	bile pigment	dips/o	thirst
blephar/o	eyelid	disc/o	intervertebral disc
brachi/o	arm	diverticul/o	diverticulum
bronch/o	bronchus	duoden/o	duodenum
bronchi/o	bronchus	dur/o	dura mater
bronchiol/o	bronchiole	encephal/o	brain
burs/o	fluid-filled sac in a joint	enter/o	small intestine
calc/o, calc/i	calcium	eosin/o	rosy
cardi/o	heart	epididym/o	epididymis
carp/o	carpals (wrist bones)	epiglott/o	epiglottis
cauter/o	burn	episi/o	vulva
cec/o	cecum	erythr/o, erythem/o	red

esophag/o	esophagus	mamm/o	breast
essi/o, esthesi/o	sensation	mandibul/o	mandible (lower jawbone)
estr/o	female	mast/o	breast
femor/o	thighbone	maxill/o	maxilla (upper jawbone)
fet/o	fetus	meat/o	meatus
fibul/o	fibula	melan/o	black
galact/o	milk	men/o	menstruation, month
gangli/o	ganglion	mening/o, meningi/o	meninges
ganglion/o	ganglion	menisc/o, menisci/o	meniscus
gastr/o	stomach	ment/o	mind
gingiv/o	gum	metacarp/o	metacarpals (hand)
glomerul/o	glomerulus	metatars/o	metatarsals (foot)
gloss/o	tongue	metr/o	uterus, measure
gluc/o	sugar	metr/i	uterus
glyc/o	sugar	mon/o	one
glycos/o	sugar	muc/o	mucus
gonad/o	ovaries and testes	my/o, muscul/o	muscle
gyn/o	female	myc/o	fungus
gynec/o	female	myel/o	bone marrow, spinal cord
hepat/o	liver	myring/o	ear drum
herni/o	hernia	myx/o	mucus
heter/o	different	nas/o	nose
hidr/o	sweat	nat/a, nat/i	birth
home/o	same	natr/o	sodium
hormon/o	hormone	necr/o	death
humer/o	humerus (upper arm bone)	nephr/o	kidney
hydr/o	water	neur/o	nerve
hymen/o	hymen	noct/i	night
hyster/o	uterus	ocul/o	eye
ichthy/o	dry/scaly	olecran/o	olecranon (elbow)
ile/o	ileus	olig/o	scant, few
ili/o	ilium (upper pelvic bone)	onych/o	nail
immun/o	immune	oo/o	egg
inguin/o	groin	oophor/o	ovary
ir/o	iris	ophthalm/o	eye
irid/o	iris	opt/o	eye, vision
ischi/o	ischium (posterior pelvic bone)	optic/o	eye
jaund/o	yellow	or/o	mouth
jejun/o	jejunum	orch/i, orch/o, orchi/o, orchid/o	testicle
kal/i	potassium		
kerat/o	hard, cornea	orth/o	straight
kinesi/o	movement	oste/o	bone
kyph/o	hump	ot/o	ear
lacrim/o	tear	ov/o	egg
lact/o	milk	ovari/o	ovary
lamin/o	lamina	ovul/o	ovulation
lapar/o	abdomen	ox/i, ox/o	oxygen
laryng/o	larynx	oxy/o	oxygen
lingu/o	tongue	pachy/o	thick
lip/o	fat	palat/o	palate
lith/o	stone	palpebr/o	eyelid
lob/o	lobe	pancreat/o	pancreas
lord/o	curve	papill/o	optic nerve
lumb/o	lower back	patell/o	patella (kneecap)
lute/o	yellow	pelv/i	pelvis (hip)
lymph/o	lymph	pericardi/o	pericardium
lymphaden/o	lymph gland	perine/o	perineum

peritone/o	peritoneum	sperm/o, spermat/o	sperm
petr/o	stone	sphygm/o	pulse
phac/o	eye lens	spir/o	breath
phak/o	eye lens	splen/o	spleen
phalang/o	phalanges (finger or toe)	spondyl/o	vertebra
pharyng/o	pharynx	staped/o	middle ear, stapes
phas/o	speech	staphyl/o	clusters
phleb/o	vein	steat/o	fat
phren/o	mind, diaphragm	ster/o, stere/o	solid, having three dimensions
phys/o	growing	stern/o	sternum (breast bone)
pil/o	hair	steth/o	chest
pituitar/o	pituitary gland	stomat/o	mouth
pleur/o	pleura	strept/o	twisted chain
pneumat/o	lung/air	synovi/o	synovial joint membrane
pneumon/o	lung/air	tars/o	tarsal (ankle)
poli/o	gray matter	ten/o	tendon
polyp/o	polyp	tend/o, tendin/o	tendon (connective tissue)
pont/o	pons	test/o	testicle
proct/o	rectum	thorac/o	thorax
prostat/o	prostate gland	thromb/o	clot
psych/o	mind	thym/o	thymus gland
pub/o	pubis	thyr/o, thyroid/o	thyroid gland
pulmon/o	lung	tibi/o	shin bone
pupill/o	pupil	toc/o	childbirth
py/o	pus	tonsill/o	tonsil
pyel/o	renal pelvis	top/o	place
pylor/o	pylorus	tox/o, toxic/o	poison
quadr/i	four	trache/o	trachea
rachi/o	spine	trich/o	hair
radi/o	radius (lower arm)	tympan/o	eardrum
radic/o, radicul/o	nerve root	uln/o	ulna (lower arm bone)
rect/o	rectum	ungu/o	nail
ren/o	kidney	ur/o	urine
retin/o	retina	ureter/o	ureter
rhin/o	nose	urethr/o	urethra
rhiz/o	nerve root	urin/o	urine
rhytid/o	wrinkle	uter/o	uterus
rube/o	red	uve/o	uvea
sacr/o	sacrum	uvul/o	uvula
salping/o	uterine tube, fallopian tube	vagin/o	vagina
scapul/o	scapula (shoulder)	valv/o, valvul/o	valve
scler/o	sclera	vas/o, vascul/o	vessel
scoli/o	bent	ven/o	vein
seb/o	sebum/oil	ventricul/o	ventricle
semin/i	semen	vertebr/o	vertebra
sept/o	septum	vesic/o	bladder
sial/o	saliva	vesicul/o	seminal vesicles
sigmoid/o	sigmoid colon	vitre/o	glass/glassy
sinus/o	sinus	vulv/o	vulva
somat/o	body	xanth/o	yellow
son/o	sound	xer/o	dry

Appendix E

Prefixes

a-	not	neo-	new
an-	not	nulli-, nulti-	none
ante-	before	oxy-	sharp, oxygen
audi-	hearing	pan-	all
bi-	two	para-	beside
brady-	slow	per-	through
de-	lack of	peri-	surrounding
dys-	difficult, painful	poly-	many
ecto-	outside	post-	after
endo-	in	primi-	first
epi-	on/upon	pseudo-	false
eso-	inward	quadri-	four
eu-	good/normal	retro-	behind
exo-	outward	sub-	under
extra-	outside	supra-	above
hemi-	half	sym-	together
hyper-	excess, over	syn-	together
hypo-	under	tachy-	fast
in-	into	tetra-	four
inter-	between	tri-	three
intra-	within	tropin-	act upon
meta-	change, after	uni-	one
multi-	many		

Appendix F

Suffixes

-agon	assemble	-oid	resembling
-algesia	pain sensation	-oma	tumor
-algia	pain	-omia	smell
-ar	pertaining to	-one	hormone
-arche	beginning	-opia	vision
-ary	pertaining to	-opsy	view of
-asthenia	weakness	-orrhexis	rupture
-blast	embryonic	-osis	condition
-capnia	carbon dioxide	-oxia	oxygen
-cele	hernia	-para	woman who has given birth
-centesis	puncture to remove (drain)	-paresis	incomplete paralysis
-chezia	defecation	-parous	to bear
-clast, -clasia, -clasis	break	-penia	deficient
-coccus	spherical bacterium	-pexy	fixation
-cyesis	pregnancy	-phagia	eating
-desis	fusion	-phonia	sound
-dilation	widening, expanding	-phylaxis	protection
-drome	run	-physis	to grow
-dynia	pain	-plasty	repair
-eal	pertaining to	-plegia	paralysis
-ectasis	stretching	-pnea	breathing
-ectomy	removal	-poiesis	production
-edema	swelling	-poly	many
-emia	blood	-porosis	passage
-esthesis	feeling	-retro	behind
-gram	record	-rrhagia	bursting of blood
-graph	recording instrument	-rrhaphy	suture
-graphy	recording process	-rrhea	discharge
-gravida	pregnancy	-schisis	split
-ia	condition	-sclerosis	hardening
-iatrist	physician specialist	-scopy	to examine
-iatry	medical treatment	-spasm	contraction of muscle
-ical	pertaining to	-steat/o	fat
-ictal	pertaining to	-stenosis	blockage, narrowing
-in	a substance	-stomy	opening
-ine	a substance	-thorax	chest
-itis	inflammation	-tocia	labor
-listhesis	slipping	-tom/o	to cut
-lithiasis	condition of stones	-tome	an instrument that cuts
-lysis	separation	-tomy	cutting, incision
-malacia	softening	-tripsy	crush
-megaly	enlargement	-tropia	to turn
-meta	change	-tropin	act upon
-meter	measurement; instrument that measures	-uria	urine
		-version	turning
-metry	measurement of		

Appendix G

Abbreviations

ABG	arterial blood gas
ABN	Advanced Beneficiary Notice; used by CMS to notify beneficiary of payment of provider services
ACL	anterior cruciate ligament
AD	right ear
AFB	acid-fast bacillus
AFI	amniotic fluid index
AGA	appropriate for gestational age
AGCUS	atypical glandular cells of undetermined significance
AKA	above-knee amputation
ANS	autonomic nervous system
APCs	Ambulatory Payment Classifications, patient classification that provides a payment system for outpatients
ARDS	adult respiratory distress syndrome
ARF	acute renal failure
ARM	artificial rupture of membrane
AS	left ear
ASCUS	atypical squamous cells of undetermined significance
ASCVD	arteriosclerotic cardiovascular disease
ASD	atrial septal defect
ASHD	arteriosclerotic heart disease
AU	both ears
AV	atrioventricular
BCC	benign cellular changes
BiPAP	bi-level positive airway pressure
BKA	below-knee amputation
BP	blood pressure
BPD	biparietal diameter
BPH	benign prostatic hypertrophy
BPP	biophysical profile
BUN	blood urea nitrogen
BV	bacterial vaginosis
bx	biopsy
C1-C7	cervical vertebrae
ca	cancer
CABG	coronary artery bypass graft
CBC	complete blood (cell) count
CF	conversion factor, national dollar amount that is applied to all services paid on the Medicare Fee Schedule basis
CHF	congestive heart failure
CHL	crown-to-heel length
CK	creatine kinase
CMS	Centers for Medicare and Medicaid Services, formerly HCFA, Health Care Financing Administration
CNM	certified nurse midwife
CNS	central nervous system
COB	coordination of benefits, management of payment between two or more third-party payers for a service
COPD	chronic obstructive pulmonary disease
CPAP	continuous positive airway pressure
CPD	cephalopelvic disproportion
CPK	creatine phosphokinase
CPP	chronic pelvic pain
CSF	cerebrospinal fluid
CTS	carpal tunnel syndrome
CVA	cerebrovascular accident, stroke
CVI	cerebrovascular insufficiency
D&C	dilation and curettage
D&E	dilation and evacuation
derm	dermatology
DHHS	Department of Health and Human Services
DLCO	diffuse capacity of lungs for carbon monoxide
DRGs	Diagnosis Related Groups, disease classification system that relates the types of inpatients a hospital treats (case mix) to the costs incurred by the hospital
DSE	dobutamine stress echocardiography
DUB	dysfunctional uterine bleeding
ECC	endocervical curettage
EDC	estimated date of confinement
EDD	estimated date of delivery
EDI	electronic data interchange, exchange of data between multiple computer terminals
EEG	electroencephalogram
EFM	electronic fetal monitoring
EFW	estimated fetal weight
EGA	estimated gestational age
EGD	esophagogastroduodenoscopy
EGJ	esophagogastric junction
EMC	endometrial curettage
EOB	explanation of benefits, remittance advice

EPO	Exclusive Provider Organization, similar to a Health Maintenance Organization except that the providers of the services are not prepaid but rather are paid on a fee-for-service basis	MDI	metered dose inhaler
		MI	myocardial infarction
		MRI	magnetic resonance imaging
		MSLT	multiple sleep latency testing
		MVV	maximum voluntary ventilation
EPSDT	Early and Periodic Screening, Diagnosis, and Treatment	NCPAP	nasal continuous positive airway pressure
		NSR	normal sinus rhythm
ERCP	endoscopic retrograde cholangiopancreatography	OA	osteoarthritis
		OD	right eye
ERT	estrogen replacement therapy	OS	left eye
ESRD	end-stage renal disease	OU	each eye
FAS	fetal alcohol syndrome	PAC	premature atrial contraction
FEF	forced expiratory flow	PAT	paroxysmal atrial tachycardia
FEV_1	forced expiratory volume in 1 second	PAWP	pulmonary artery wedge pressure
FEV_1:FVC	maximum amount of forced expiratory volume in 1 second	PCWP	pulmonary capillary wedge pressure
		PEAP	positive end-airway pressure
FHR	fetal heart rate	PEEP	positive end-expiratory pressure
FI	fiscal intermediary, financial agent acting on behalf of a third-party payer	PEG	percutaneous endoscopic gastrostomy
		PERL	pupils equal and reactive to light
FRC	functional residual capacity	PERRL	pupils equal, round, and reactive to light
FSH	follicle-stimulating hormone	PERRLA	pupils equal, round, and reactive to light and accommodation
FVC	forced vital capacity		
fx	fracture	PFT	pulmonary function test
GERD	gastroesophageal reflux disease	pH	symbol for acid/base level
GI	gastrointestinal	PICC	peripherally inserted central catheter
H or E	hemorrhage or exudate	PID	pelvic inflammatory disease
HCFA	Health Care Financing Administration, now known as Centers for Medicare and Medicaid Services (CMS)	PND	paroxysmal nocturnal dyspnea
		PNS	peripheral nervous system
		PROM	premature rupture of membranes
HCVD	hypertensive cardiovascular disease	PSA	prostate-specific antigen
HD	hemodialysis	PST, PSVT	paroxysmal supraventricular tachycardia
HDL	high-density lipoprotein	PT	prothrombin time
HEA	hemorrhage, exudate, aneurysm	PTCA	percutaneous transluminal coronary angioplasty
HHN	handheld nebulizer		
HJR	hepatojugular reflux	PTT	partial thromboplastin time
H&P	history and physical (examination)	PVC	premature ventricular contraction
HPV	human papillomavirus	RA	remittance advice, explanation of services
HSG	hysterosalpingogram	RA	rheumatoid arthritis
HSV	herpes simplex virus	RBBB	right bundle branch block
I&D	incision and drainage	RDS	respiratory distress syndrome
IO	intraocular	REM	rapid eye movement
IOL	intraocular lens	RLQ	right lower quadrant
IPAP	inspiratory positive airway pressure	RSR	regular sinus rhythm
IRDS	infant respiratory distress syndrome	RUQ	right upper quadrant
IVF	in vitro fertilization	RV	respiratory volume
IVP	intravenous pyelogram	RVG	*Relative Value Guide*
JBP	jugular blood pressure	RVH	right ventricular hypertrophy
KUB	kidneys, ureter, bladder	RVS	relative value studies, list of procedures with unit values assigned to each
L1-L5	lumbar vertebrae		
LBBB	left bundle branch block	RV:TLC	ratio of respiratory volume to total lung capacity
LEEP	loop electrosurgical excision procedure		
LGA	large for gestational age	SHG	sonohysterogram
LLQ	left lower quadrant	sp gr	specific gravity
LP	lumbar puncture	SROM	spontaneous rupture of membranes
LUQ	left upper quadrant	subcu, subq, SC, SQ	subcutaneous
LVH	left ventricular hypertrophy		
MAT	multifocal atrial tachycardia	SUI	stress urinary incontinence

SVT	supraventricular tachycardia	UA	urinalysis
T1-T12	thoracic vertebrae	UCR	usual, customary, and reasonable—third-party payers' assessment of the reimbursement for health care services: usual, that which would ordinarily be charged for the service; customary, the cost of that service in that locale; and reasonable, as assessed by the payer
TAH	total abdominal hysterectomy		
TEE	transesophageal echocardiography		
TENS	transcutaneous electrical nerve stimulation		
TIA	transient ischemic attack		
TLC	total lung capacity		
TLV	total lung volume		
TM	tympanic membrane	UPJ	ureteropelvic junction
TMJ	temporomandibular joint	URI	upper respiratory infection
TPA	tissue plasminogen activator	UTI	urinary tract infection
TSH	thyroid-stimulating hormone	V/Q	ventilation/perfusion scan
TST	treadmill stress test	VBAC	vaginal birth after cesarean
TURBT	transurethral resection of bladder tumor	WBC	white blood (cell) count
TURP	transurethral resection of prostate		

Appendix H

Further Text Resources

Anatomy and Physiology

Book Title	Author	Imprint	Copyright Date	ISBN-13
Medical Terminology & Anatomy for Coding, 3rd Edition	Shiland	Mosby	2018	978-0-323-42795-1
The Anatomy and Physiology Learning System, 4th Edition	Applegate	Saunders	2011	978-1-4377-0393-1
Gray's Anatomy for Students, 3rd Edition	Drake, Vogl, Mitchell	Churchill Livingstone	2014	978-0-702-05131-9
Anthony's Textbook of Anatomy and Physiology, 20th Edition	Thibodeau, Patton	Mosby	2012	978-0-323-09600-3

Coding

Book Title	Author	Imprint	Copyright Date	ISBN-13
Step-by-Step Medical Coding, 2018 Edition	Buck	Elsevier	2018	978-0-323-43081-4
2018 ICD-10-CM Hospital Professional Edition	Buck	Elsevier	2018	978-0-323-43072-2
2018 ICD-10-CM Physician Professional Edition	Buck	Elsevier	2018	978-0-323-43071-5
2018 ICD-10-PCS Professional Edition	Buck	Elsevier	2018	978-0-323-43069-2
2018 HCPCS Level II Professional Edition	Buck	Elsevier	2018	978-0-323-43075-3
The Next Step: Advanced Medical Coding and Auditing, 2017/2018 Edition	Buck	Elsevier	2017	978-0-323-43077-7
Simulated Medical Coding Internship, 2017/2018 Edition	Buck	Elsevier	2017	978-0-323-49772-5
Practice Management with Auditing for Coders Powered by SimChart® for the Medical Office		Elsevier	2016	978-0-323-43011-1
ICD-10-CM/PCS Coding: Theory and Practice, 2018 Edition	Lovaasen	Elsevier	2018	978-0-323-52445-2

Pathophysiology

Book Title	Author	Imprint	Copyright Date	ISBN-13
Pathology for the Health Professions, 5th Edition	Damjanov	Saunders	2017	978-0-323-35721-0
Essentials of Human Diseases and Conditions, 6th Edition	Frazier, Drzymkowski	Saunders	2016	978-0-323-22836-7
Gould's Pathophysiology for the Health Professions, 5th Edition	VanMeter, Hubert	Saunders	2015	978-1-4557-5411-3
Introduction to Human Anatomy and Physiology, 4th Edition	Solomon	Saunders	2016	978-0-323-23925-7
The Human Body in Health and Illness, 5th Edition	Herlihy	Saunders	2014	978-1-4557-7234-6
The Human Body in Health and Disease, 7th Edition	Thibodeau, Patton	Mosby	2017	978-0-323-40211-8

Medical Terminology

Book Title	Author	Imprint	Copyright Date	ISBN-13
The Language of Medicine, 11th Edition	Chabner	Saunders	2017	978-0-323-37081-3
Mastering Healthcare Terminology, 5th Edition	Shiland	Mosby	2016	978-0-323-29858-2
Jablonski's Dictionary of Medical Acronyms & Abbreviations, 6th Edition	Jablonski	Saunders	2008	978-1-4160-5899-1
Exploring Medical Language, 10th Edition	LaFleur Brooks, LaFleur Brooks	Mosby	2018	978-0-323-39645-5
Building a Medical Vocabulary: with Spanish Translations, 9th Edition	Leonard	Saunders	2015	978-1-4557-7268-1
Quick & Easy Medical Terminology, 7th Edition	Leonard	Saunders	2014	978-1-4557-4070-3
Mosby's Dictionary of Medicine, Nursing & Health Professions, 10th Edition		Mosby	2017	978-0-323-22205-1
Dorland's Illustrated Medical Dictionary, 32nd Edition		Saunders	2011	978-1-4160-6257-8

Computers & Electronic Health Record

Book Title	Author	Imprint	Copyright Date	ISBN-13
SimChart® for the Medical Office		Elsevier	2014	978-0-323-24195-3
SimChart® for the Medical Office: Learning the Medical Office Workflow, 2017 Edition		Elsevier	2017	978-0-323-49792-3
The Electronic Health Record for the Physician's Office with SimChart® for the Medical Office, 2nd Edition	Pepper		2017	978-0-323-51146-9
Computerized Medical Office Procedures: A Worktext, 4th Edition	Larsen	Saunders	2014	978-1-4557-2620-2

Medical Transcription

Book Title	Author	Imprint	Copyright Date	ISBN-13
Medical Transcription Guide: Do's and Don'ts, 3rd Edition	Diehl	Saunders	2005	978-0-7216-0684-2
Medical Transcription: Techniques and Procedures, 7th Edition	Diehl	Saunders	2012	978-1-4377-0439-6

Professionalism

Book Title	Author	Imprint	Copyright Date	ISBN-13
Job Readiness for Health Professionals: Soft Skills Strategies for Success, 2nd Edition		Elsevier	2016	978-0-323-43026-5
Health Careers Today, 6th Edition	Gerdin	Mosby	2016	978-0-323-28050-1
Career Development for Health Professionals: Success in School and on the Job, 4th Edition	Haroun	Saunders	2016	978-0-323-31126-7

Basic Math

Book Title	Author	Imprint	Copyright Date	ISBN-13
Saunders Math Skills for Health Professionals, 2nd Edition	Hickey	Saunders	2016	978-0-323-32248-5

Medical Billing/Insurance

Book Title	Author	Imprint	Copyright Date	ISBN-13
Health Insurance Today: A Practical Approach, 5th Edition	Beik	Saunders	2015	978-0-323-18817-3
Insurance Handbook for the Medical Office, 14th Edition	Fordney	Saunders	2017	978-0-323-31625-5

Law and Ethics

Book Title	Author	Imprint	Copyright Date	ISBN-13
Legal and Ethical Issues for Health Professions, 3rd Edition		Elsevier	2015	978-1-4557-3366-8

Index

Page numbers followed by "*f*" indicate figures, and "*b*" indicate boxes.

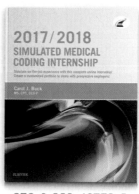